Special Type of Finger Replantation

Jian Lin • He-Ping Zheng
Yong-Qing Xu • Tian-Hao Zhang

Special Type of Finger Replantation

Techniques and Cases

Springer

Jian Lin
Department of Orthopaedic Surgery
Xin-hua Hospital (ChongMing)
Shanghai, Shanghai
China

He-Ping Zheng
Clinical Anatomic Center
Nanjing District General Hospital of PLA
Fuzhou, Fujian
China

Yong-Qing Xu
Orthopaedic Department
Kunming General Hospital of PLA
Kunming, Yunnan
China

Tian-Hao Zhang
Department of Orthopaedic Surgery
Xin-hua Hospital (ChongMing)
Shanghai, Shanghai
China

ISBN 978-981-10-6228-5 ISBN 978-981-10-6229-2 (eBook)
https://doi.org/10.1007/978-981-10-6229-2

Library of Congress Control Number: 2018931169

Printed on acid-free paper

This Springer imprint is published by Springer Nature
The registered company is Springer Nature Singapore Pte Ltd.
The registered company address is: 152 Beach Road, #21-01/04 Gateway East, Singapore 189721, Singapore

Content Summary

Special Types of Finger Replantation is a monograph of clinical cases and pictures. The authors have referred to the latest international literature, combined with their own valuable clinical experience and research results. The book consists of more than 200,000 words and includes more than 150 color pictures and drawings and over 500 photos of clinical surgery. The book is divided into two parts. One is the pandect part of finger replantation, mainly referring to the development of the history of replantation, hand anatomy, commonly used equipment and materials, frequently used medicines, preoperative treatment, selection of anesthesia, regular replantation methods, postoperative treatment and management, and methods of functional recovery after finger replantation. The other part focuses on the concepts of 13 special types of finger replantation, case introductions, surgical key points and precautions, etc., along with more than 60 representative cases including photos. Compared with similar books published all over the world, this book focuses more on the combination of systematic and thematic, basic theory and clinical practice, case photos and text description.

This book is rich in illustrations, suitable for hand surgeons, foot surgeons, micro- and reconstructive surgeons, trauma surgeons, orthopedic surgeons, and plastic surgeons to read, follow, and carry out. We hope that this book promotes the technology of finger replantation.

Preface

The human hands are the most valuable and a universal tool of labor. They are very easily damaged in everyday life, study, and work. The most serious damage to the hands is the severances. Without timely and effective treatment of replantation or reconstruction of the hand function, especially the special types of replantation, life-long harm to the patients may be caused. Thus, referring to the latest literature at home and abroad, combined with our own long years of clinical experience and research results, we have written this monograph, *Special Types of Finger Replantation*. We hope that this book plays a role in promoting this technology.

Special Types of Finger Replantation consists of more than 200,000 words, more than 150 specimens, and over 500 photos of clinical surgery. The book is divided into two parts. The first part is general, introducing the history of the development of finger replantation; the anatomy of the hands; commonly used drugs, equipment, and materials; relevant matters of replantation before treatment; selection of anesthesia; routine replantation methods; treatment and management after replantation surgery; and postoperative functional rehabilitation methods and their significance. The second part focuses on the thirteen special types of replantation concepts, case introductions, and surgical key points and precautions. We try do our best to achieve a systematic and thematic combination of basic theory and clinical practice as well as sample photos and text descriptions.

The book is rich in content and illustrations; it is suitable for surgeons who specialize in hand surgery, microsurgery, trauma surgery, orthopedics, plastic surgery, etc. It is a valuable reference book for finger replantation and research. Because of our limited level of English, mistakes and errors in this book are inevitable. Please let us know of any such errors, so that they can be further corrected.

As soon as the idea of a "special type" of replantation was put forward, it was supported and guided by Professor Hou Chunlin, who is the director of Chinese rehabilitation medicine and reconstructive surgery and director of the Chinese Medical Association. Famous clinical anatomist and Chinese academician, Professor Zhong Shizhen; the hand surgery expert and academician at the Chinese Academy of Engineering, Professor Gu Yudong; and the chief editor of the *Chinese Journal of Clinical Anatomy*, Professor Xu Chuanda, carefully reviewed and revised the manuscript.

Shanghai, China	Jian Lin
Fuzhou, China	He-Ping Zheng
Kunming, China	Yong-Qing Xu
Shanghai, China	Tian-Hao Zhang

Contents

About the Authors

Jian Lin was born in October 1973, Anhui, China. He is associate chief physician of the Department of Orthopedics, Xinhua Hospital Affiliated to Shanghai Jiao Tong University School of Medicine (Chongming); academic leader of the micro- and reconstructive surgery of the hands and feet; Chinese Youth League Committee member of the Asia Pacific micro- and reconstructive surgery; committee member for injury prevention and treatment and tissue injury repair of the Association of Chinese Research Hospitals; member of the microsurgical branch of the Chinese Medical Doctor Association; member of the national orthopedic surgeons in the Chinese Health Association; member of the Chinese repair, reconstructive, and flap surgeons; member of the Microsurgical League of the East China Microsurgery Commission; member of the microsurgery branch of the Shanghai Medical Association; academic reviewer for the *Chinese Journal of Trauma* and *Local Anatomy and Surgery*; and editor of *Microsurgery*, *Chinese Journal of Plastic Surgery*, and *Journal of Practical Hand Surgery*. Dr. Lin has a long-term focus on limb trauma and reconstructive microsurgery and is especially skilled at limb (finger) replantation, reconstruction, skin flap repair, and functional reconstruction with large areas of skin and soft-tissue defects, hand and foot deformity, etc. Dr. Lin has also managed more than ten provincial and local funding projects, worth more than one million yuan. He has published more than 70 scientific research papers, achieving the first and second place for more than ten papers. In addition, he is the editor of more than six medical books and chief editor of *Perforator Flaps*, *Surgical Illustration of Perforator Flaps*, and *Surgical Atlas of Perforator Flaps* and has won second place for a grant more than twice. He has also won funding for national science and progress twice and successfully obtained five grants for scientific research and progress and two national patents.

Xu Yongqing, born in May 1962, is director of the Orthopaedic Center of the Kunming General Hospital of PLA Chengdu Military Region, chief physician, doctoral tutor, and postdoctoral mentor. He has held major academic positions at the International Committee of Microsurgical Reconstruction and SICOT Trauma Committee of the China Branch of the Chinese Medical Association and served as Vice Chairman of Microsurgery of the Chinese Medical Association Society, Chairman of Microsurgery of the PLA Medical Association Society, Yunnan branch Chairman of Orthopaedics of Yunnan Province Medical Association, member of AO Alumni Association, Standing

Committee member of Hand Surgery Association of China, and Chairman of Orthopedics of the Committee of the Chengdu Military Region. He has published over 300 academic papers in the *SCI* and the statistics of the source magazine, edited and published 25 academic monographs, and won eight times the national and provincial second prize for his achievements in the field and three national patents. In addition, he is the deputy editor and editor of 15 books.

Tian-Hao Zhang, born in July 1982, is surgeon-in-charge. He graduated from Shanghai Jiao Tong University School of Medicine. He worked in Xinhua Hospital (Chongming), affiliated to Shanghai Jiao Tong University School of Medicine. He is capable of clinical work, scientific research, and teaching and is an expert in trauma, microsurgery, and plastic and reconstructive surgery. His current focus is on the application of modified perforator flaps in the extremities and the treatment of severe fracture of soft tissue defect. He is a member of the *Journal of Practical Hand Surgery*. He participates in three research projects on provincial and ministerial issues. He has published over 30 academic papers in the *SCI* and the statistics of the source magazine, achieving the third place for two scientific research papers. He has edited two academic monographs and has contributed in five academic monographs.

He-Ping Zheng, born in February 1962, is chief physician, Master Supervisor of Fujian Medical University, China; Incumbent Nanjing Military Area Command of Fuzhou General Hospital of Department of Comparative Medicine Director; member of the Professional Committee of Reparative and Reconstructive Surgery of China; many times member and secretary general of the Chinese Journal of Clinical Anatomy Society; member of the Standing Committee of the Army Association for Laboratory Animal Science, Fujian Province Microsurgical Society; deputy director of the committee, Fujian Province Experiment; deputy director of the Institute of Zoology, Nanjing Military Area Command of Experimental Animal Science; deputy director of the professional committee members; and member of the editorial boards of the *Chinese Journal of Microsurgery*, *Chinese Journal of Clinical Anatomy, Joint Surg* (electronic edition; editor), and *Image of Function and Molecular Medicine Learn* (electronic version; editorial board). He has been engaged in basic research into microsurgery for more than 20 years. He presided over eight finance subjects of the army and the Natural Science Foundation of Fujian Province and received more than two million yuan of scientific research funds. He has published over 100 academic papers in the *SCI* and the statistics of the source magazine, edited and published seven academic monographs, and won eight times the national and provincial second prize for his achievements in the field and three national patents. In addition, he is the deputy editor and editor of ten books.

Part I

Finger Replantation

Finger transection is the most serious trauma to the hands. Finger replantation after hand injury is the most difficult but effective treatment, during which the surgeons perform a sophisticated and technically difficult operation using microscopy and microscopic equipment. At the same time, the surgeons perform a complete debridement for completely or incompletely severed fingers from the hand, the bone, and carry out re-anastomosis of the injured nerves, tendons, skin resurrection, and blood vessels. After the surgery, all aspects of comprehensive treatment are necessary. The purpose is to repair the tissues from the severely wounded finger and enhance the functional reconstruction, save the injured and transected fingers, and to restore function as far as possible. With the continuous improvement in microsurgical techniques and the continuous efforts of microsurgical surgeons, the finger replantation technique has evolved from simple and general finger replantation to a serious and complex special type of replantation for use after finger tissue damage.

1 The History of the Replantation of Amputated Fingers

The hand is an organ related to labor and beauty that distinguishes humans from other animals. As human civilization progresses, the hands play an irreplaceable role in the process when human activities shift from handicraft to light industry, heavy industry, and electronic technology information. Hands are most susceptible to damage during daily life and work. During industrial production in particular, with relatively low automaticity, it is not uncommon for severe traumas caused by high energy damage in hands to result in finger mutilation, leading to life-long disability. Surgeons face the arduous task of attempting to repair and reconstruct the injuries, reduce the patient's disability and improve their quality of life. Human efforts to carry out studies of hand trauma have never ceased, whether the study be fundamental or clinical. The simple trauma care of hand injuries has been directed to evolve toward the complicated replantation of mutilated fingers and the recovery of hand functions. Long-term clinical practice has demonstrated that patient cooperation and reasonable functional exercise is also of vital significance during the treatment of hand trauma, in addition to the doctor's accurate judgment, skill proficiency, and proper management. Satisfying results can be achieved in the recovery of hand trauma only after the joint efforts of both doctors and patients.

Replantation of amputated fingers is a difficult technique that is performed by surgeons under a surgical microscope using microscopic instruments. Its aim is to repair the tissues and reconstruct the functions of severely traumatized fingers. Its development involves four stages, namely the starting stage (1960s), the growing stage (1970s), the fruiting stage (1980s), and the stage of improving functional recovery (1990s). The earliest replantation work was published by Hopfner in 1903 (Chen, 1997) tried limb replantation in animals that did survive for a short period of time. Thereafter, with the further exploration and improvement of surgical methods, an increasing number of successful cases have been reported that constantly improve and enrich our recognition of replantation. In China, Zhixian Wang (1960) and Kaiyuan Tu (1963) were the first to begin replantation in animals. Professor Tu's successful replantation of a dog's amputated leg set a precedent. In 1963, Zhongwei Chen et al. first reported successful replantation in a patient who underwent complete amputation because of forearm trauma and achieved reliable function. It was recognized worldwide as the first successful replantation, starting a new chapter of clinical study of replantation. In 1964, Shuhuan Wang et al. became the first surgeon in the world to complete the replantation of amputated fingers under a microscope, during which they replanted a rabbit's ear successfully under a magnifying glass; in May of the same year, he successfully replanted a child's finger that had been completely amputated. In 1965, Komatsu and Tanlai first successfully replanted a completely amputated

J. Lin et al., *Special Type of Finger Replantation*, https://doi.org/10.1007/978-981-10-6229-2_1

thumb. At the same time, Zhongwei Chen et al. (Shanghai Sixth People's Hospital) were the first in China to replant an amputated limb under a magnifying glass. Later, there were reports of success from Shanghai Ninth People's Hospital, the First Affiliated Hospital of Zhongshan Medical College, Beijing Jishuitan Hospital, the First Affiliated Hospital of Shanxi Medical University, PLA No. 89 Hospital and No. 401 hospital, which made China the leading country in this field in both quality and quantity. With the constant development of the microsurgical technique and the great effort made by microsurgeons, the replantation of amputated fingers has evolved from simple replantation to the complex and special replantation of the multiple fingers that often cause serious vascular injuries, etc.

Starting in the 1980s, China's special amputated finger replantation is the cutting-edge technique that has been developed from the simple normal amputated finger replantation with its further evolution and innovation. After 30 years of endeavor, special amputated finger replantation has achieved remarkable progress in treatment, in-depth development ,and eye-catching accomplishments, which is evidence for the continuous improvement in comprehensive capacity of Chinese microsurgery and in the skill level of Chinese surgeons.

References

Chen HC. New era of reconstructive microsurgery. Changgeng Yi Xue Za Zhi. 1997;20(3):153–62.

Tu K. Replantation of severed limbs in animal experiment. Chin J Surg. 1963;10:1–3.

Wang Z. Replantation of limbs in animal experiment. Shandong Med J. 1960;3:36.

2 Applied Anatomy of the Hand

2.1 Holistic View

2.1.1 Hand Surface Landmarks

Hand surface landmarks include skin landmarks, bony landmarks, and tendon (muscle) landmarks. These landmarks are exposed to varying extents when the hand has different statuses. Therefore, they can appear more apparent when moving different joints during clinical applications.

2.1.1.1 Skin Landmarks (Fig. 2.1)

1. Palmar creases: The skin of the palmar surface has a proximal palmar crease, a middle palmar crease, and a distal palmar crease.

   Proximal palmar crease: Also called a thenar pattern, it is located at the ulnar side of the thenar; obliquely running toward the outer and lower direction, it almost circulates transversely at the distal end and reaches the radial margin of the palm, and its deep surface corresponds to the second metacarpal bone. This crease caters for the thumb's need to engage in separate activities.

   Middle palmar crease: This crease overlaps with the thenar pattern at the distal end, extends to the ulnar side of the palm, and inserts at the lateral border of the hypothenar; it mainly caters for the need of the index finger to engage in activities.

   Distal palmar crease: Starting from the site 1.5 cm away from the proximal side of the second finger web, it circulates transversely inward until the palmar ulnar margin is reached; this transverse crease corresponds to the third to fifth metacarpophalangeal joint lines and is located at a site about 2 cm away from the proximal side of the palm/finger crease. It caters for the needs of the middle finger, ring finger, and little finger to engage in activities. Under normal circumstances, the distal end of the finger pulp can touch the palmar distal transverse crease in the case of finger flexion, which can clinically serve as a simple method of measuring the degree of finger flexion.
2. Finger palmar crease: The proximal transverse crease, middle transverse crease (the thumb lacks of the middle transverse crease), and the distal transverse crease can be found at the palmar surface of the finger, and they are generated to cater for the finger's need to engage in activities. All transverse creases are attached to the deep sheath, so they move less; they become accumulated into a deep groove in the case of finger flexion, so it can serve as a body surface landmark and the mark for surgical incision. The two ends of the transverse creases reach the dorsoventral boundaries of the hands (i.e., the juncture between the finger palmar side and the dorsal side). The distal transverse crease is parallel and level to the finger-web margin; the middle transverse crease directly faces the proximal interphalan-

J. Lin et al., *Special Type of Finger Replantation*, https://doi.org/10.1007/978-981-10-6229-2_2

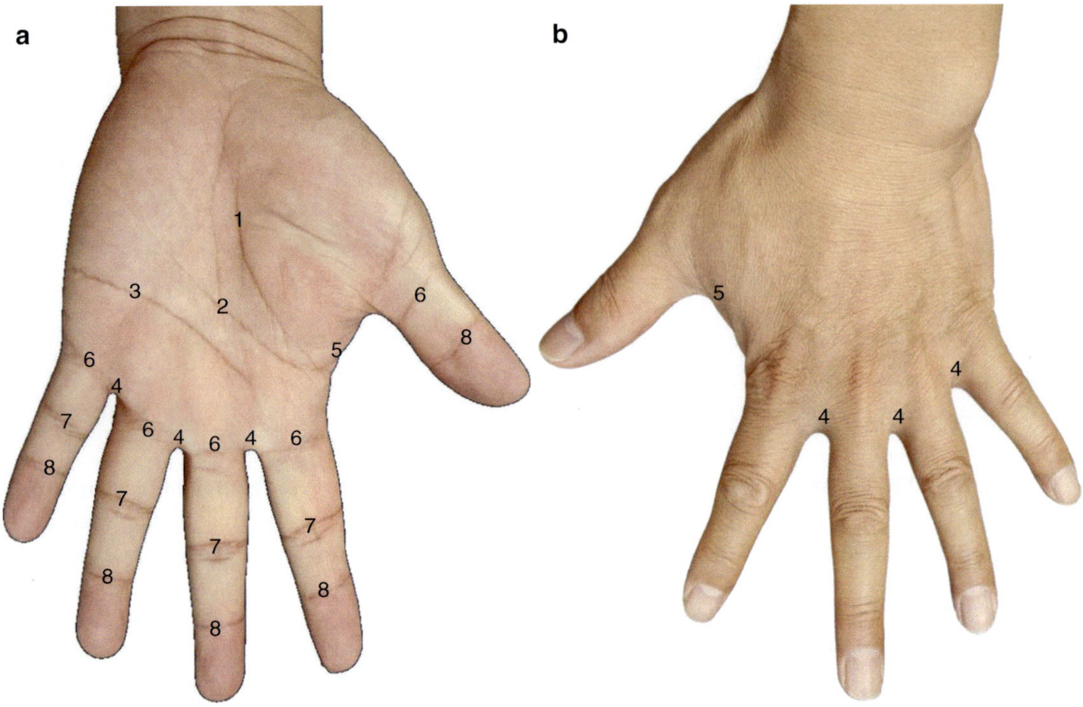

Fig. 2.1 Hand surface landmarks. (**a**) Palmar surface view. (**b**) Dorsal surface view. *1* Proximal palmar crease. *2* Middle palmar crease. *3* Distal palmar crease. *4* Finger web. *5* First web space. *6* Proximal transverse crease. *7* Middle transverse crease. *8* Distal transverse crease

geal joint line; the distal transverse crease is located in the position slightly above the distal interphalangeal joint line.

3. Finger dorsal crease: Several transverse creases and annular eminences can be found at the proximal side of the finger's dorsal surface and the distal interphalangeal joint because this can cater for the dorsal extension of the interphalangeal joint.
4. Finger web: Finger web refers to the skin fold formed by the mutual migration of the palmar and dorsal skin between the adjacent finger roots at the distal end of the palm, and it is level with the middle part of the proximal phalanx. The margins of the finger webs are in the same plane as the hand's palmar skin, and it is connected to the dorsal skin to form an inclined plane. The finger web between the thumb and index finger is the largest, and is called the first web space. Under normal circumstances, the angle of the first web space is maximally greater than 90° when the thumb is fully abducted. In the case of the deformity of scarring and contracture in the first web space, this angle shrinks to varying degrees, having an impact on the thumb function; therefore, repair and reconstruction must be performed.
5. Finger nail: Located at the dorsal side of the fingertip, this refers to a derived structure of skin at the digital dorsum, which is generated because of the thickening of the dermis (Fig. 2.2). The exposed part of the nail is called the nail body and is connected to the deep skin, and there is a white half moon region at its basal part, called the lunula of the nail. The part in which the proximal end of the nail body is hidden below the skin is called the nail root, and the skin germinal layer of the nail root is the growing point of the finger nail, which should be protected during surgery. The periungual skin fold is called the nail fold. The horny layer of the nail root extends toward the distal end into a thin layer of epidermal fold, which is called the

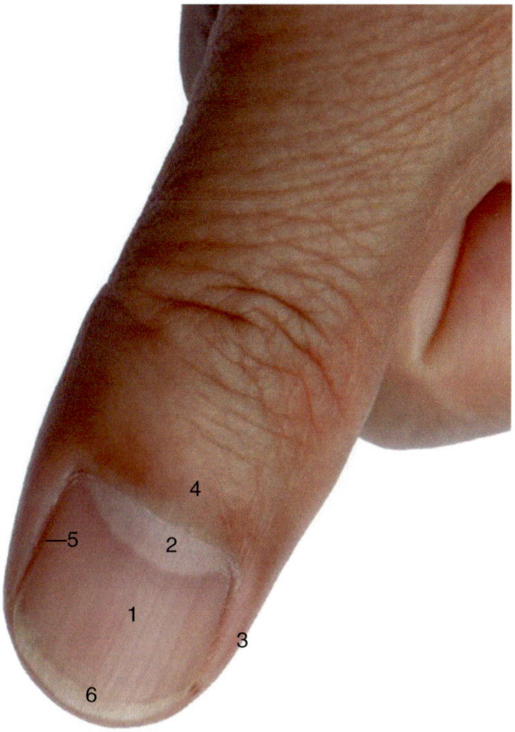

Fig. 2.2 Nail appearance: *1* Nail body. *2* Lunula of the nail. *3* Nail fold. *4* Eponychium. *5* Nail groove. *6* Hyponychium

eponychium. The groove between the nail lateral margin and the nail fold is called the nail groove. The hyponychial dermis is called the nail bed. The horny layer of the epidermis below the nail's free margin is very thick, and the part that is extended to the subungual region is called the hyponychium. The finger nail has the role of supporting the distal pulp space and also beautifying the finger; however, it is the most vulnerable part.

2.1.1.2 Bony Landmarks

The tubercle of the scaphoid bone is palpable at the lateral side of the distal transverse crease of the wrist, and at the slightly distal end of the tubercle of the scaphoid bone is the tubercle of the trapezium bone. They constitute the radial eminence of the wrist. Lentiform bone is palpable at the medial side of the distal transverse crease, and at the slightly distal end of the lentiform bone is the hook of hamate bone. Together, they constitute the ulnar eminence of the wrist. At the bilateral margins of the carpal canal, the radial eminence and the ulnar eminence, with the wrist transverse ligament and carpal canal groove, constitute the carpal canal.

At the hand's dorsal surface, the metacarpus and phalange are located subcutaneously and are easily palpable; in the case of flexion of the metacarpophalangeal joint, the metacarpal bone is obviously visible.

2.1.1.3 Muscle (Tendon) Landmarks (Fig. 2.3)

Thenar: This is the fish-abdomen-shaped eminence, mainly formed of the thenar muscles at the radial side of hand's palmar surface. Injuries of the median nerve can cause paralysis and atrophy of the thenar muscles, causing the thenar to be flat.

Hypothenar: This is the fish-abdomen-shaped eminence mainly formed of the hypothenar muscles at the ulnar side of the hand's palmar surface. Injuries of the ulnar nerve can cause paralysis and atrophy of the hypothenar muscles and interosseous muscles, causing the hypothenar to be flat, and the intermetacarpal spaces to become deepened.

Center of the palm: The triangular pit at the center of palm, on the deep surface of which lie the large vessels, nerves, finger flexor tendon, lumbrical muscle, interosseous muscles, etc.

Tendon eminence: In the case of the extension of the thumb, the thumb extensor tendon is palpable from the dorsal aspect of the thumb and the base of the distal phalanx. In the case of the extension of the remaining fingers, it is clearly visible that the finger extensors run toward all the fingers. When the thumb and the index finger are close to each other, an eminence formed by the first dorsal interosseous muscle is visible at the first intermetacarpal space.

Anatomist's snuff-box: This is a pit visible at the dorsal aspect below the radial bone in the case of thumb abduction and dorsal extension. At the lateral border lie the short extensor tendon of the thumb and the extensor tendon of the thumb, at the medial border lies the long extensor tendon of the thumb, and at the fossa base lie the navicular bone of the hand, the larger multangular bone,

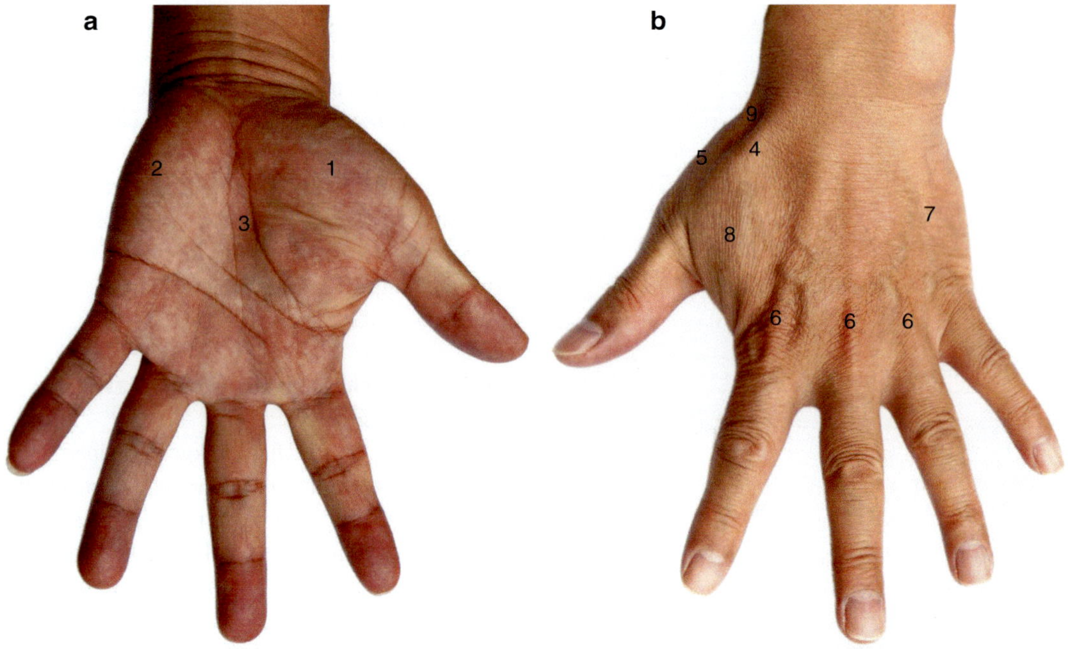

Fig. 2.3 Muscle (tendon) landmarks of hand. (**a**) Palm of the hand. (**b**) Dorsal aspect of the hand. *1* Thenar. *2* Hypothenar. *3* Center of the palm. *4* Extensor pollicis longus tendon. *5* Extensor pollicis brevis tendon. *6* Extensor digitonum. *7* Extensor digiti minimi. *8* First dorsal interosseous muscle. *9* Anatomical snuffbox

and the first base of the metacarpal bone. The radial styloid process is located in the fossa, and the radial artery runs through this fossa until the first intermetacarpal space. The cephalic vein is one of the important contents of the superficial layer structure in the nasopharyngeal fossa, and its course runs from inner to outer, obliquely across the long extensor tendon of the wrist on the radial side, and then upward.

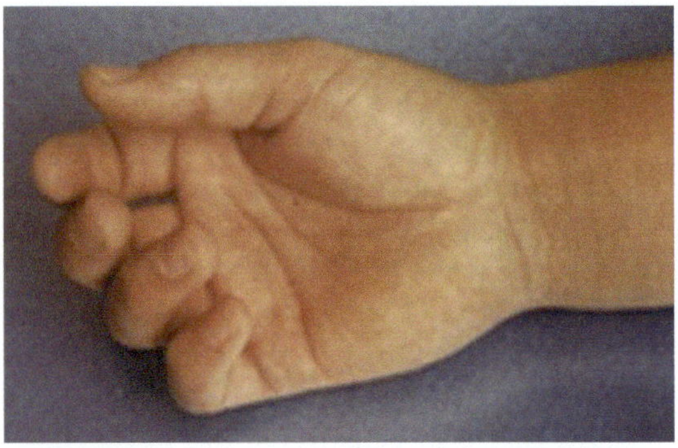

Fig. 2.4 Resting position of the hand

2.1.2 Hand Posture

2.1.2.1 Resting Position of the Hand

The resting position of the hand consists of a kind of natural and half-fisted position during sleep or general anesthesia (Fig. 2.4). The wrist joint is in the position of dorsiflexion (10–15°) with mild ulnar inclination; the thumb has a mild abduction, and the radial margins of the distal interphalangeal joint of the index finger is palpable at the finger pulp. The fingers from the index finger to the little finger, the metacarpophalangeal joint and the interphalangeal joint are in the semi-flexed position; a trend toward the ulnar side means a larger flexion, the index finger becomes mildly inclined toward the ulnar side, and the little finger becomes mildly inclined toward the radial side. In this position, the muscular tensions of the flexor and extensor are relatively balanced. If the hand is damaged, this balanced status is destroyed.

2.1.2.2 Functional Position of the Hand

The functional position of the hand is like the position of holding a cup, which is also the position for performing most functions of the hand (Fig. 2.5). The wrist joint is in the position of dorsiflexion (about 30°) with mild ulnar inclination (about 10°), the thumb is fully abducted, and the thumb metacarpophalangeal joint and interphalangeal joint have a slight flexion. All fingers are separated by flexion of varying degrees; i.e., the metacarpophalangeal joint becomes flexed by 30–45°, the proximal interphalangeal joint by 60–80°, and the distal interphalangeal joint by 10–15°. In the functional position, the hand can perform maximal functions. Thus, for hand fractures following injury, it is generally necessary to fix the hand in the functional position.

2.1.2.3 Pinching Position of the Hand

The pulps of the thumb and index finger (sometimes including the middle finger) have close contact to pinch a thin and small object (such as writing and pinching a needle), which is the pinching position. At this time, the wrist becomes obviously dorsiflexed, the first metacarpal bone is rotated and abducted, the thumb metacarpophalangeal joint and interphalangeal joint have mild flexion, the index finger metacarpophalangeal joint and interphalangeal joint also have flexion, the thumb tip can touch the index finger tip, the thumb and the index finger resemble the two arms of a forceps, and the thumb adductor and the first and second dorsal interosseous muscles provide strong muscular strength. During needle threading, the thumb's interphalangeal joint and the index finger's distal interphalangeal joint turn to the extension position to exert maximal muscle strength (Fig. 2.6).

2.1.2.4 Grasping Position of the Hand

Grasping is an important function of the hand, in the following two forms: strong grasping (such as grasping a hammer handle) and fine grasping (such as unscrewing a cap). In the case of strong grasping, the wrist becomes dorsiflexed, the metacarpophalangeal joint and the interphalangeal joint become flexed by 90° and adducted so that the long flexor of the finger can solidly compress the object onto the palm; the thumb becomes opposed and adducted, the thumb's carpometacarpal joint, metacarpophalangeal joint, and interphalangeal joint become flexed, and the thumb is compressed onto the clenched fingers or directly clenched onto the object. In the case of fine grasping, the wrist becomes dorsiflexed or palmar flexed, the finger becomes semi-flexed, and the thumb is opposed to the semi-flexed fingers. In this position, the hand interosseous muscles can drive the fingers to engage in various kinds of movements, rapidly changing from one position to another. The above two forms also appear at the same time. For example, the middle, ring, and little fingers are used to grasp a rope, and the index finger and the thumb are used to buckle the two ends (Fig. 2.7).

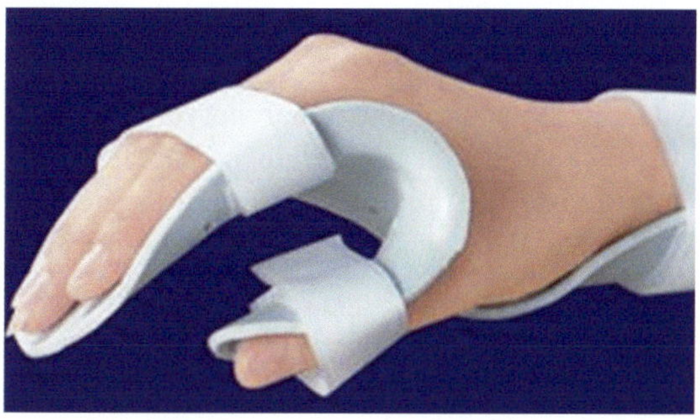

Fig. 2.5 Functional position of the hand

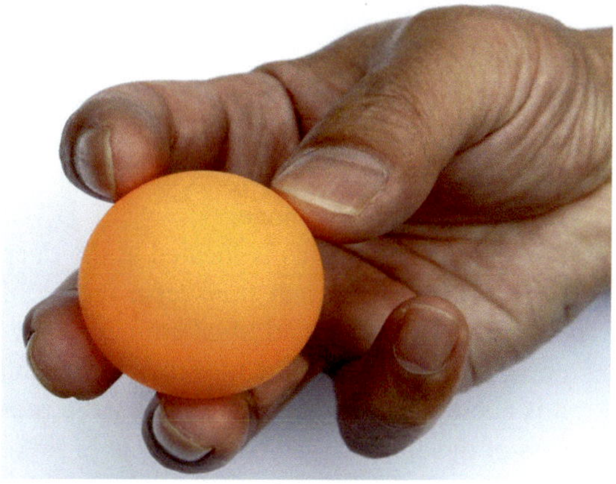

Fig. 2.6 Pinching position of the hand

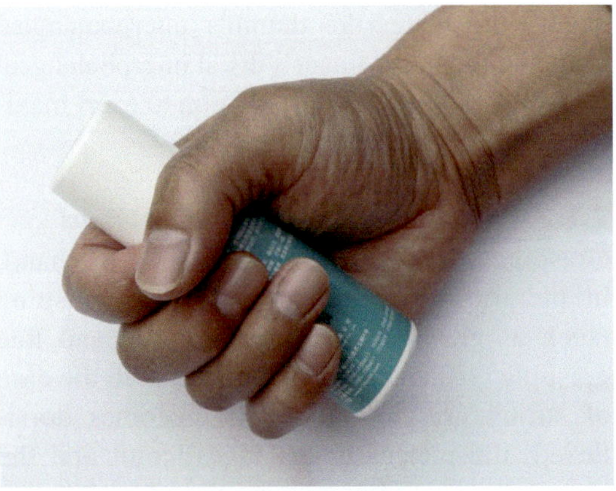

Fig. 2.7 Grasping position of the hand

2.1.3 Body Surface Projection

2.1.3.1 Bone and Joint Projection (Fig. 2.8)

1. Pisiform bone: The distal crease of the wrist happens to pass through the proximal end of the pisiform bone; after the wrist becomes extended backward, the pisiform bone is easily palpable. In the case of wrist anteflexion, there is mild activity.
2. Hamulus of hamate bone: This is located at the site about 1 cm away from the distal radial side of the pisiform bone.
3. Larger multi-angular bone: This is located at the deep surface of the distal side of the wrist. The medial side is covered by the wrist flexor at the radial side, the distal side is covered by the trapezium bone, which is difficult to palpate, and this is relatively obvious in the case of the posterior extension of the wrist.
4. Tubercle of the trapezium bone: This is adjacent to the distal end of tubercle of trapezium bone, and its proximal part is hidden on the tubercle of trapezium bone.
5. Radiocarpal joint: This is located at the deep surface of the proximal transverse crease of the wrist. The radial and tibial eminence covers nearly one third of the navicular bone, and it is about 1.2 cm longer than the styloid process of the ulna.
6. Metacarpophalangeal joint: The slight distal side of the transverse part of the thenar pattern is parallel and level to the metacarpophalangeal joint of the index finger, the slight distal side of the distal palmar crease is parallel and level with the metacarpophalangeal joint of the middle, ring, and little fingers, and the slightly distal side of the proximal crease of the thumb is parallel and level with the metacarpophalangeal joint of the thumb.
7. Interphalangeal joint: The middle crease of the finger opposes the proximal interphalangeal joint, the slightly distal side of the finger distal crease is parallel and level with the distal interphalangeal joint, and the distal crease of the thumb is parallel and level with the thumb's interphalangeal joint.

2.1.3.2 Vascular Nerve Projection (Fig. 2.8)

1. Ulnar nerve and ulnar artery: The ulnar nerve passes through the radial side of the lentiform bone, and the ulnar nerve lies on the radial side of the nerves.
2. Superficial palmar arch: An arch line is drawn from the radial side of the lentiform bone, and then connected with the median point of the palmar median line (which is the connecting line between the distal crease of the wrist and the proximal crease of the middle finger) to roughly represent the ulnar part of the superficial palmar arch.
3. Deep palmar arch: This is located at the site about 1 cm away from the proximal side of the superficial palmar arch.
4. Recurrent branch of the median nerve: The radial region at the proximal third of the thenar or ulnar region at the proximal part of thenar is where the recurrent branch is distributed. Injury or incision in this region may involve the recurrent branch.
5. Deep branch of the ulnar nerve: This runs between the distal margin of the lentiform bone and the proximal margin of the hook of hamate bone, and then surrounds the inner anterior margin of the hook of hamate bone, accompanying the deep palmar arch Figs. 2.9, 2.10, 2.11, 2.12, and 2.13.

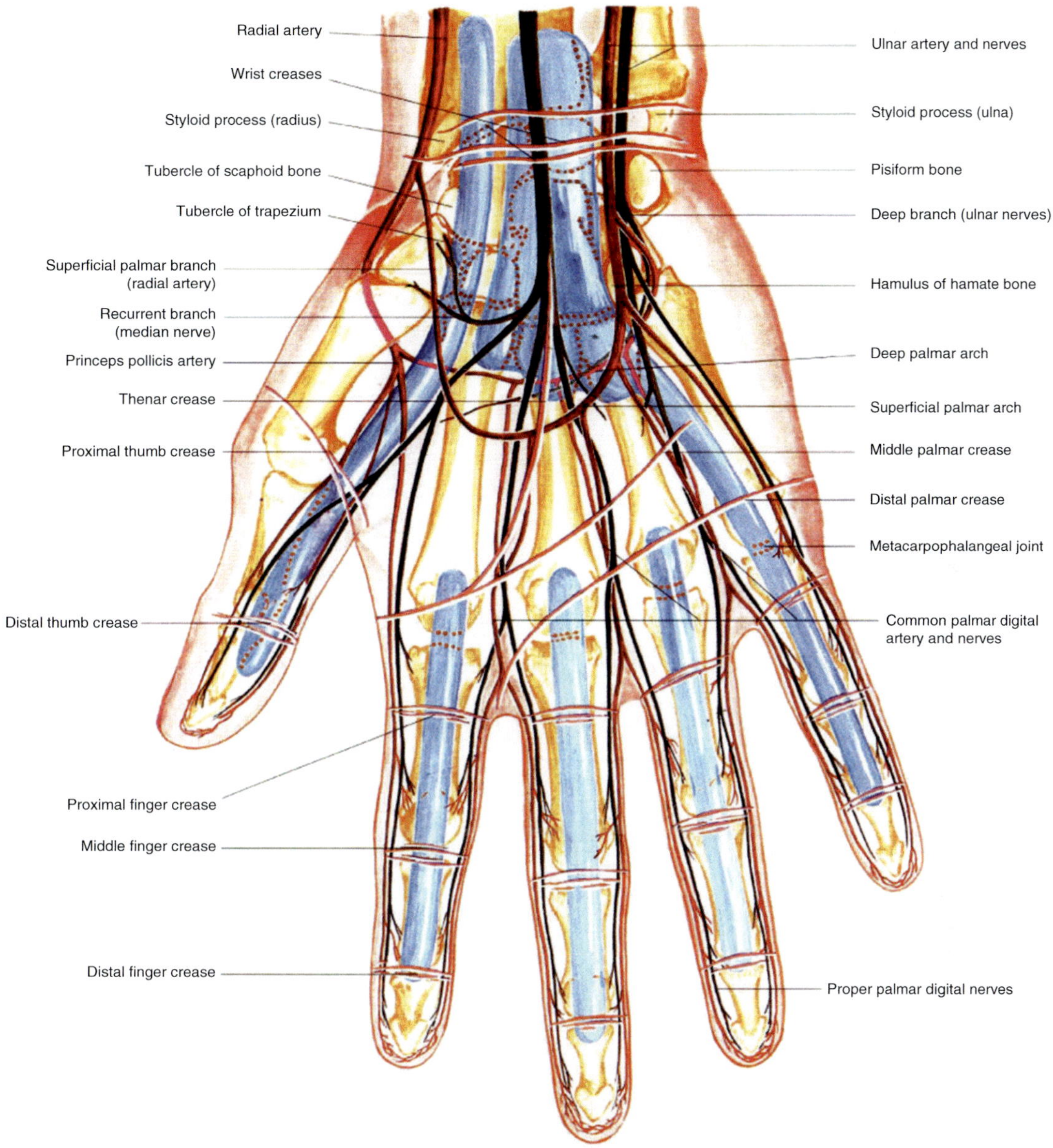

Fig. 2.8 Projection of the deep structures to the palmar surface of the hand

6. Digital arteries and nerves: The common palmar digital artery accompanies the common palmar digital nerves, and the nerves are located at the deep surface. The bifurcation at the arterial side 1.25 cm away from the finger web margin is the proper palmar digital artery, and the nerve bifurcations are located on the proximal side of the arterial bifurcations. At the plane of the metacarpophalangeal joint, the proper palmar digital artery runs along the margins of all palmar surfaces of the fingers; at the slightly ante-

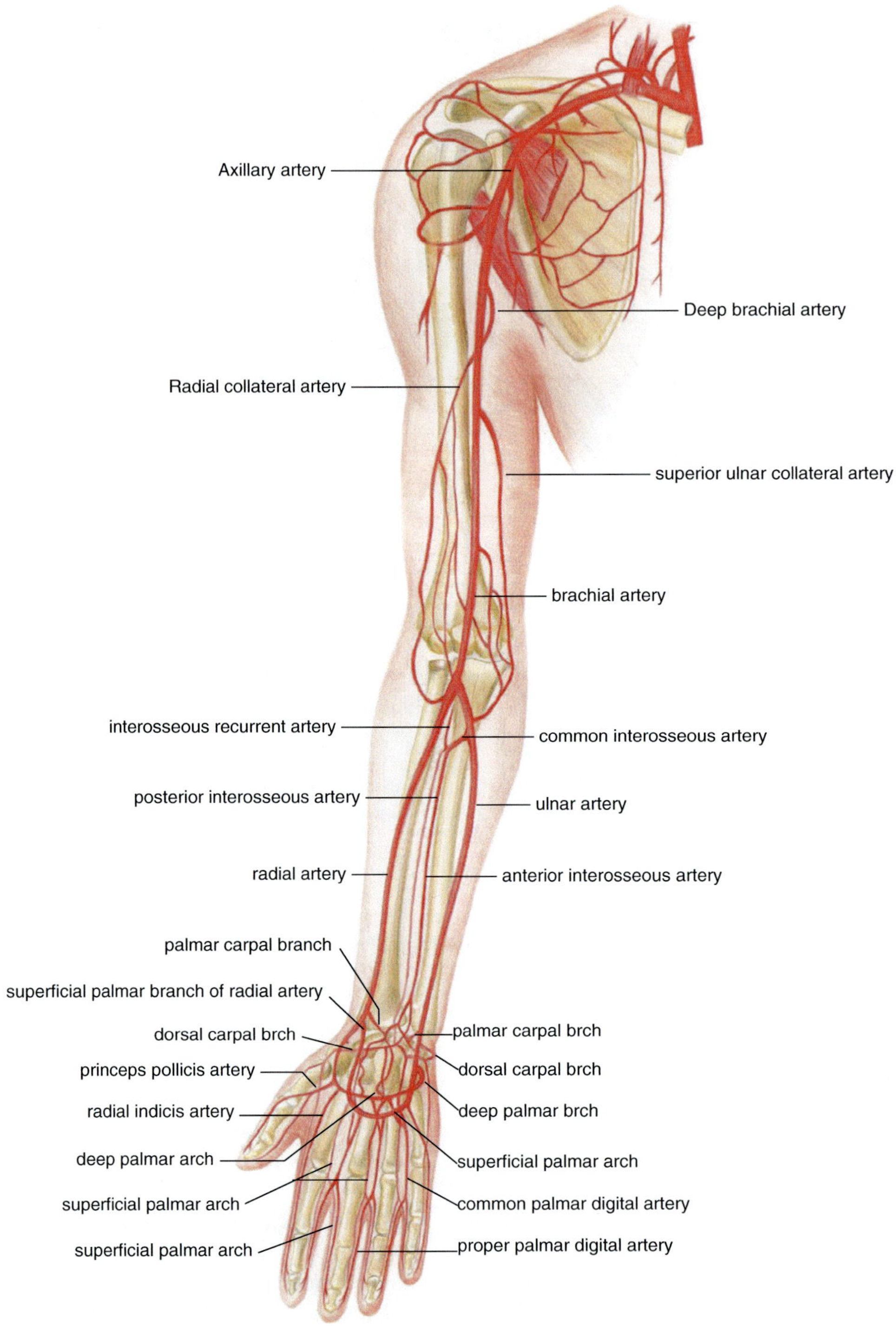

Fig. 2.9 Upper limb artery (schematic diagram)

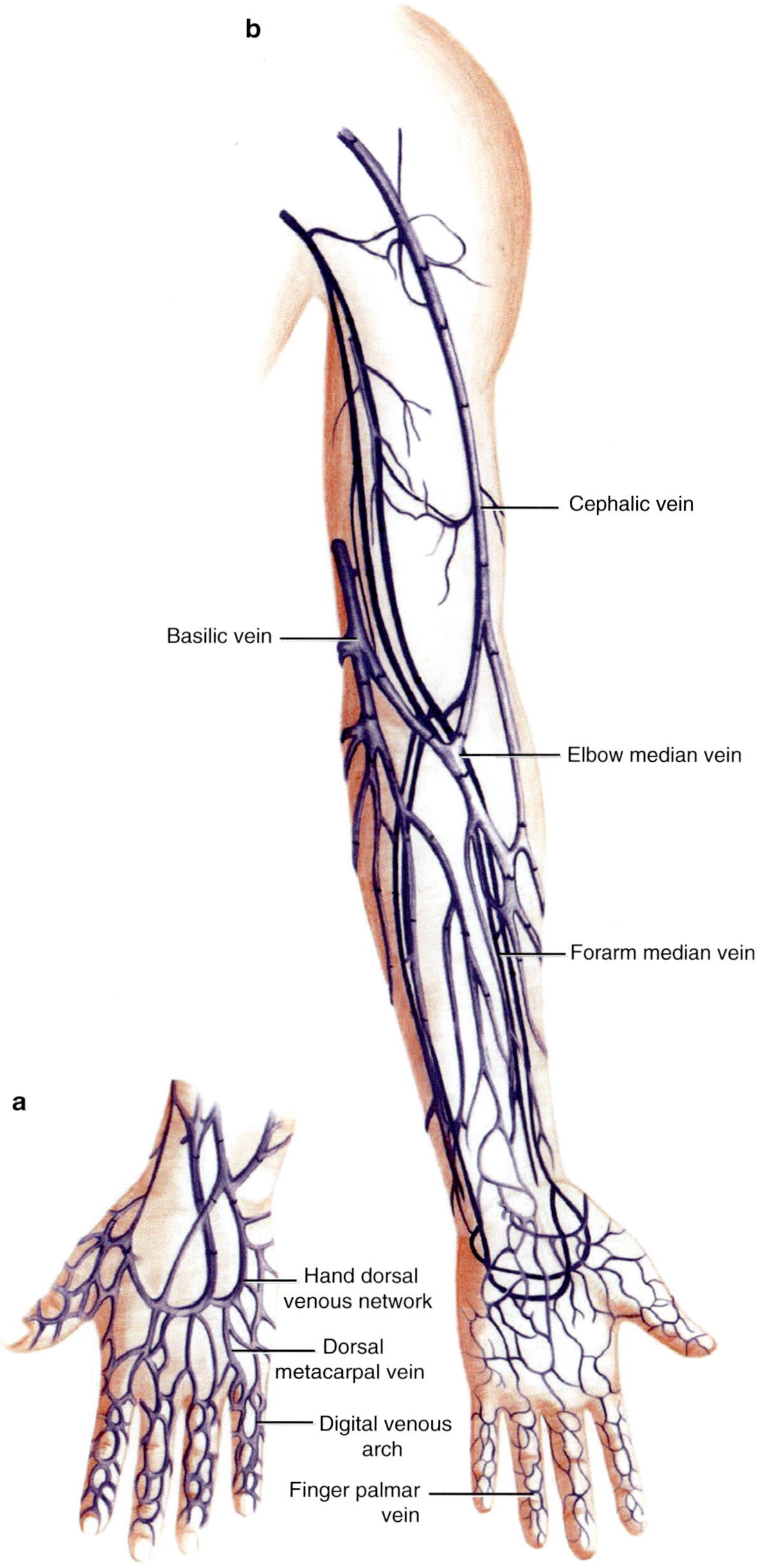

Fig. 2.10 Upper limb superficial vein (schematic diagram). (**a**) Dorsal aspect of the hand. (**b**) Upper limb anterior aspect

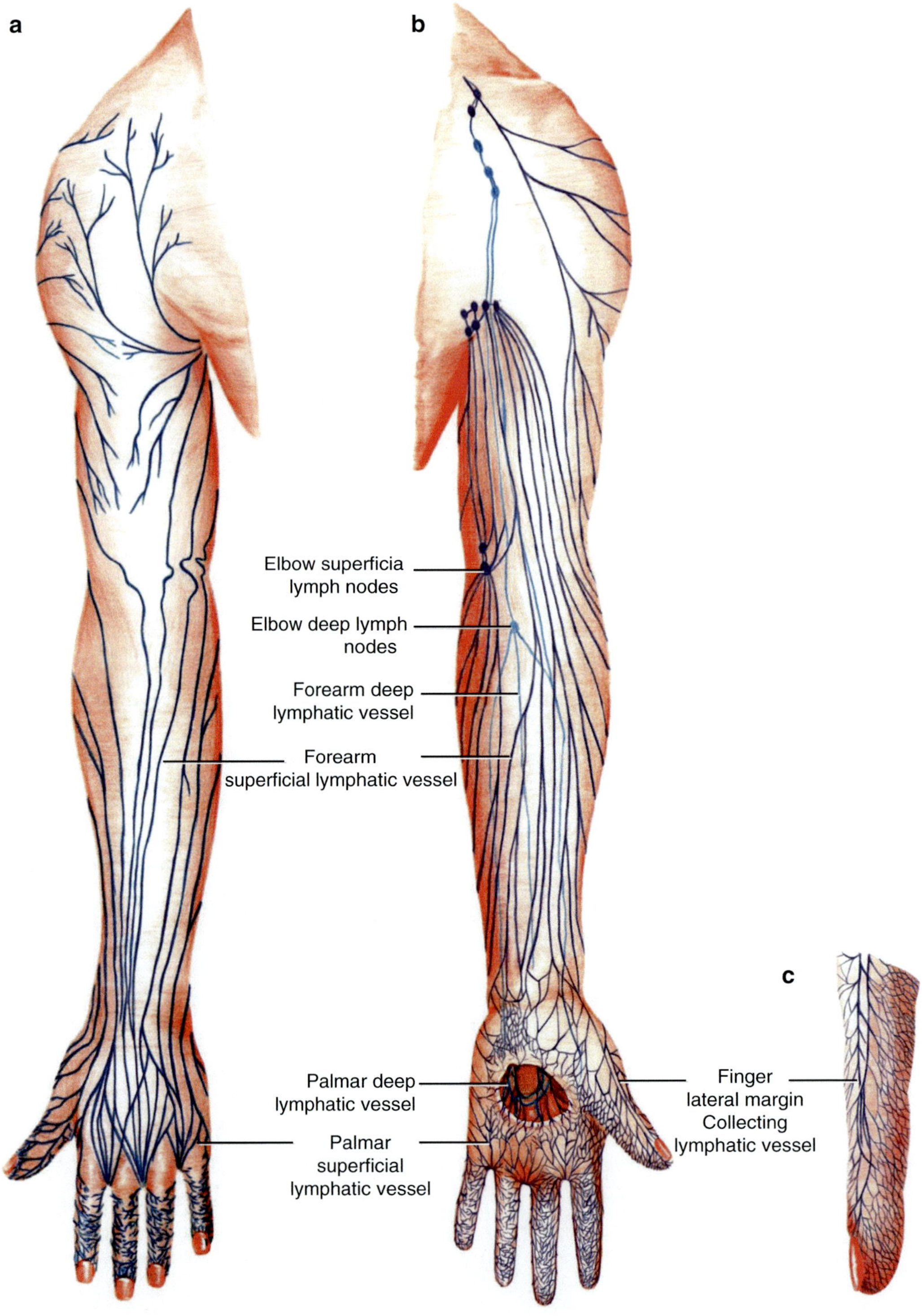

Fig. 2.11 Upper limb lymphatic vessel and lymph node (schematic diagram). (**a**) Dorsal aspect. (**b**) Anterior aspect. (**c**) Finger lateral aspect

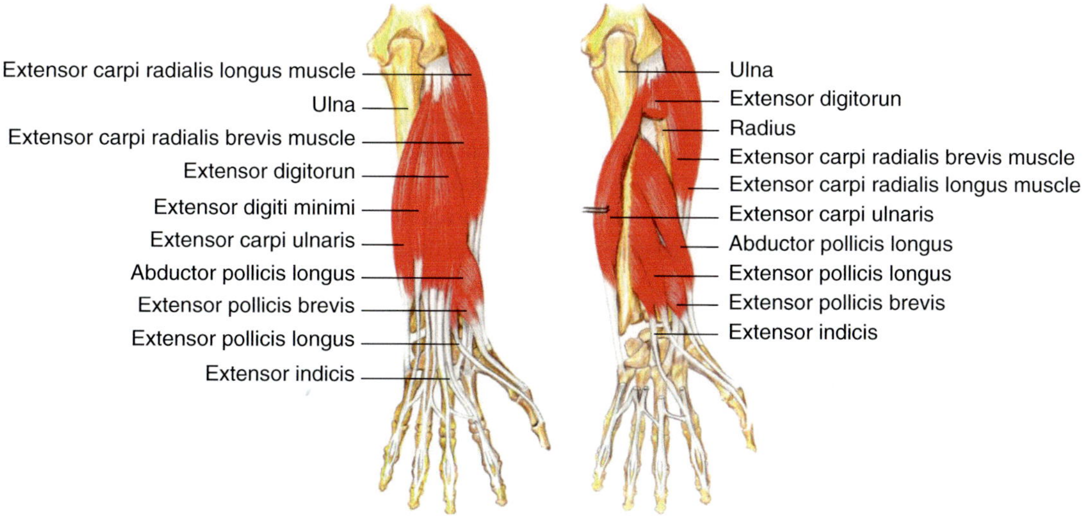

Fig. 2.12 Hand extrinsic muscle (finger extensor)

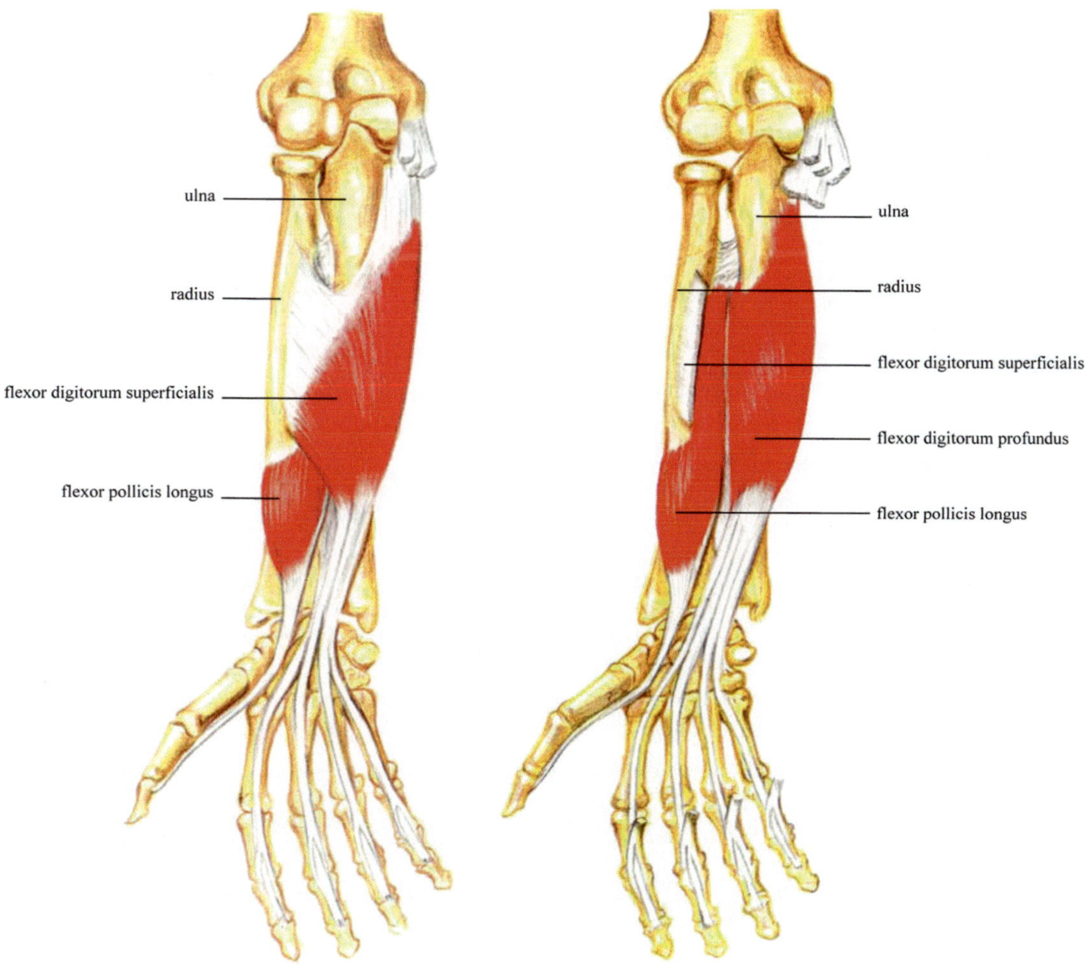

Fig. 2.13 Hand extrinsic muscle (finger flexor)

rior position of the dorso-ventral boundary of the hand, the nerves run on the palmar side of the arteries

2.2 Palm

The palm is quadrilateral and a transition region of the wrist and hand.

2.2.1 Superficial Layer Structure

1. Skin: Thick and tough, it has no elasticity; it is without hair follicles and sebaceous glands, but it has abundant sweat glands.
2. Superficial fascia: The thenar is relatively loose; the palm center is very dense, through which many fiber bundles vertical to the palmar surface pass; the superficial surface is connected to the skin and the deep surface is attached to the palmar aponeurosis, separating the superficial fascia into countless grids, and superficial vessels, inside which lymphatic vessels and cutaneous nerves run (Fig. 2.14). As the fiber bundles connect the skin and palmar aponeurosis closely, the skin has a low mobility, which facilitates the grasping of tools and facilitates labor. However, in the case of inflammation in the superficial fascia, pus is mostly local, making it difficult to spread toward four directions; the pus can be discharged smoothly only after the fiber bundles are cut down. The palmar surgical incision should be generally parallel to the palmar crease, which can reduce scarring and contracture and guarantee hand functions.

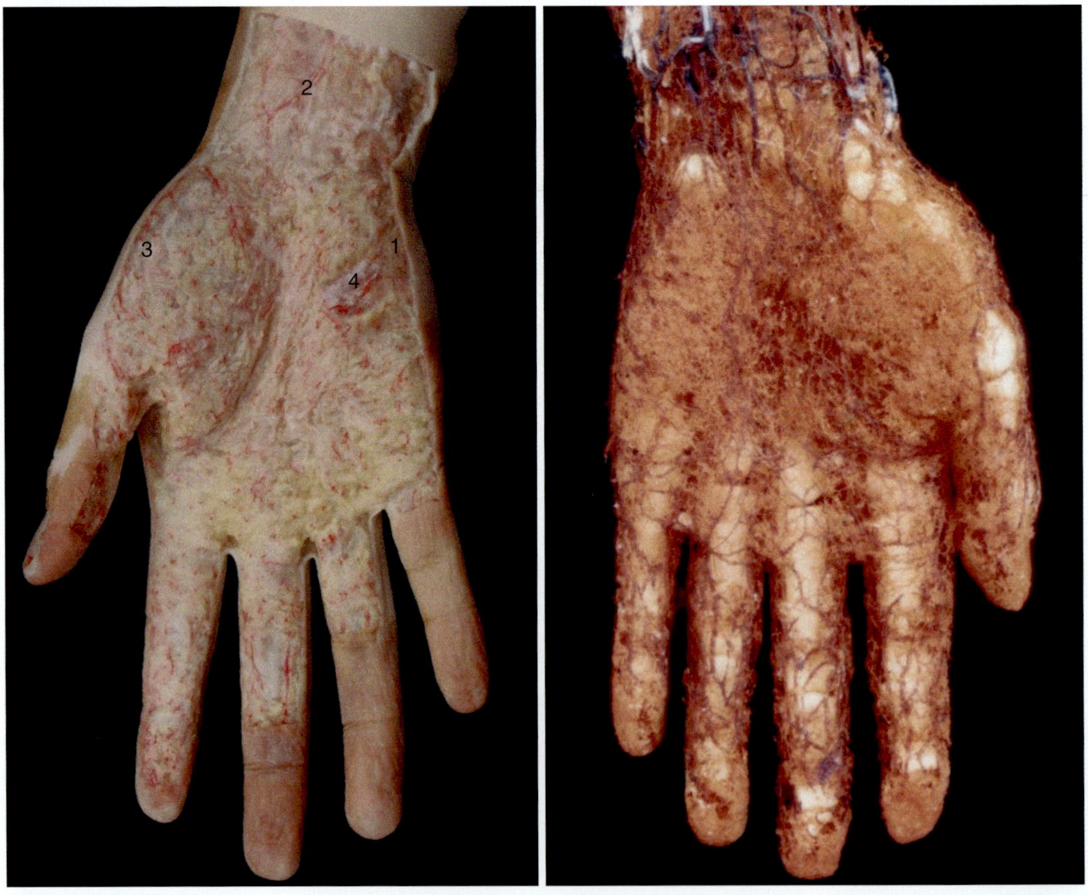

Fig. 2.14 Hand palmar superficial fascia and its structure. *1* Palmar branch of the ulnar nerve. *2* Palmar branch of the median nerve. *3* Superficial branch of the radial nerve. *4* Short palmar muscle

Palmar branch of the ulnar nerve: This descends along the anterior aspect of the ulnar nerve to the palm, penetrates the deep fascia, runs superficially from it, and is then distributed at the hypothenar skin.

Palmar branch of the median nerve: This is sent from the median nerve at the upper margin of the flexor retinaculum, penetrates and runs out from the deep fascia through the surface of the flexor retinaculum, and is finally distributed at the center of the palm and the thenar skin.

Superficial branch of the radial nerve: This is divided into four to five dorsal digital nerves after proceeding across over the extensor retinaculum, and the first dorsal digital nerve dominates the lateral skin of the thenar.

Short palmar muscle: As the degenerative cutaneous muscle, this is located in the superficial fascia at the proximal side of the hypothenar, with the effects of fixing the superficial fascia and protecting the ulnar nerves and ulnar vessels of the deep surface.

3. Deep fascia and palmar aponeurosis: The Palmar deep fasciaof the hand is relatively weak at the two sides and covers the surface of thenar and hypothenar. The middle part is very hard and thick, and the reinforced long palmar tendon is specially called palmar aponeurosis (Fig. 2.15). Palmar aponeurosis is actually composed through the mutual interweaving of the deep fascia and the tendon fiber of the long palmar muscle. The palmar aponeurosis is shaped like a triangle, the prox-

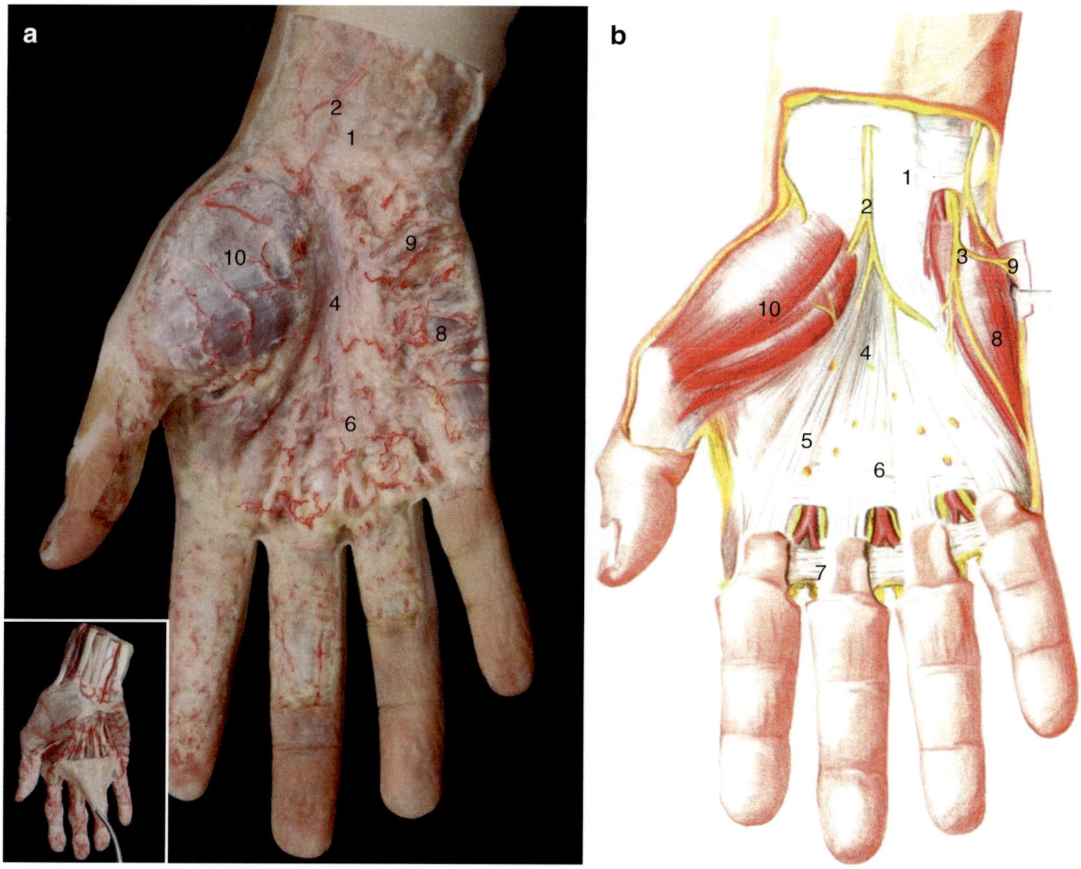

Fig. 2.15 Palmar aponeurosis and the short palmar muscle. (**a**) Specimen of a real object. (**b**) Schematic diagram. *1* Long palmar muscle. *2* Palmar branch of the median nerve. *3* Superficial transverse metacarpal ligament. *4* Palmar aponeurosis. *5* Longitudinal band. *6* Transverse band. *7* Superficial transverse metacarpal ligament. *8* Hypothenar. *9* Short palmar muscle. *10* Thenar

imal side of its apex becomes extended with the long palmar muscle tendon, the distal end of its bottom forms four bundles of fibers which run longitudinally toward the metacarpophalangeal joint, called palmar aponeurosis longitudinal band or tendon anterior bundle, it is solidly attached onto the flexor tendon fibrous sheath of the second to the fifth fingers and the lateral ligament of metacarpophalangeal joints to protect the deep surface tendon, vessels and nerves. In addition, the palmar aponeurosis is connected with skin through the vertical fibers, the connection is more apparent at the crease, and these fiber bundles are tense in case of the finger dorsiflexion.

At the site proximal to the plane of the head of the metacarpal bone, transverse bands are connected among the longitudinal bands of palmar aponeurosis and they are called palmar aponeurosis transverse bands; at the site slightly distal to the plane of the metacarpophalangeal joint, some relatively superficial transverse fibers are attached onto the finger flexor tendon sheath and can enhance the fixation on the metacarpal bone. They are called palmar superficial transverse ligaments. Further beyond, some transverse fibers are connected at the finger web spaces of the second to the fifth fingers below the interphalangeal fold skin and they are called finger web ligaments. They can become extended into the fingers and cover the digital arteries and nerves, and they are reinforced by the cutaneous ligaments. The finger web can reinforce the interphalangeal skin folds; the extension of a finger can limit the hyperflexion of the adjacent fingers, or the flexion of a finger can limit the hyperextension of adjacent fingers.

Between the proximal side of the superficial transverse metacarpal ligament and the palmar aponeurosis longitudinal band, three gaps are filled by fat, and the arteries and nerves that run to the fingers can be exposed after the fat is removed. Palmar fascia contracture syndrome (Dupuytren's contracture syndrome) refers to the flexion contracture of the palmar interphalangeal joint and proximal interphalangeal joint induced by partial or whole fibroplasia, hypertrophy, and crispation of the palmar aponeurosis. The palmar skin becomes thickened and folds appear. In severe cases, it can involve the deep structures, causing secondary contracture.

2.2.2 Middle Layer Structure

2.2.2.1 Bone Aponeurosis of Investment

A septum of fibrous tissue is sent from the lateral margin of the palmar aponeurosis, passes through the space between the thenar muscle and the index finger flexor tendon and penetrates deeper, finally attaching to the first metacarpal bone; this fibrous septum is called the lateral intermuscular septum of the palm. Similarly, a fibrous septum is also sent from the medial margin of the palmar aponeurosis, passing through the space between the hypothenar muscle and the little finger flexor tendon, penetrating deeper, and finally attaching to the first metacarpal bone. This fibrous septum is called the medial intermuscular septum of the palm. Therefore, three bone fascia grids (lateral, middle, and medial) are formed at the palm.

The lateral grid, also called the thenar grid, is formed by being surrounded by the thenar fascia, the lateral intermuscular septum of the palm and the first metacarpal bone. It contains the short abductor muscle of the thumb, the short flexor muscle of the thumb, the opposing muscle of the thumb, the long flexor tendon of the thumb and its tendon sheath, in addition to the thumb vessels and nerves.

The middle grid is formed by being surrounded by the palmar aponeurosis, the palmar medial and lateral intermuscular septum, the bone palmar fascia, and the adductor fascia of the thumb. It contains the finger and the superficial and deep flexor tendons, the lumbrical muscle, the common flexor sheath, the superficial palmar arch, the digital arteries and nerves, etc.

The medial grid, also called the hypothenar grid, is formed by being surrounded by the hypothenar fascia, the palmar medial intermuscular septum, and the fifth metacarpal bone. It contains the little finger's abductor, breviflexor, and opposing muscle, and the vessels and nerves that reach the little finger.

In addition, the thumb adductor sheath can also be found at the lateral side of the posterior aspect of the middle grid and is formed by being surrounded by the thumb adductor sheath, the

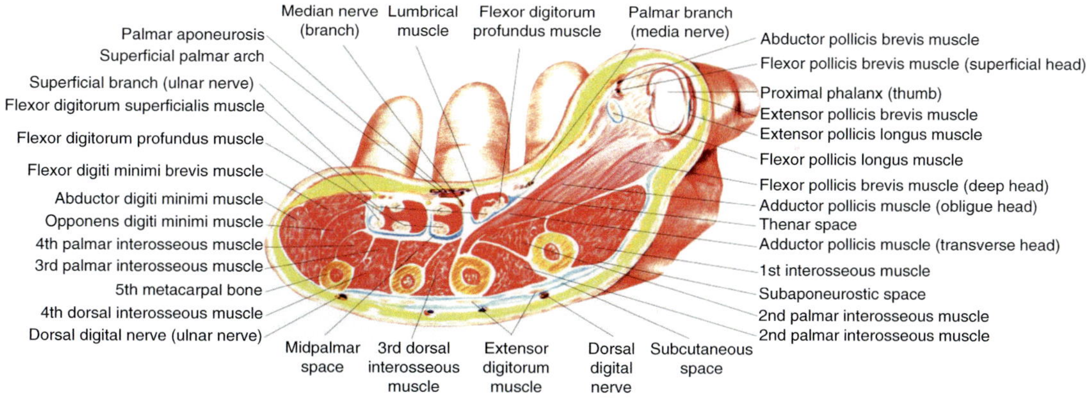

Fig. 2.16 Transverse section through the metacarpophalangeal joint of the thumb

interosseous palmar fascia, the first metacarpal bone, and the third metacarpal bone, and this sheath surrounds the thumb's adductor. The space between the thumb's adductor and the interosseous palmar fascia is called the thumb's retro-adductor space Fig. 2.16.

2.2.2.2 Fascial Space

Located at the deep part of the palmar middle grid, the fascial space contains loose connective tissues, including the lateral thenar space and the medial palmar middle space. The two spaces are separated by the palmar septum. The palmar septum is the fibrous tissue that connects the palmar fascia and interosseous palmar fascia; after it surrounds the index finger flexor tendon and the first lumbrical muscle, it is attached to the third metacarpal bone, separating the hand palmar fascia space into the midpalmar space and the thenar space (Fig. 2.17).

1. Midpalmar Space: This is located at the deep part of the ulnar (hemi) side of the palmar middle grid. The anterior border originates from the radial side and sequentially meets the third to fifth finger flexor tendons, the second to fourth lumbrical muscles; the posterior borders are at the posterior aspect of the palmar septum and meet the third to fourth metacarpal bones, interosseous muscles, and the interosseous palmar fascia at the anterior aspect; the medial border is the medial intermuscular septum, and the lateral border is the palmar septum. The distal side of the midpalmar space is connected to the second to fourth finger web spaces along the second to fourth lumbrical muscle canals, and its proximal side continues to the back of the hand. The proximal side of the midpalmar space can reach the deep surface of the common flexor sheath, and it can be connected to the forearm retro-flexor space through the carpal canal. Infection at this space can spread along the above channel.
2. Thenar Space: This is located in the radial (hemi) deep direction of the palmar middle grid. The anterior border is the anterior aspect of the intermuscular septum, index finger flexor tendon, and the first lumbrical muscle; the posterior border is the thumb adductor fascia; the lateral border is the lateral intermuscular septum; the medial border is the posterior aspect of palmar septum. The thenar space runs distally and is connected with the digital dorsum through the first lumbrical muscle, and its proximal end is the cecum.

2.2.2.3 Synovial Tendon Sheath of the Palm

The tendon is wrapped in a synovial sheath of tendon when running below the ligament or passing through the bone fibrous canal to reduce the friction and facilitate the tendon's activities. The synovial sheath of the tendon is an enclosed sleeve-shaped structure in two layers: the visceral layer and the parietal layer. The visceral layer is closely attached to the tendon, the wall layer is lined at the inner face of the peripheral structures, the potential space between the two layers is filled with a small amount of synovia, and the two layers are connected by synovial folds; those with wide synovial folds are

Fig. 2.17 Fascial space and synovial sheath of the tendon. (**a**) Projection. (**b**) Fascial space cross section (schematic diagram). *1* Palmar septum. *2* Thenar space. *3* Midpalmar space. *4* Digital common flexor sheath. *5* Long flexor muscle tendon sheath of the thumb. *6* Lumbrical muscle canal. *7* Digital synovial sheath

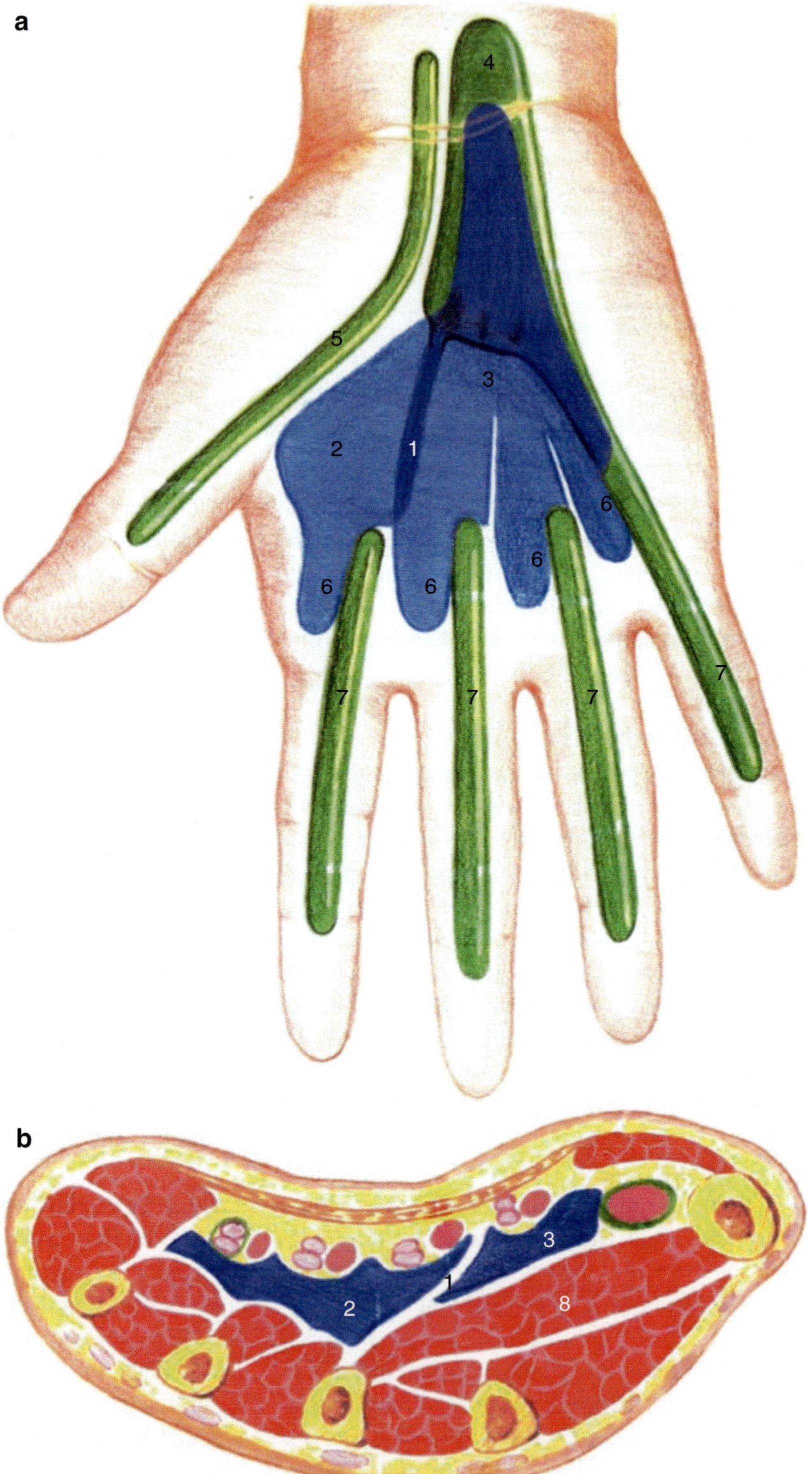

mesotendineum and those with narrow synovial folds are tenaculum tendinum, through which vessels and nerves pass. The palmar surface has the fingers' common flexor sheath and long flexor muscle tendon of the thumb (Fig. 2.18).

1. Digital common flexor sheath: Also called the ulnar synovial bursa, this wraps the digital superficial and deep flexor tendons, and most of it is located in the carpal canal. Its proximal end reaches the site two fingers above the flexor retinaculum, and its distal end is parallel and level to the ulnar margin when the thumb is abducted. The ultra side of the distal end is constantly connected with the little finger's synovial sheath (about 80–90%); when viewed at the cross-section, the bursa runs deep into the space between the digital superficial and deep flexor tendons, the ulnar margins are connected, the radial margins are separated, and it is "E"-shaped. The ulnar nerve runs along the superficial surface of the ulnar bursa, and the bursa should be incised with great caution to avoid the ulnar nerves.

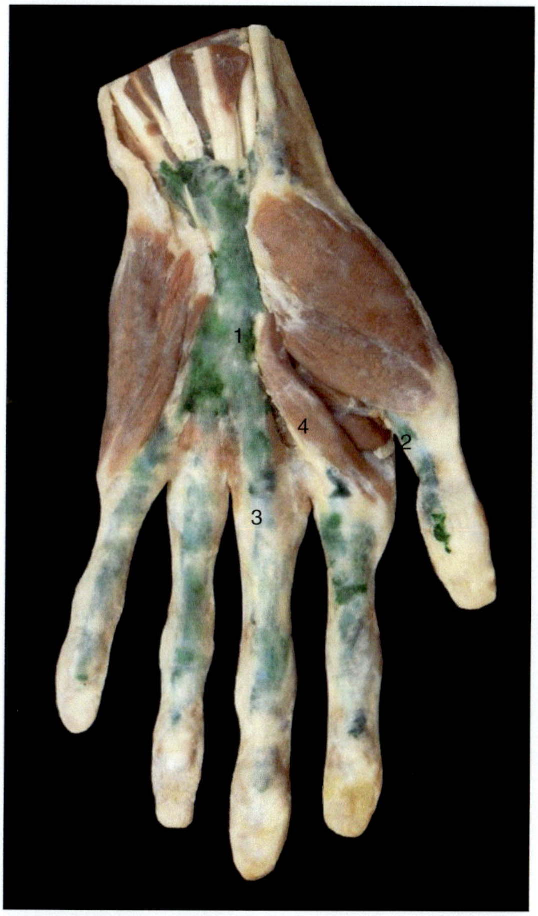

Fig. 2.18 Synovial fluid sheath of the palmar surface. *1* Digital common flexor sheath. *2* Long flexor muscle tendon sheath of the thumb. *3* Digital synovial tendon sheath. *4* The first lumbrical muscle

2. Long flexor muscle tendon sheath of the thumb: Also called the radial bursa, this is located on the lateral side and wraps the long flexor muscle tendon of the thumb; its proximal end also reaches the site two fingers above the flexor retinaculum, and its distal end is constantly connected to the thumb's Synovia. As the medial side is close to the ulnar bursa, the suppuration of one bursa is prone to cause the rupture of another bursa. At this time, the thumb and the little finger can be mutually infected. The median nerve runs along the superficial surface between the radial bursa and the ulnar bursa, the recurrent branch runs along the anterior lateral aspect of the radial bursa, and the bursa should be incised with great cautions to avoid injury to the recurrent branch Fig. 2.19.
3. Digital Synovial Tendon Sheath

   This wraps the digital flexor tendons of all fingers and is attached onto the two sides of the phalanges and is covered by the digital fiber bundles. Its proximal end reaches the distal palmar crease or metacarpophalangeal joint, and its distal end inserts at the bases of the distal phalanxes of all the fingers. The digital vessels and nerves run along the two sides of the palmar surface of the synovial tendon sheath, which should be incised as appropriate closely along the lateral margins of the phalanges.
4. Hand's Internal Muscles

   These include the lateral group, middle group, and medial group (Fig. 2.20).

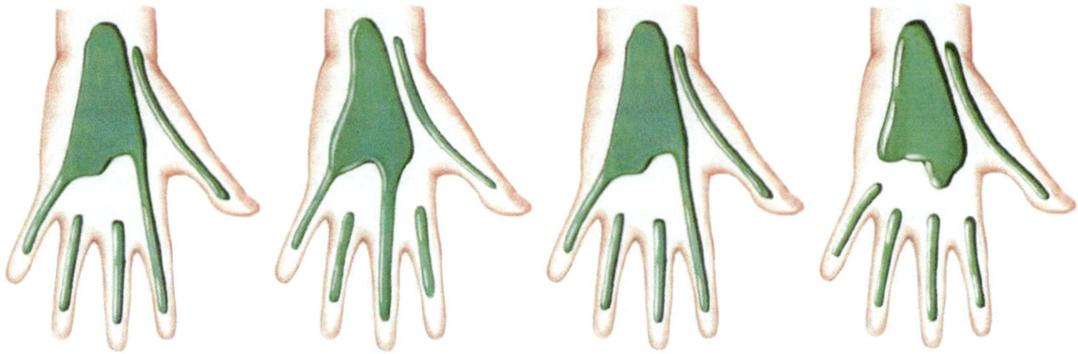

Fig. 2.19 Variation type of synovial bursa and digital flexor tendon sheath

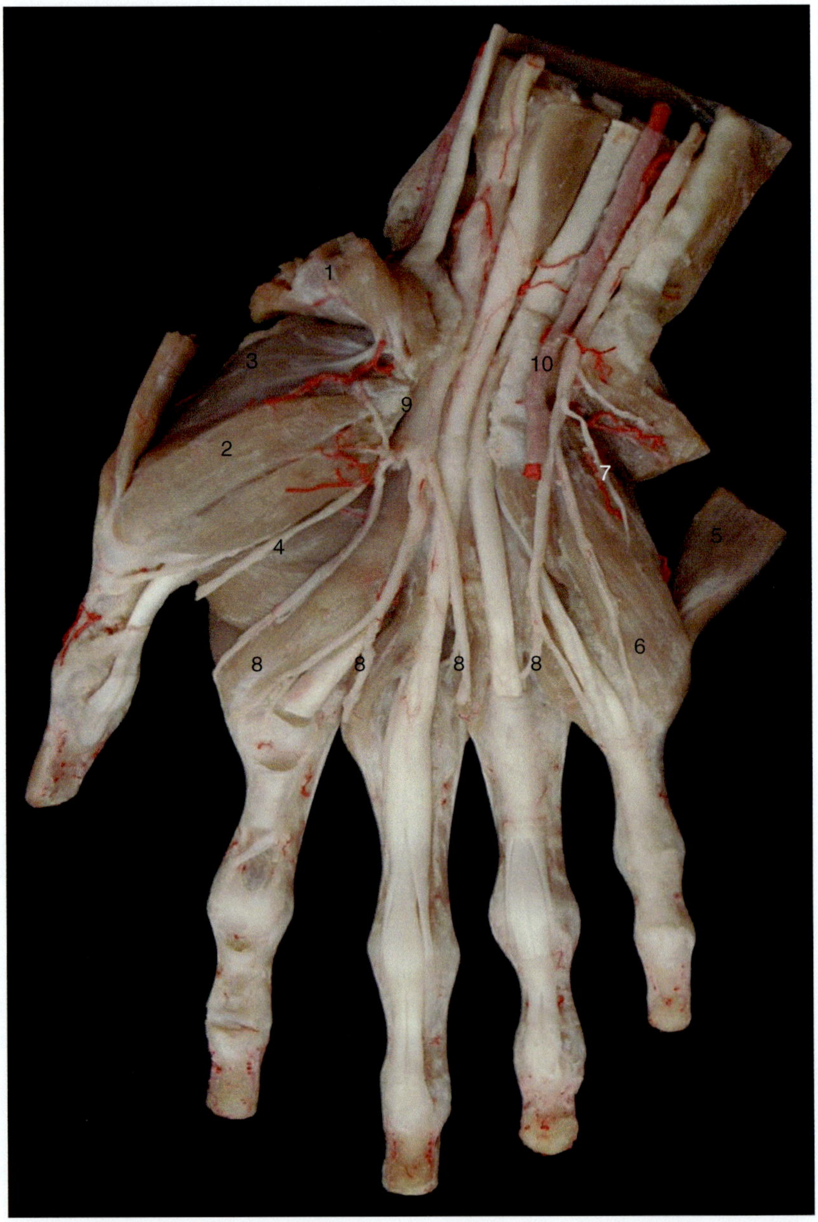

Fig. 2.20 Hand internal muscle. *1* Short abductor muscle of the thumb. *2* Short flexor muscle of the thumb. *3* Opposing muscle of the thumb. *4* Transverse head of the thumb adductor. *5* Little finger abductor. *6* Little finger breviflexor. *7* Little finger opposition. *8* Lumbrical muscle. *9* Median nerve. *10* Ulnar nerve

Lateral Group

Short abductor muscle of the thumb: This originates from the flexor retinaculum, tubercle of the scaphoid bone, and long palmar muscle tendon, and 79% of it originates from the long flexor muscle tendon of the thumb. Muscle fibers pass the metacarpophalangeal joint and end at the radial side of the base of the thumb's proximal phalanx, lateral sesamoid bone and articular capsule, and the thumb's dorsal aponeurosis (Fig. 2.21). Abduct the thumb.

Short flexor muscle of the thumb: Its superficial head originates from the distal margin of the flexor retinaculum, the radial carpal flexor tendon sheath, and the tubercle of the trapezium bone, and inserts at the radial side of the base of the thumb's proximal phalanx, lateral sesamoid bone and dorsal aponeurosis; the lateral side is often fused with the opposing muscle of the thumb. The appearance rate of the deep head is 85%; it appears together with the oblique head of the thumb's adductor and inserts together with the superficial

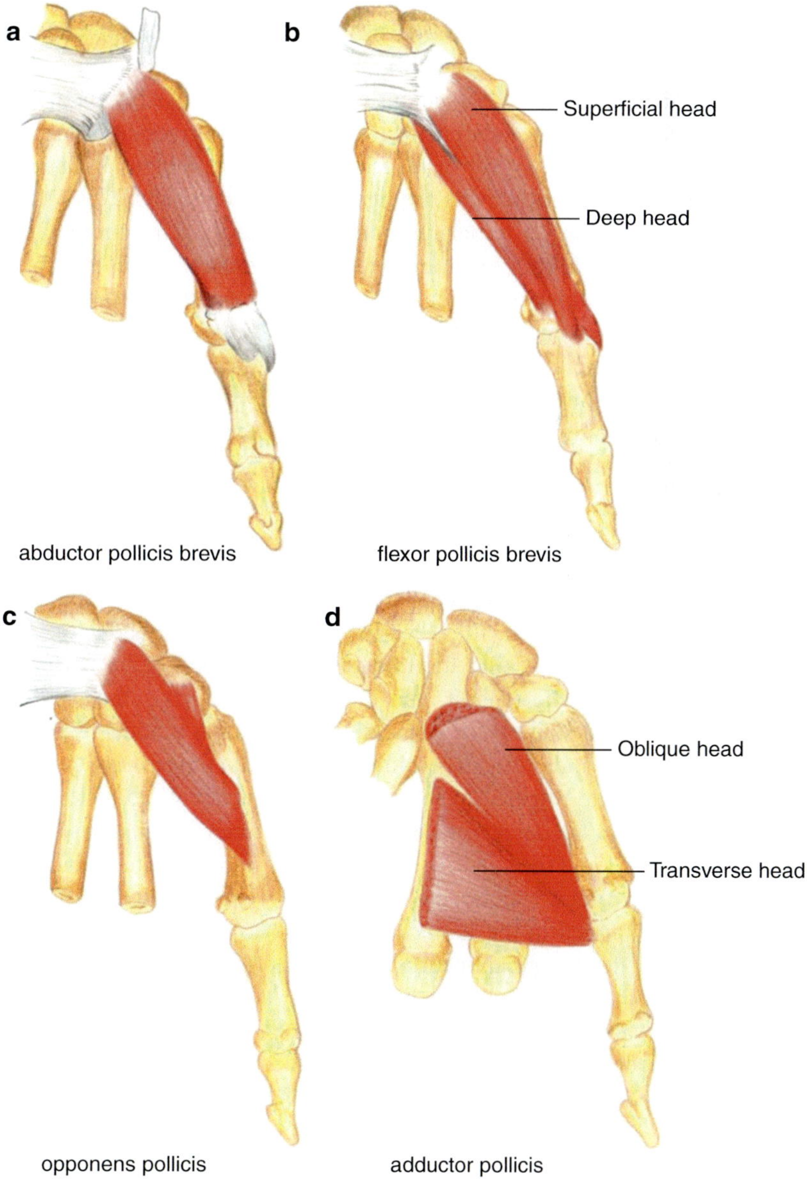

Fig. 2.21 Lateral group (thenar muscle)

head; a long flexor muscle tendon of the thumb is inserted between the two ends (Fig. 2.21). Flex the thumb's metacarpophalangeal joint.

Opposing muscle of the thumb: This is located at the deep surface of the short abductor muscle of the thumb. It originates from the carpal transverse ligament, the tubercle of the trapezium bone, and the carpometacarpal joint (the muscle fiber becomes inclined toward the outer lower direction) and inserts at the radial full length of the first metacarpal bone until the head of the metacarpal bone is reached (Fig. 2.21). It opposes the thumb.

Thumb adductor: This is located on the ulnar side of the thumb, and the deep surface of the short flexor muscle of the thumb and the long flexor muscle tendon of thumb. Oblique head and transverse head can be found. The oblique head originates from the capitate bone, and inserts into the position between the metacarpal neck and the metacarpal base; the transverse head originates from the capitate bone and covers the ligaments of capitate bone and lesser trapezium bone, and the muscle bundles of both ends are integrated into a short tendon, which inserts at the base and volar plate of the thumb's proximal phalanx (Fig. 2.21). It adducts and flexes the thumb, mildly flexing the metacarpophalangeal joint, and extending the interphalangeal joint.

Middle Group

Lumbrical muscle is located at the center of the palm and at the deep surface of the palmar aponeurosis; it corresponds to the radial side of the digital deep flexor tendon. It is earthworm-shaped, the muscle fibers that migrate toward the fingertip become the tendon, and then the fibers skip the radial side of the metacarpophalangeal joint of the index finger, middle finger, ring finger, and little finger to reach the digital dorsum. They lie at the deep surface of the neurovascular bundles and the superficial surface of the palmar deep transverse ligament. In addition, they are wrapped in the lumbrical muscle canal formed by the palmar aponeurosis and end at the fingers. Finally, they migrate to the radial side of the dorsal aponeurosis of the index finger, middle finger, ring finger, and little finger to reach the plane of the proximal interphalangeal joint. In the case of muscle contraction, the metacarpophalangeal joints of the index finger, middle finger, ring finger, and little finger are flexed, and the distal interphalangeal joints are extended (Fig. 2.22).

The first lumbrical muscle is unipennate, originating from the radial side of the digital deep flexor tendon of the index finger. It is the most constant, and 2.3% have an additional head at the origin. The second lumbrical muscle is also unipennate, originating from the radial side of the deep flexor tendon of the middle finger, but there are many variations. Those that are bipennate and originate from the deep flexor tendon of the index finger and the middle finger account for 23.1%. The third lumbrical muscle is bipennate in most cases, originating from the deep flexor tendons of the two adjacent fingers; 4.17% are unipennate and originate from the deep flexor tendon of the ring finger. It inserts when tendon splitting occurs, and 27.8% end at the dorsal aponeurosis of the adjacent two fingers. The fourth lumbrical muscle is bipennate in most cases, originating from the deep flexor tendons of the two adjacent fingers; 13.6% are unipennate and originate from the deep flexor tendon of little finger or those with an additional head account. It inserts when tendon splitting occurs, and 22.7% insert at the adjacent dorsal aponeuroses.

Interosseous muscles: The interosseous muscles are divided into palmar interosseous muscle and dorsal interosseous muscle (Fig. 2.23). The former is the adductor of the fingers, and the latter is the abductor. The so-called adduction and abduction are performed with the middle finger as the axis, the act of drawing close to the middle finger is adduction and the act of leaving the middle finger is abduction. As the thumb has an independent adductor and abductor, no matched interosseous muscle grows; the little finger has an independent abductor; thus, there are no interosseous muscles, either.

Palmar interosseous muscles: There are three pieces of palmar interosseous muscles (all are single-headed), which lie at the deep surface of the digital deep flexor tendon and lumbrical muscle and at the volar side of the second to fifth intermetacarpal spaces. The first to third palmar interosseous muscles originate from one side of the second, fourth, and fifth metacarpal bone bodies near the middle finger, pass along the dorsal side of the palmar deep transverse ligament, and insert at the dorsal side of the base of the proximal phalanxes of the middle finger, ring finger, and little finger; they are involved in the formation of the dorsal aponeurosis. In the case of contraction, the index finger, middle ringer, and ring finger are adducted, the metacarpophalangeal joint is flexed, and the proximal interphalangeal joint is extended.

Dorsal interosseous muscle: There are four pieces of dorsal interosseous muscle, which are both double-headed, and lie at the dorsal side of the second to fifth intermetacarpal spaces. They originate from the body of the metacarpal bone, which borders the intermetacarpal space, pass along the dorsal side of the palmar deep transverse ligament, and insert at the base of the proximal phalanxes of the digital radial side, two sides of the middle finger, and the ulnar side of the ring finger; they are involved in the formation of the dorsal aponeurosis. In the case of contraction, it abducts the index finger, middle finger (radial and ulnar deviation), and ring finger, and assists the flexion of the metacarpophalangeal joint and the extension of the interphalangeal joint.

Medial Group

Little finger abductor: This is located in the proximal subcutaneous adipose tissues of the hypothenar and lies at the ulnar side of the palmar aponeurosis; it originates from the lentiform bone and inserts at the ulnar side of the proximal phalanx of little finger and the dorsal aponeurosis (Fig. 2.24). It flexes and abducts the little finger joints.

Little finger breviflexor: This is located at the radial side of the little finger abductor; it originates from the hook of hamate bone and carpal transverse ligaments and inserts at the ulnar side

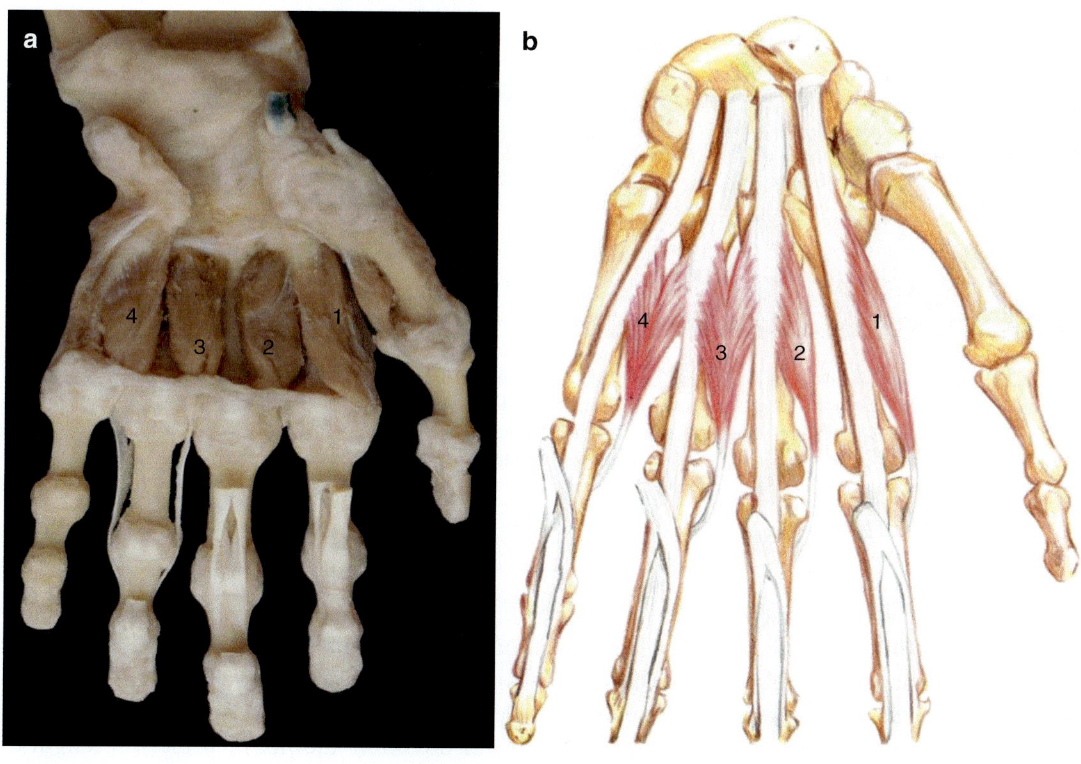

Fig. 2.22 Shape of lumbrical muscle. (**a**) Specimen of real object. (**b**) Schematic diagram. *1* The first lumbrical muscle. *2* The second lumbrical muscle. *3* The third lumbrical muscle. *4* The fourth lumbrical muscle

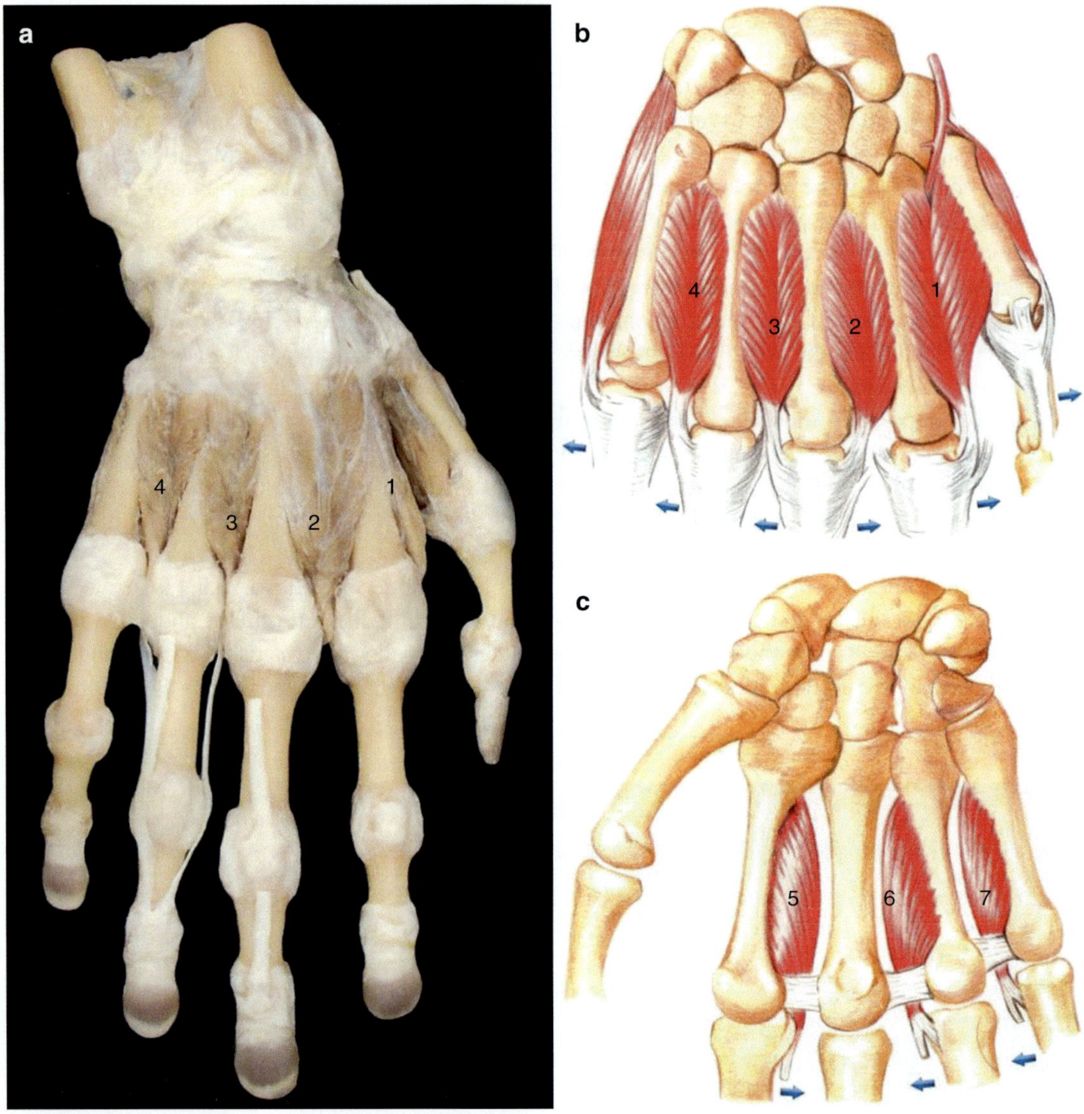

Fig. 2.23 Shape of interosseous muscles. (**a**) Dorsal interosseous muscle (specimen of real object). (**b**) Dorsal interosseous muscle (schematic diagram). (**c**) Palmar interosseous muscles (schematic diagram). *1* The first dorsal interosseous muscle. *2* The second dorsal interosseous muscle. *3* The third dorsal interosseous muscle. *4* The fourth dorsal interosseous muscle. *5* The first palmar interosseous muscles. *6* The second palmar interosseous muscles. *7* The third palmar interosseous muscles

of the base of the little finger proximal phalanx and the dorsal aponeurosis. Sometimes, it is absent. The ulnar artery and the deep branch of the ulnar nerve passes through the space between this muscle and the little finger abductor (Fig. 2.24). It has the effect of flexing the metacarpophalangeal joint of the little finger and abducting the little finger.

Opposing muscle of little finger: This is located at the deep surface of the above two muscles. It originates from the hook of hamate bone and carpal transverse ligament; the muscle fibers become inclined toward the inner and lower direction and insert at the full length of the ulnar margin of the fifth metacarpus. In the case of contraction, it can tract the fifth meta-

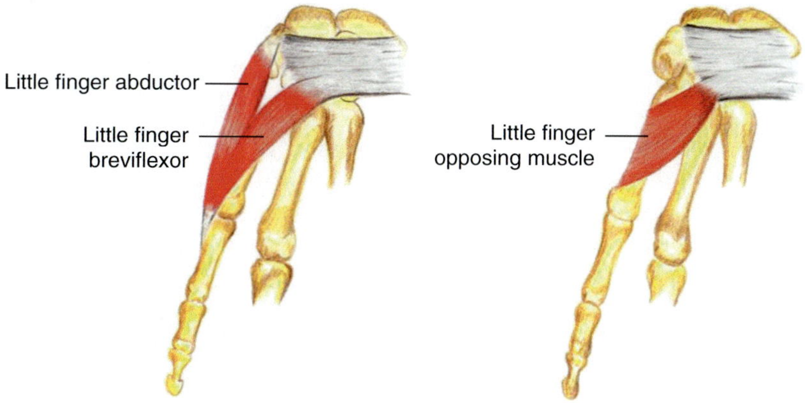

Fig. 2.24 Medial group (hypothenar muscle)

carpus to produce opposition along the direction of the thumb. It can draw the fifth metacarpus in an anterior direction to make the palm pit deeper.

2.2.2.4 Vessels

The main blood supply of the hand is directly from the branches of the radial and ulnar arteries, and they become anastomosed mutually into the superficial palmar arch and deep palmar arch. The anterior interosseous artery and posterior interosseous artery of the forearm are involved in the formation of the carpal arterial network. Some individuals still have relatively developed medial arteries, which are distributed at the proximal side of the palm or involved in the formation of the superficial palmar arch.

Superficial Palmar Arch

This is located at the deep surface of the palmar aponeurosis and short palmar muscle and at the superficial surface of the little finger breviflexor, the common palmar digital nerve, the finger flexor tendon and lumbrical muscle, and the convex side of the arch points to the fingers. The body surface projection line is generally at the arch line drawn from the median point of the palm's central line to the radial side of the lentiform bone.

The superficial palmar arch is formed by the anastomosis between the end branch of the ulnar artery and the arteries such as the superficial palmar branch of the radial arteries (Fig. 2.25). The medial outer diameter of the superficial palmar arch is 2.2 mm. The convex side of the superficial palmar arch sends three common palmar digital arteries and little finger ulnar palmar arteries, and the pit side sends several small recurrent branches to the wrist to participate in the formation of rete carpi volare. The superficial palmar arch and its branches are accompanied by the veins of the same name.

Common palmar digital artery: the appearance rate is almost 100%, and the outer diameter of the origin of all arteries is 1.2–1.5 mm. The proper palmar digital artery is accompanied by the common palmar digital nerve after being sent out, passing along the second to the fourth intermetacarpal spaces and below the surfaces of the corresponding lumbrical muscles, and inserting near the metacarpophalangeal joint, where it receives the palmar metacarpal artery and the branches from the dorsal metacarpal artery. It is divided into two proper palmar digital arteries at the site 1.2 cm away from the finger web margin.

Ulnar palmar artery of little finger: This originates from the ulnar margin of the convex side of the superficial palmar arch, descends along the surface of the hypothenar muscle, and is distributed at the ulnar margin of the little finger.

According to the source of the arteries anastomosed with the end branch of the ulnar arteries, the superficial palmar arch is classified into four categories:

(a) Ulnar arterial type (51.72%), composed of the end branch of the arterial artery, without the involvement of the radial artery

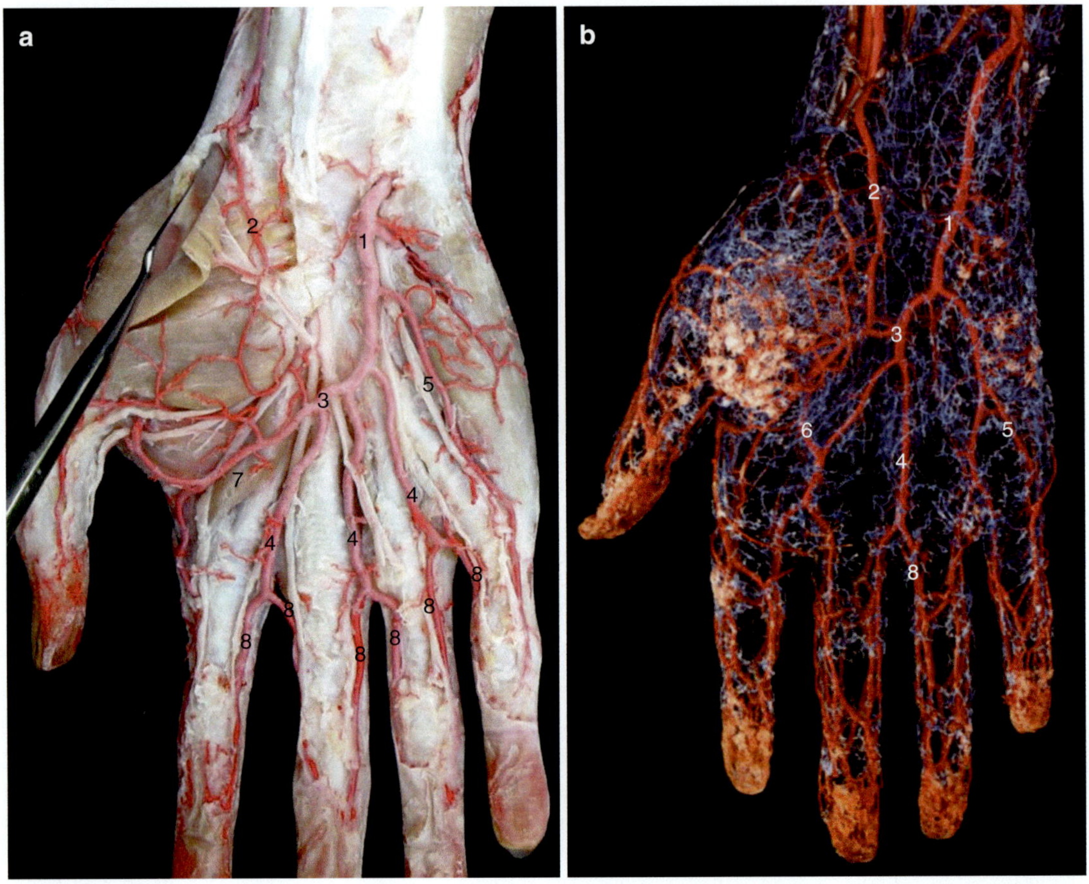

Fig. 2.25 Position, composition, and branches of the superficial palmar arch. (**a**) Specimen of the real object. (**b**) Cast specimen. *1* End branch of the ulnar artery. *2* Superficial palmar branch of the radial artery. *3* Superficial palmar arch. *4* Common palmar digital artery. *5* Ulnar palmar artery of the little finger. *6* Common palmar digital nerve. *7* Lumbrical muscle. *8* Proper palmar digital artery

(b) Ulnar arterial type (37.31%), composed of the end branch of the ulnar artery and superficial palmar branch of the radial artery
(c) Medial ulnar arterial type (4.51%), composed of the end branch of the ulnar artery and medial artery
(d) Radioulnar medial arterial type (0.96%), composed of the end branch of the ulnar artery, the superficial palmar branch of the radial artery, and the medial artery (Fig. 2.26)

Deep Palmar Arch

This is located at the digital deep and superficial flexor tendons, lumbrical muscles, superficial head of the short flexor muscle of the thumb, and the space between the little finger breviflexor and the interosseous muscle. The transverse position ranges from the fundus of the first intermetacarpal space to the fundus of the fifth metacarpal bone. The arch body surface projection line is equal to the connecting

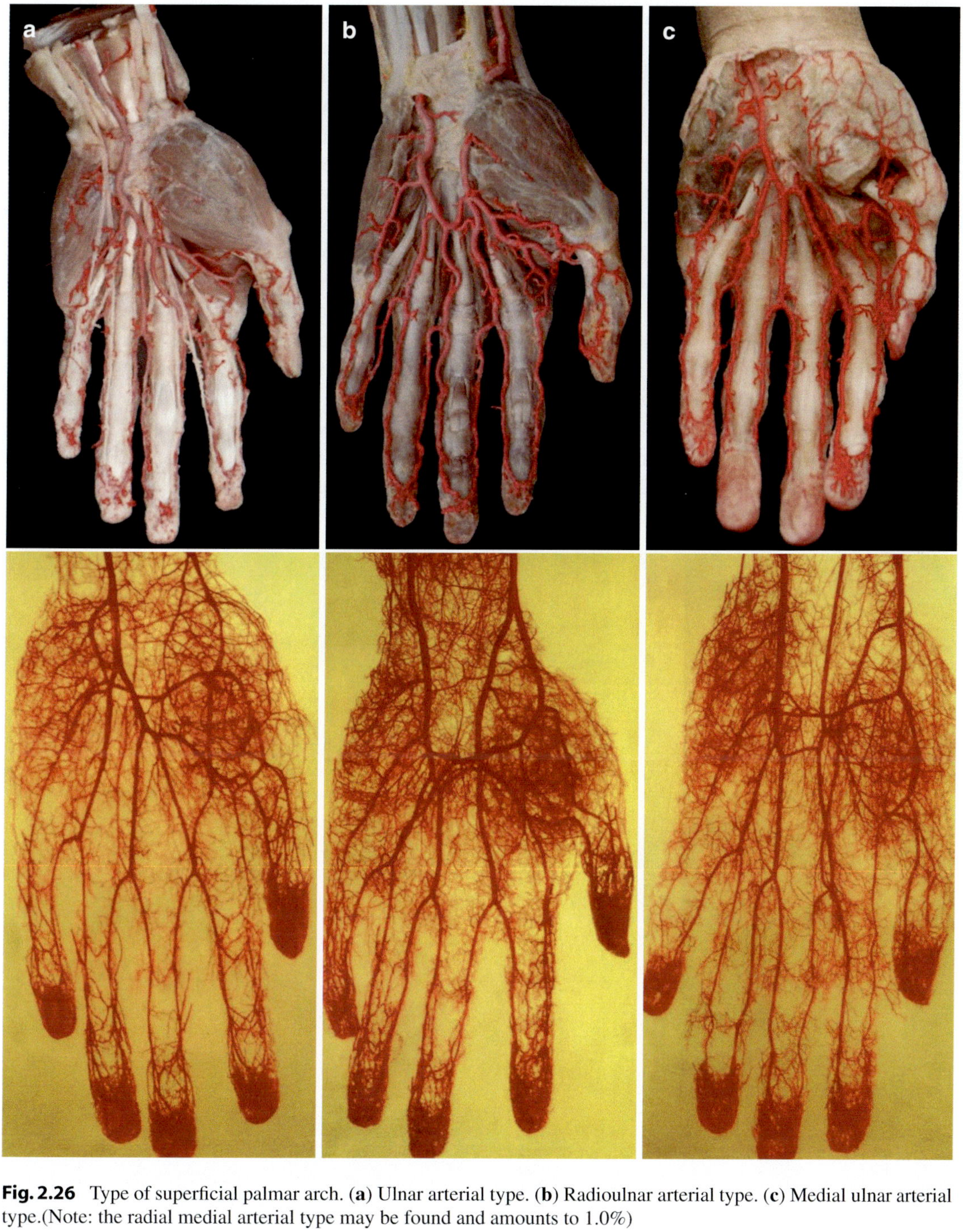

Fig. 2.26 Type of superficial palmar arch. (**a**) Ulnar arterial type. (**b**) Radioulnar arterial type. (**c**) Medial ulnar arterial type.(Note: the radial medial arterial type may be found and amounts to 1.0%)

line between the proximal end of the first intermetacarpal space to the hamate bone. The deep palmar arch is accompanied by the vein of the same name.

The deep palmar arch is mainly composed of the end branch of the radial artery and the middle outer diameter of the arch is 2.0 mm. The deep palmar arch is divided into complete type and incomplete type based on whether the end branch of the arterial branch is anastomosed with other arteries (Fig. 2.27).

1. The complete type accounts for about 95%, and is formed by the anastomosis between the end branch of the radial artery and the deep palmar branch or other branch of the ulnar artery. The arch formed by the anastomosis between the end branch of the radial artery and the upper or lower deep palmar branch of ulnar artery accounts for 55%, the arch formed by the anastomosis with the third common palmar digital artery or the branch of the little finger ulnar palmar artery accounts for 30%, and the arch formed by the anastomosis with another nonconstant branch accounts for 10%.
2. The remaining 5% are of the incomplete type and the end branch of the radial artery runs inward and does not become anastomosed with another branch. Actually, the end branch of the radial artery is widely anastomosed with other peripheral branches, which are merely small. The end branch can become a perforating branch to pass through

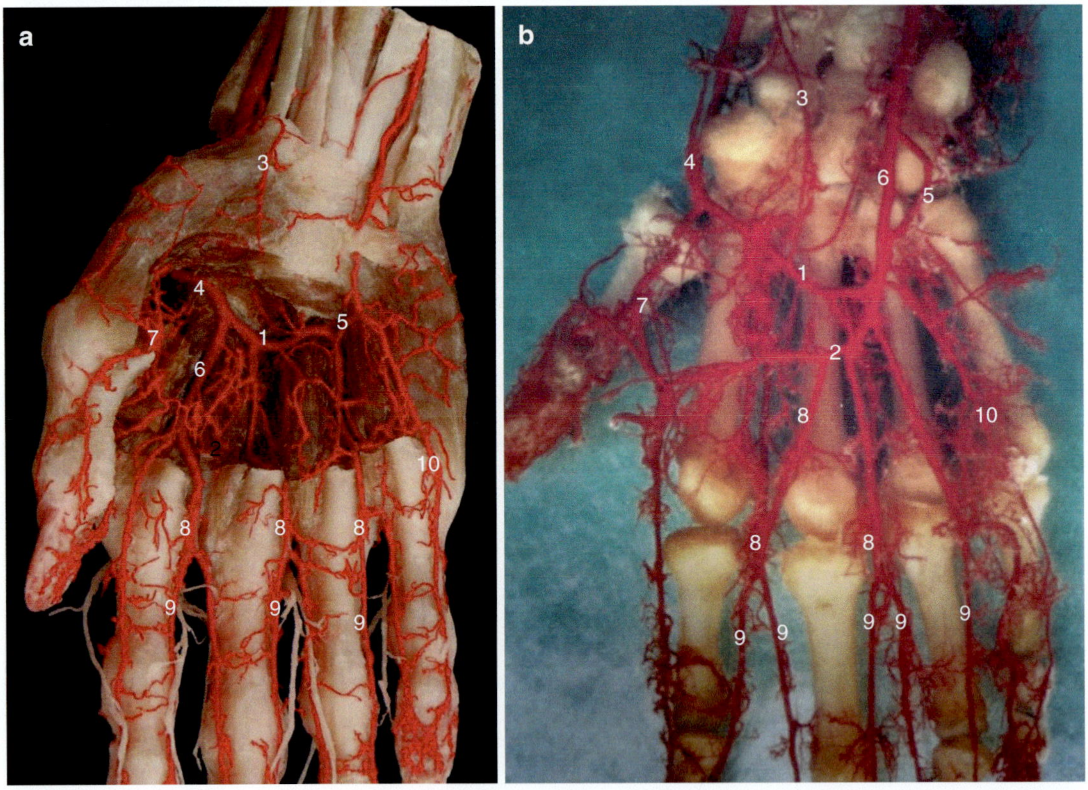

Fig. 2.27 Position, composition, and branches of the deep palmar arch. (**a**) Specimen of the real object. (**b**) Cast specimen. *1* Deep palmar arch. *2* Superficial palmar arch. *3* Superficial palmar branch of the radial artery. *4* End branch of the radial artery. *5* Deep palmar arch of the ulnar artery. *6* End branch of the ulnar artery. *7* Principal artery of the thumb. *8* Common palmar digital artery. *9* Proper palmar digital artery. *10* Ulnar palmar artery of the little finger

the fourth intermetacarpal space, forming the fourth dorsal metacarpal artery, and it can also insert at the fourth intermetacarpal space.

The convex side of the deep palmar arch sends three palmar metacarpal arteries toward the fingers, the concave side of the deep palmar arch sends two to four recurrent branches toward the wrist to participate in the lateral rete carpi volare, and the dorsal side of the arch sends three perforating branches toward the back of hand.

2.2.2.5 Nerves

Ulnar nerve, median nerve, and their branches are distributed on the palmar surface of the hand.

Ulnar Nerve

Its main trunk passes along the superficial surface of the flexor retinaculum, runs downward closely along the space between the radial side of the lentiform bone and the ulnar nerve, and then it passes along the deep surface of the short palmar muscle to the palm. The ulnar nerve is divided into two branches (superficial and deep) after running to the outer lower direction of the lentiform bone.

Superficial branch of the ulnar nerve: This runs along the medial side of the ulnar artery, sends branches to the short palmar muscle, and is divided into the digital palmar proper nerve and the common palmar digital nerve at the deep surface of this muscle. The digital palmar proper nerve is distributed at the ulnar margin of the little finger's palmar surface; the common palmar digital nerve is divided into two digital palmar proper nerves when reaching the finger web space, and they are distributed in the skin of the margins that correspond to the little finger and ring finger (Fig. 2.28).

Deep branch of the ulnar nerve: accompanied by the deep palmar branch of ulnar nerve, it passes by the origin of the hypothenar muscles and accompanies the deep palmar arch, then it sends branches to the hypothenar muscles, all interosseous muscles, the third and fourth lumbrical muscles, and the thumb adductor (Fig. 2.29). The position of the segment from the lentiform bone to the hamate bone passing by the deep branch is superficial, and vulnerable to injuries. After injury, the paralysis of the thumb adductor, interosseous muscle, and little finger abductor make the fingers incapable of adduction and abduction, causing the manifestation of "claw hand."

Median Nerve

This enters the palm through the carpal canal and runs at the deep surface (slightly prone to being on the radial side) and the superficial surface of the flexor tendon; it is immediately divided into two branches after running in the carpal canal.

Lateral branch: Relatively small, this branch first sends a recurrent branch and is then divided into three digital palmar proper nerves, which are distributed at the two sides of thumb, and the palmar skin of the radial side of the index finger. The recurrent branch is sent from the inferior margin of the flexor retinaculum, then draws and circles the medial margin of the short flexor muscle of the thumb toward the proximal end, and the branches dominate the short flexor muscle of the thumb, the short abductor muscle of the thumb, and the opposing muscle of the thumb. The surface of the median nerve's recurrent branch is located at the median point of the thenar medial margin, equivalent to the site about 2.5 cm below the carpal anterior transverse crease. No incision can be made arbitrarily during the operation to avoid nerve injuries; otherwise, the thumb function may be partially lost.

Medial branch: Relatively large, it is immediately divided into two common palmar digital nerves. Accompanied by the vessel with the same name, at the finger web space, it is divided into two digital palmar proper nerves at the proximal side of the arterial branch with the same name, and they are distributed in the skin of the margins that correspond to the second to fourth fingers.

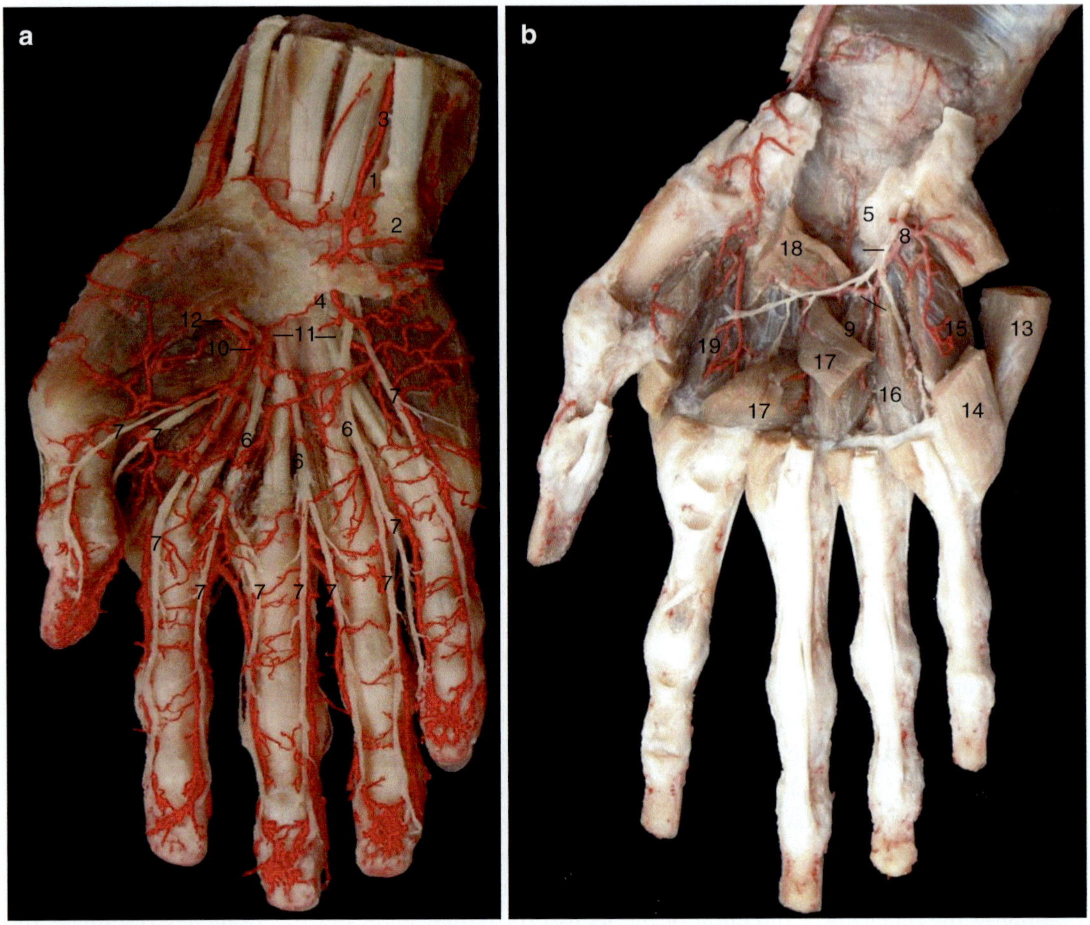

Fig. 2.28 Median nerve, ulnar nerve, and branches. *1* The ulnar nerve. *2* Pisiform bone. *3* Ulnar artery. *4* Ramus superficialis nervi ulnaris. *5* Profundus nervi ulnaris. *6* The palm side always nervous. *7* Nervi digitales volares proprii. *8* Metacarpal artery, volar, deep. *9* Arcus palmaris profundus. *10* Rami lateralis. *11* Rami medialis. *12* Recurrent branch. *13* Abductor muscle of little finger. *14* Flexor digitorum brevis brevis. *15* Musculi opponens digiti quinti manus. *16* Musculi lumbricales. *17* Adductor pollicis (horizontal head). *18* Adductor pollicis (oblique head). *19* Interosseus

The median nerve also sends muscular branches to dominate the first and second lumbrical muscles (Fig. 2.30).

2.3 Dorsum of the Hand

2.3.1 Superficial Layer Structure

The skin at the dorsum of the hand is relatively thin; with hair and sebaceous glands, it has a high elasticity. As its combination with superficial fascia is relatively loose, it is easy to move. In the case of clenching the fist, the skin is tense; in the case of finger extension, the skin appears to be excessively flaccid; therefore, trauma is prone to causing skin tear. It is distributed in the superficial veins, superficial lymphatic vessels, and cutaneous nerves.

2.3.1.1 Venous Network of the Dorsum of the Hand

The rich superficial veins in the superficial fascia are mutually anastomosed to form the venous network of the dorsum of the hand (Fig. 2.31), and they can be divided into five categories (Fig. 2.32). Located at the superficial surface, it receives the veins originating from the finger and

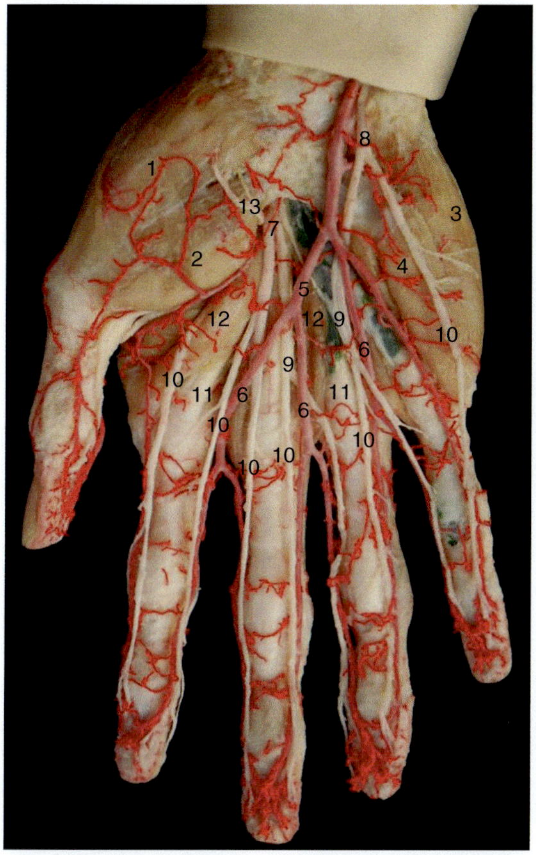

Fig. 2.29 Median nerves. The branches and distribution of the ulnar nerve. *1* Abductor pollicis brevis. *2* Flexor pollicis brevis (caput Superficial). *3* Abductor digiti Minimi. *4* Flexor digiti Minimi brevis. *5* Superficialis palmar arch. *6* Common palmar digital artery. *7* Median nerve. *8* Ulnar nerve. *9* Nervi digitales palmares communes. *10* Nervi digitale palmares proprii. *11* Superficial flexor tendon of finger. *12* Musculi lumbricales. *13* Recurrent branch of median nerve

palm superficial layers in addition to the deep part of the hand. The dorsal veins of the hand have many thick branches, and most hand veins gather there to reflux to the forearm. The digital radial vein and digital ulnar vein are distributed at the two sides of each digital dorsum; in addition to the effects of gathering the small branches at the digital palmar surface, they are also mutually anastomosed to form the digital venous arch. There are three rows of venous arches, arranged at the dorsal aspect of each phalanx, including the single arches and compound arches.

The digital radial and ulnar veins of the adjacent fingers mutually converge at the metacarpophalangeal joints to form the second to fourth palmar dorsal veins. At the convergence, the veins between the metacarpal heads also converge. The second palmar dorsal veins receive the index finger ulnar veins and middle finger radial veins, and the palmar dorsal veins run toward the proximal side along the intermetacarpal space, forming venous arches or a venous network at the dorsum of the hand. At the dorsum of the wrist, the radial and ulnar ends of the arch or network are continued to the starting part of the cephalic vein and basilic vein.

The blood reflux of the hand mainly involves the hand's dorsal veins; in the case of replantation for the amputated part below the wrist, the hand dorsal veins should be carefully recanalized so that the survival of the broken hand can be guaranteed.

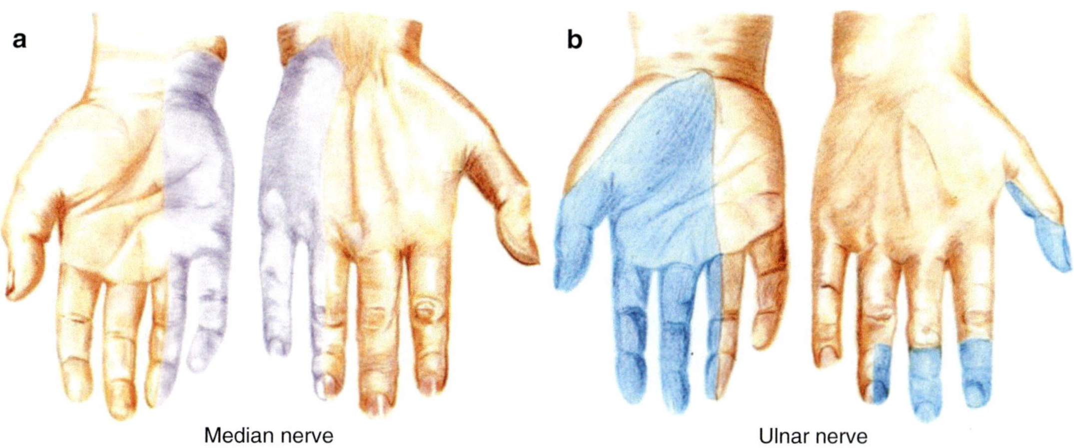

Fig. 2.30 Cutaneous innervation. (**a**) Palmar view. (**b**) Posterior (dorsal) view

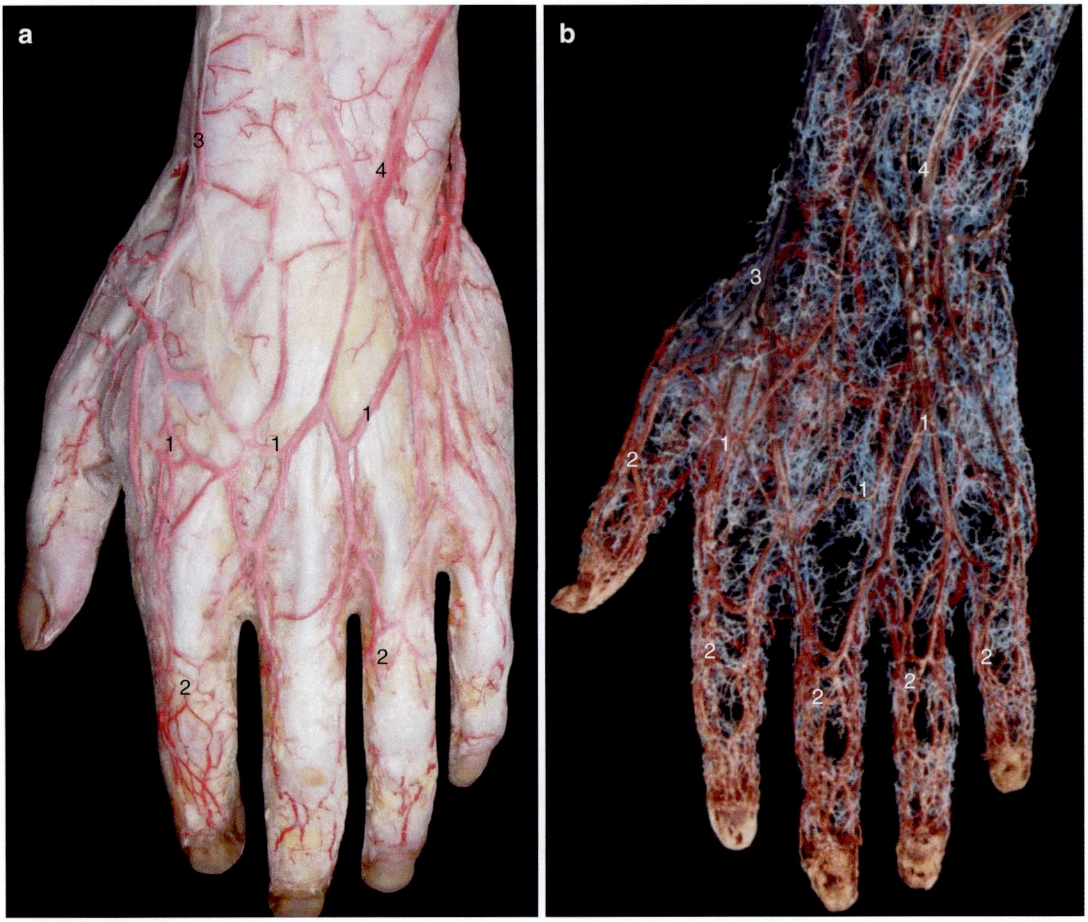

Fig. 2.31 Hand's dorsal vein network. (**a**) Specimen of a real object. (**b**) Cast specimen. *1* Hand dorsal vein network. *2* Digital dorsal vein. *3* Cephalic vein. *4* Basilic vein

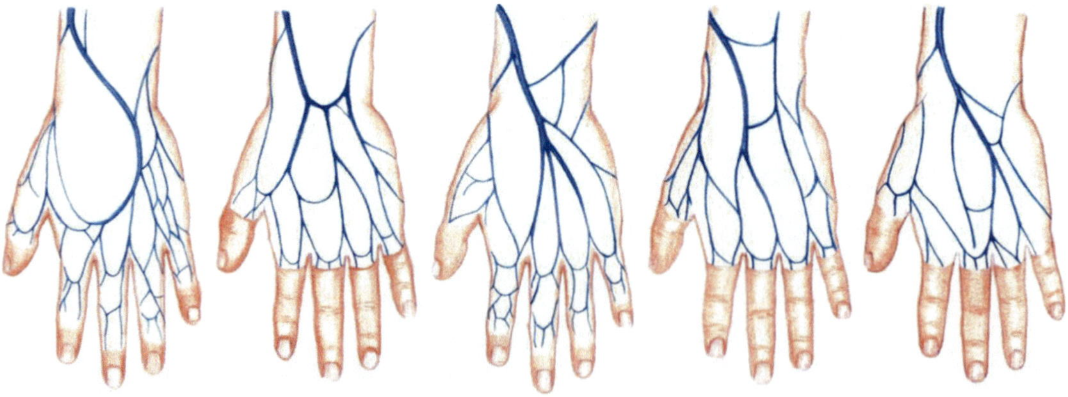

Fig. 2.32 Main types of hand dorsal veins. *I* Arch type. The palmar dorsal veins form a large venous arch at the dorsum of the hand. *II* Arch type. The palmar dorsal veins form a large venous arch at the dorsum of the wrist, and sometimes form a grade II and grade III venous arch at the dorsum of the hand. *III* Net type. The second to fourth palmar dorsal veins are relatively thick and gradually converge toward the proximal side, forming a thick venous trunk. *IV* Net type. The second to third palmar dorsal veins are relatively thick and form a thick venous trunk, and the remaining veins are relatively thin and net-shaped. *V* Net type. The third and fourth palmar dorsal veins are relatively thick and gradually converge toward the proximal side, and the remaining veins are relatively thin

2.3.1.2 Dorsal Cutaneous Nerves of the Hand (Fig. 2.33)

Superficial branch of the radial nerve: This penetrates the deep fascia at the site three fingers above the wrist, and then runs downward to pass the thumb's long abductor and short extensor superficial surfaces to reach the dorsum of the hand. It is distributed in the radial hemi-skin of the digital dorsum and sends five digital dorsal cutaneous nerves, which are distributed in the skin of the margins that correspond to the proximal segments of the thumb, index finger, and middle finger.

Dorsal branch of the ulnar nerve: This penetrates the deep fascia at the site 4–5 cm above the wrist, is distributed in the ulnar hemi-skin of the dorsum of the hand, and then sends five digital cutaneous nerves, which are distributed in the skin of the margins that correspond to the little finger, ring finger, and middle finger.

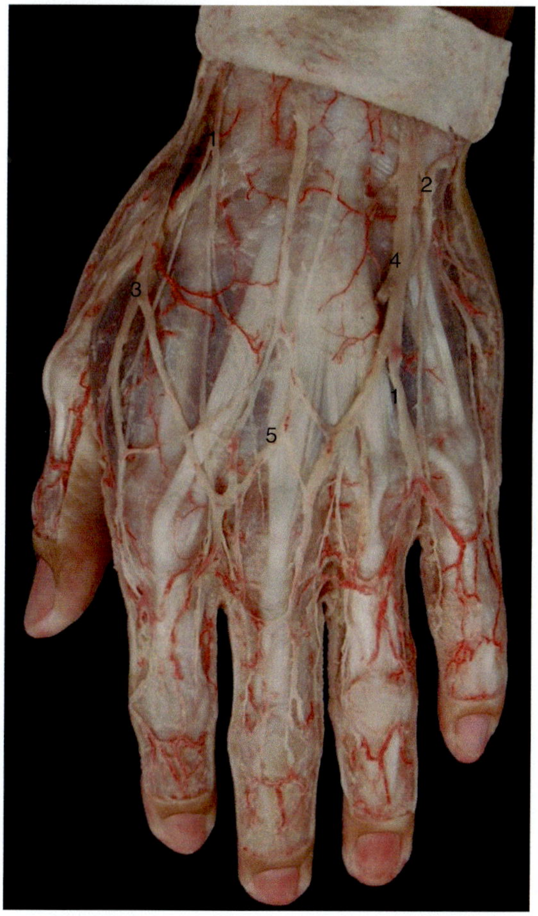

Fig. 2.33 Dorsal cutaneous nerves of the hand

Digital palmar proper nerve (median nerve): The branches sent by the dorsal ramus are distributed in the skin at the distal position of the dorsal aspect of three and a half radial fingers.

Forearm lateral cutaneous nerve: This is distributed in the skin on the radial side of the carpal dorsal aspect.

The distribution and typing of the hand's dorsal cutaneous nerves (Fig. 2.34) are as follows:

Type I: The superficial branch of the radial nerve and the hand's dorsal branch of the ulnar nerve are distributed in two and a half fingers on the radioulnar sides, and this type accounts for 60.92%.

Type II: Its distribution is the same as for type I, thick anastomotic branches are attached between the two nerves, and this type accounts for 2.46%.

Type III: The hand's dorsal branches of the ulnar nerve outnumber the superficial branches of the radial nerve, and this type accounts for 3.28%.

Type IV: The superficial branches of the radial nerve outnumber the hand's dorsal branches of the ulnar nerve, and this type accounts for 28.69%.

Type V: The superficial branches of the radial nerve are distributed in the entire arm, only one hand's dorsal branch of the ulnar nerve remains or the branch is absent, and this type accounts for 1.92%.

Type VI: The forearm's lateral cutaneous nerve, in place of the superficial branch of the radial nerve, is distributed in the dorsum of the hand, only one superficial branch of the radial nerve remains or the branch is absent, and this type accounts for 2.73%.

2.3.2 Deep Layer Structure

1. Extensor retinaculum: This is formed after the antebrachial fascia becomes thickened on the carpal dorsal side, and it is also called the carpal dorsal ligament (Fig. 2.35). It is about 2–3 cm wide; its fibers run transversely and obliquely. On the radial side, it is attached to the lateral margin of the lower end of the radius and the radial styloid process. On the

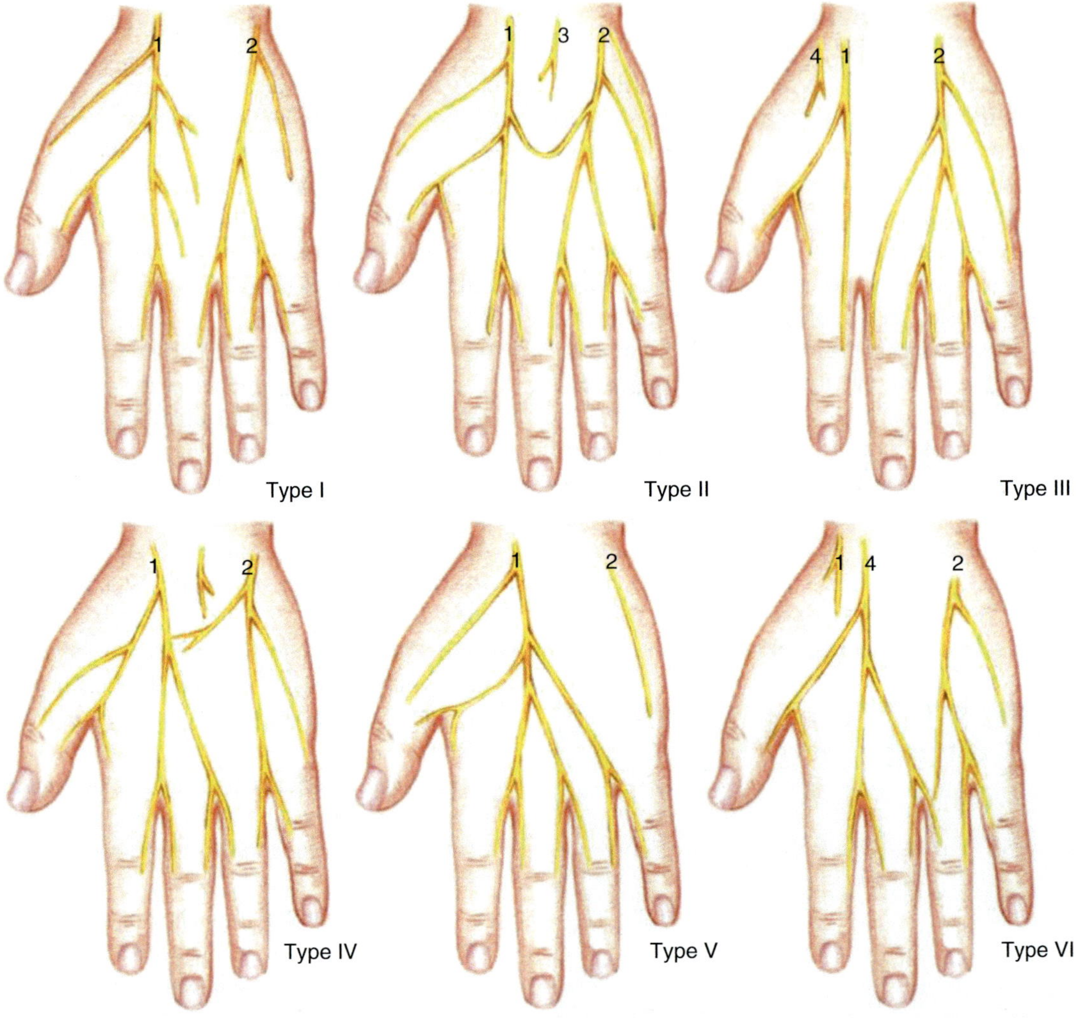

Fig. 2.34 Distribution and typing of the hand's dorsal cutaneous nerves. *1* Superficial branch of the radial nerve. *2* Hand's dorsal branch of the ulnar nerve. *3* Forearm's posterior cutaneous nerve. *4* Forearm's lateral cutaneous nerve

ulnar side, it passes through the ulnar styloid process and its distal end and continues to the flexor retinaculum. In addition, it is attached to the lentiform and triangular bones.

2. Dorsal deep fascia of the hand: This can be divided into the superficial and deep layers. The superficial layer is relatively thick, and it is the continuation of the carpal dorsal ligament (extensor retinaculum); together with the extensor tendon, it forms the hand dorsal aponeurosis. The second and fifth metacarpal bones are attached to both sides. The deep layer covers the deep surfaces from the second to fifth metacarpal bones and from the second to the fourth dorsal interosseous muscles, and it is called interosseous dorsal fascia. It is connected with hand dorsal fascia through the fiber grid at the proximal end of metacarpal bone, and at its distal end, the two layers of fasciae are mutually combined at the site of finger web.
3. Fascial space: Because the hand's dorsal fasciae are mutually combined at the proximal and distal ends of the metacarpal bone, the

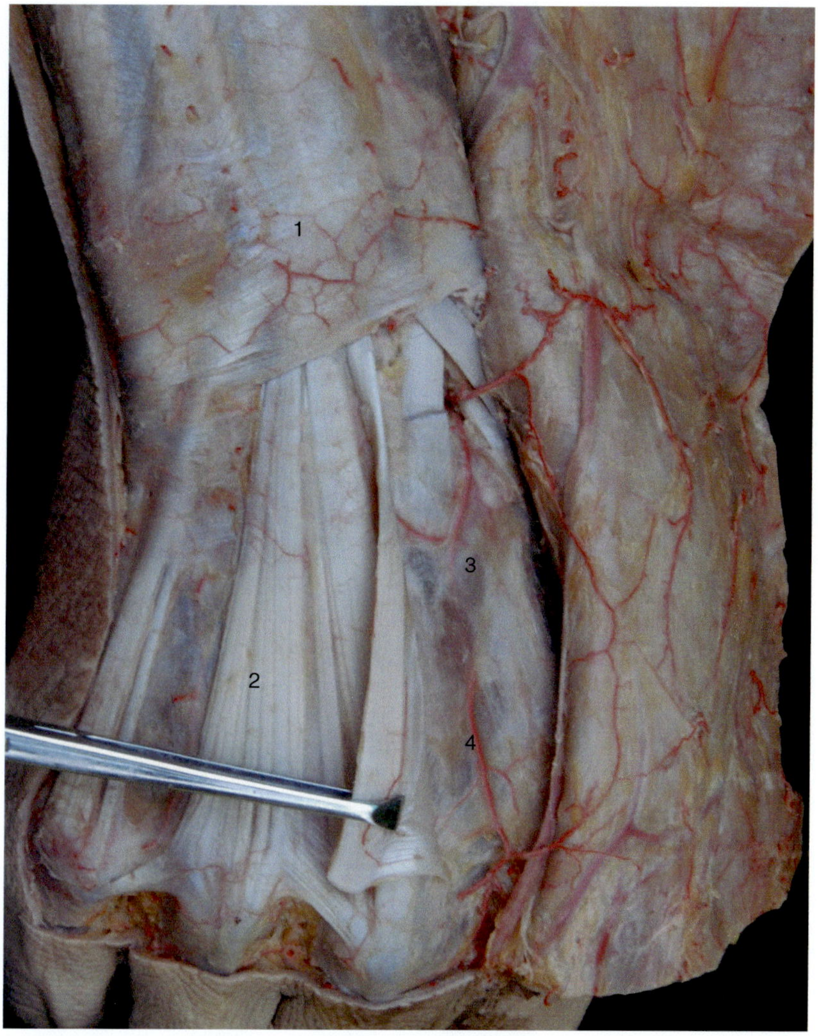

Fig. 2.35 Deep layer structure of the dorsum of the hand. *1* Extensor retinaculum. *2* Extensor tendon. *3* Interosseous dorsal fascia. *4* Second dorsal metacarpal artery

hand's dorsal subcutaneous space and the subaponeurotic space are formed between the superficial fascia and the dorsal aponeurosis pf the hand (the interosseous dorsal fascia). The former is the space between the superficial fascia and the hand's dorsal aponeurosis; the latter is the space between the hand's dorsal aponeurosis and the interosseous dorsal fascia. The two spaces communicate mutually; in the case of the infection of hand's dorsum, the swelling of the entire hand's dorsum is obvious.

4. Digital extensor tendon: The digital extensor tendon can be divided into the radial group and the ulnar group (Fig. 2.36). The radial group, including the thumb's long extensor tendon and the thumb's short extensor tendon, is related the movement of the thumb.

The ulnar group, including the digital extensor tendon, the index finger's extensor tendon, and the little finger's extensor tendon, is related to the extension of the second to fourth fingers. At the site near the head of the metacarpal bone, the four extensor tendons are connected by three bundles of tendon fibers of different categories, and this connection is called the intertendinous connection.

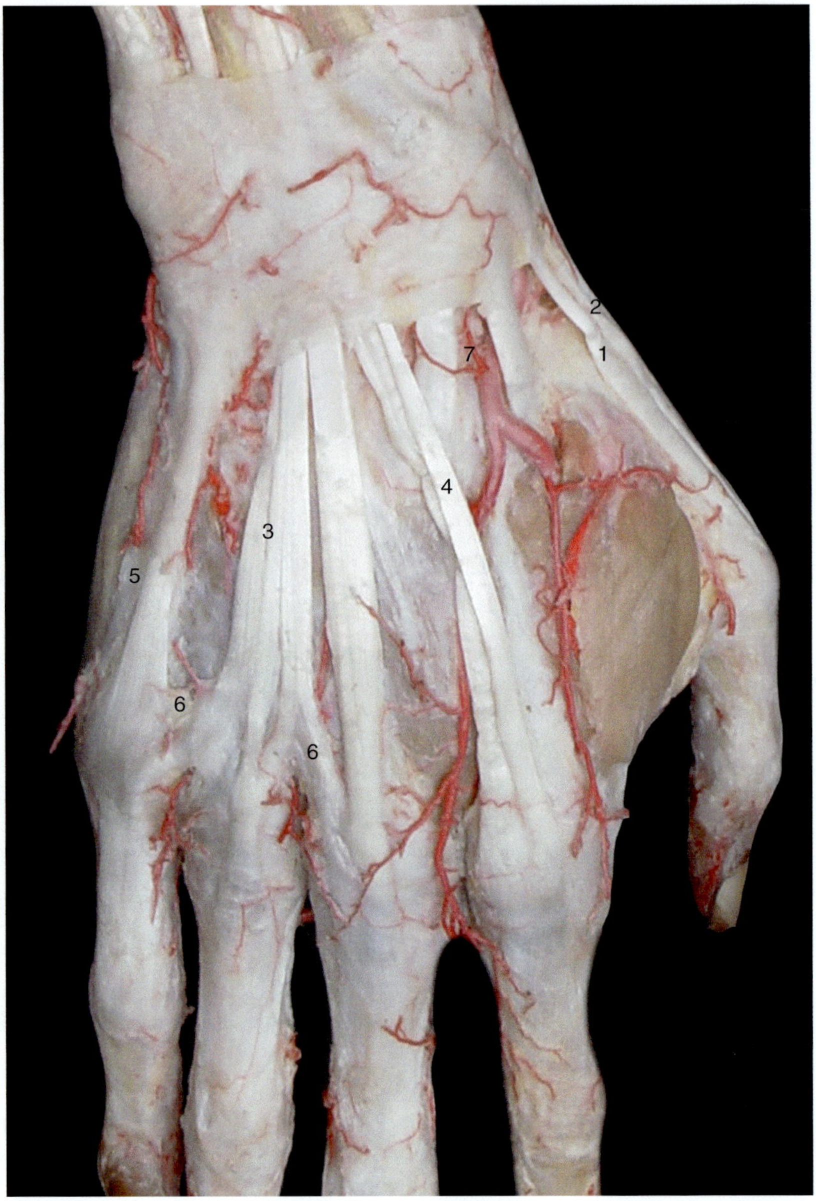

Fig. 2.36 Digital extensor tendon. *1* Long extensor tendon of thumb. *2* Short extensor tendon of thumb. *3* Digital extensor tendon. *4* Extensor tendon of index finger. *5* Extensor tendon of little finger. *6* Intertendinous connection. *7* Radial artery

The intertendinous connection has the function of consolidating the stability of digital extension and limiting the separate activities of each finger. In particular, it should be mentioned that the intertendinous connection of the middle, ring, and little fingers is more obvious; when a certain extensor digitorum tendon becomes ruptured at the proximal end of the intertendinous connection, there is no obvious disorder in finger extension function. The middle finger and the ring finger have one extensor tendon, and the remaining fingers

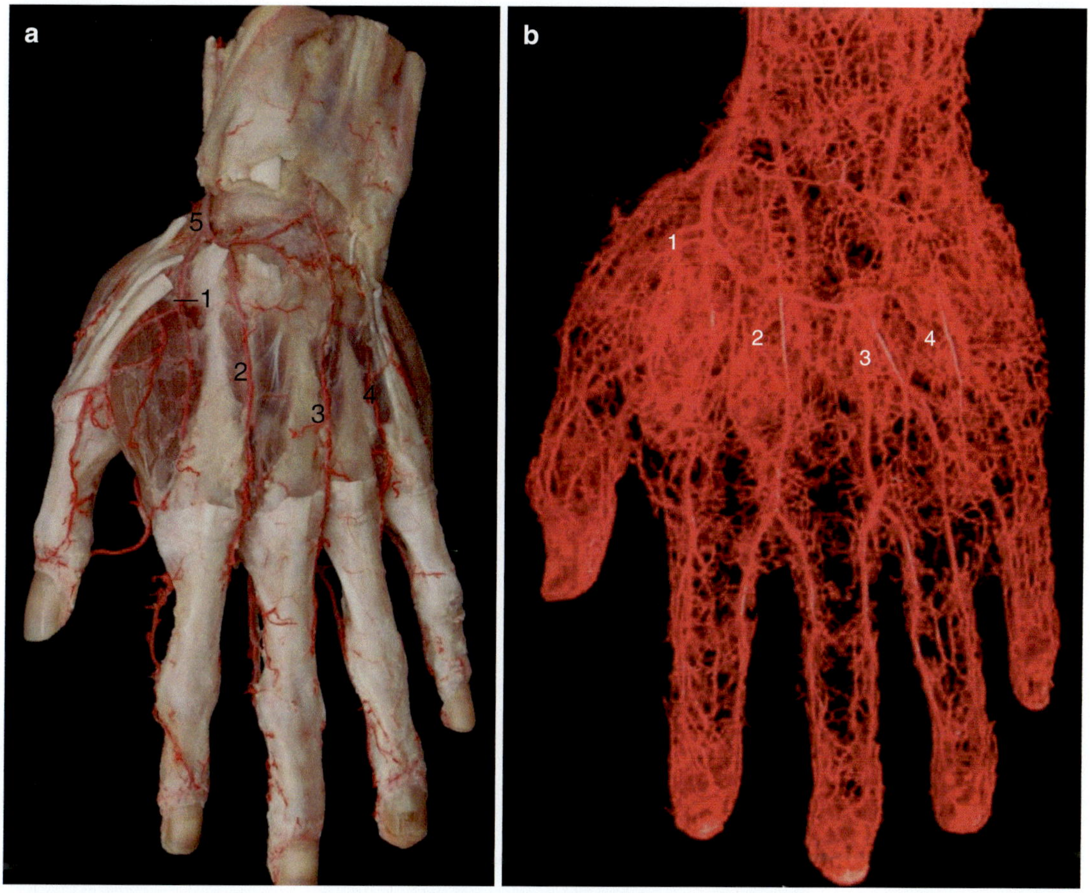

Fig. 2.37 Origin, running, and distribution of dorsal metacarpal arteries. (**a**) Specimen of a real object. (**b**) Cast specimen. *1* The first dorsal metacarpal artery. *2* The second dorsal metacarpal artery. *3* The third dorsal metacarpal artery. *4* The fourth dorsal metacarpal artery. *5* Radial artery

have two tendons. The extensor tendons of the index finger and the little finger are combined with the digital extensor tendons that reach the two fingers; except for the fact that the two extensor tendons of the thumb run in different directions, there is no obvious difference in their insertions and formed structures.

5. Dorsal Metacarpal Artery

There are four dorsal metacarpal arteries, which lie in the corresponding intermetacarpal spaces and run between the digital extensor tendon and the dorsal interosseous muscle (Fig. 2.37).

The first dorsal metacarpal artery is directly sent by the arterial artery, and then divided into three end branches (Fig. 2.38).

Radial branch: This runs along the dorsal side of the first metacarpal bone and continues to the dorsal digital artery at the ulnar side of the thumb, and it is accompanied by the cutaneous nerve with the same name sent by the superficial branch of the radial nerve.

Ulnar branch: This runs along the radial side of the second metacarpal bone and continues to the dorsal digital artery on the radial side of index finger. It is accompanied by the dorsal

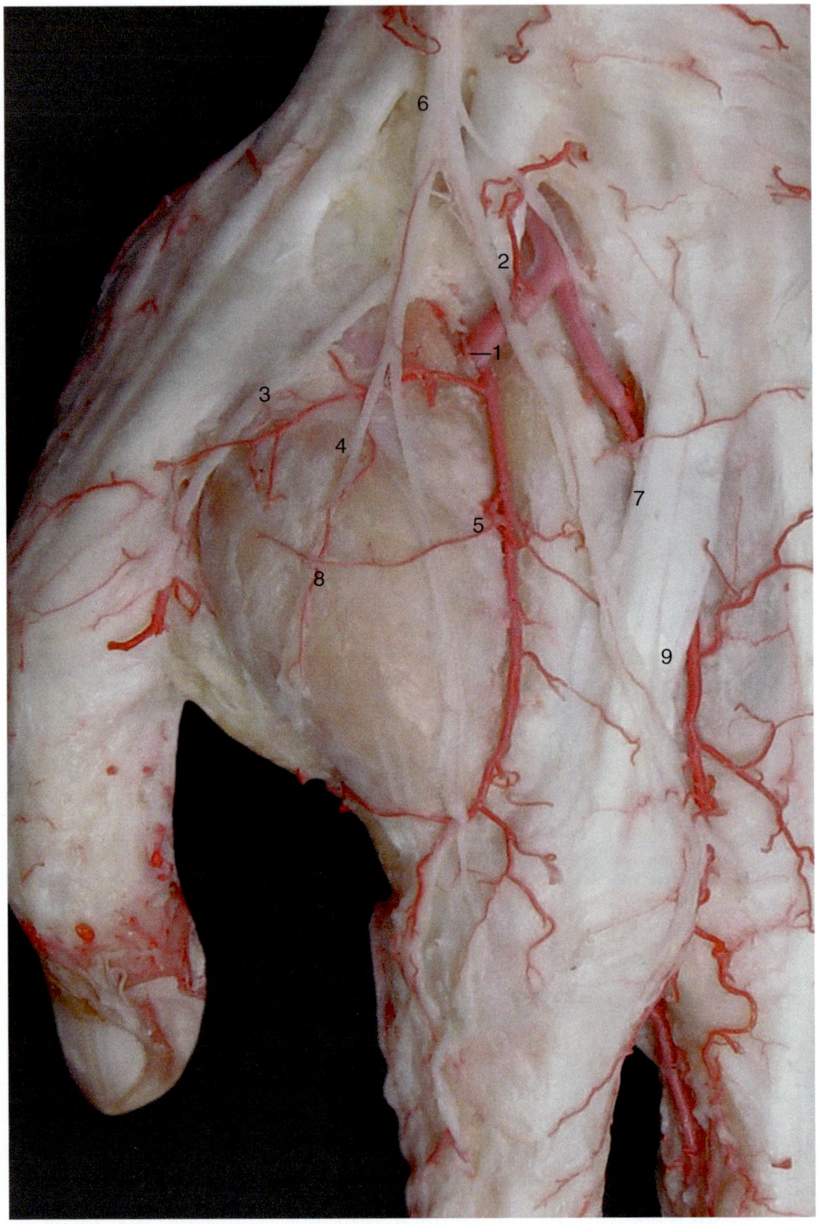

Fig. 2.38 Origin, course, and distribution of the first dorsal metacarpal artery. *1* First dorsal metacarpal artery. *2* Radial artery. *3* Radial branch. *4* Middle branch. *5* Ulnar branch. *6* Superficial branch of the radial nerve. *7* Digital extensor (tendon). *8* Dorsal interosseous muscle. *9* The second dorsal metacarpal artery

digital cutaneous nerve of the same name sent by the superficial branch of the radial nerve. Middle branch: This runs along the fascia surface of the first dorsal interosseous muscle and is distributed in this area, and it is accompanied by the first inter-finger web cutaneous nerve of the same name sent by the superficial branch of the radial nerve.

The second dorsal metacarpal artery usually has a good development, originating from three positions (Fig. 2.39): the deep palmar arch (40%), the dorsal carpal rete (30%) or the trunk of the radial artery (30%). The second dorsal metacarpal artery, sent by the dorsal carpal rete and the trunk of radial artery, is often connected to a proximal perforating branch (superior perforat-

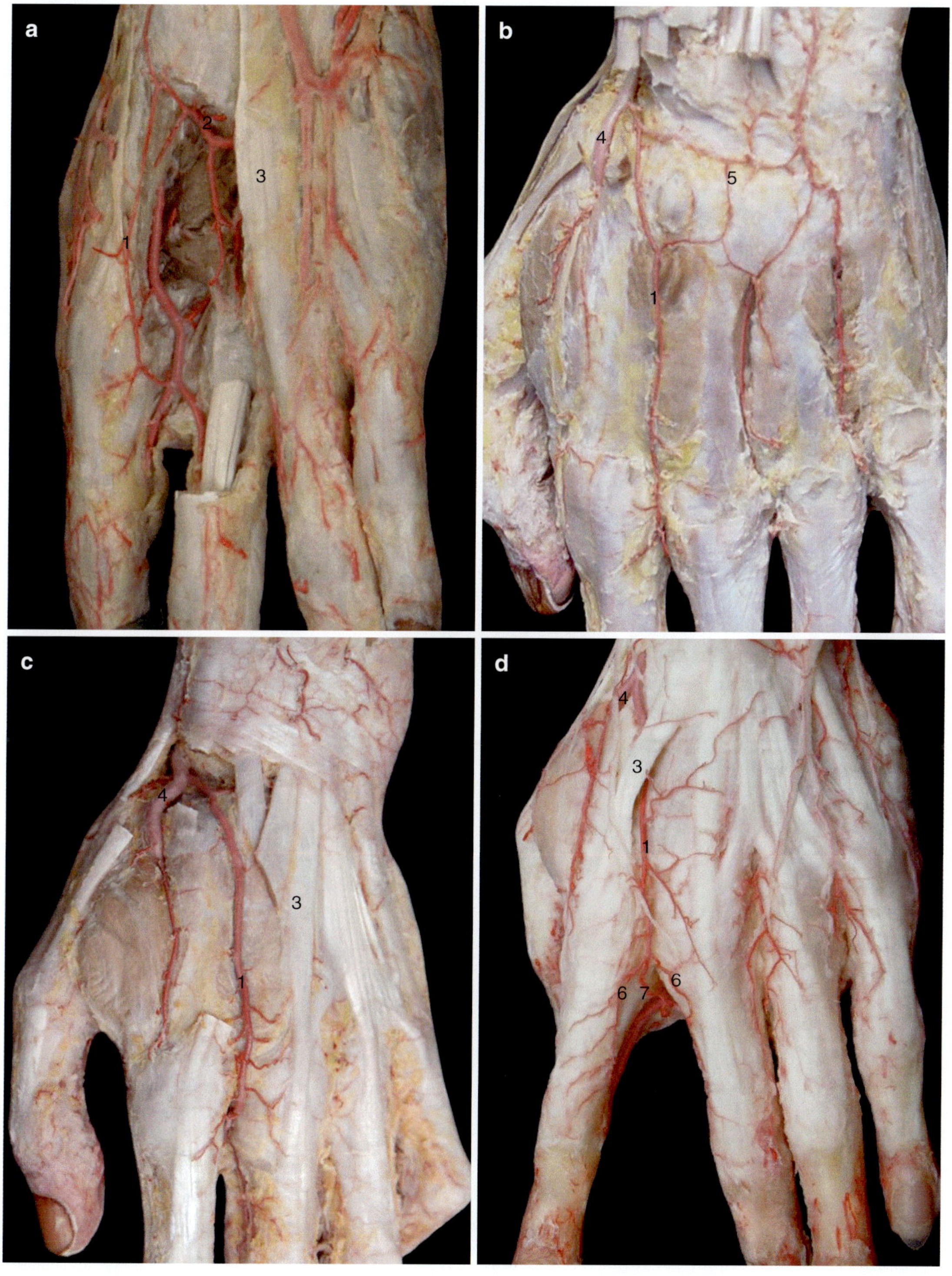

Fig. 2.39 Origin, course, and distribution of the second dorsal metacarpal artery. (**a**) Deep palmar arch type (40%). (**b**) Dorsal carpal rete type (30%). (**c**) Trunk of the radial artery (30%). (**d**) Branch and anastomosis. *1* The second dorsal metacarpal artery. *2* Deep palmar arch. *3* Digital extensor (tendon). *4* Radial artery. *5* Dorsal carpal rete. *6* Dorsal digital artery. *7* Communicating branch

ing artery) and deep palmar arch at the second intermetacarpal space, occurring in 52%. The third and fourth dorsal metacarpal arteries are sent from two sites, meaning that they are formed by the proximal perforating branches sent by the dorsal carpal rete or by the deep palmar arch at the third and fourth intermetacarpal spaces. The fourth dorsal metacarpal artery is absent in 30%. The dorsal metacarpal arteries are often divided into three end branches (two dorsal metacarpal arteries at the dorsal sides of the adjacent margins of the digital proximal segments, and one communicating branch with the common digital artery) at the metacarpophalangeal joint. The outer diameter at the origin of the dorsal metacarpal artery is about 0.8 mm. The diameter and the number of dorsal metacarpal arteries is inversely proportional to the size and number of distal perforating branches; i.e., a lower quantity and the smaller diameter of the dorsal metacarpal artery means a higher quantity and larger diameter of the perforating branches, showing a positive proportion to the size and the number of the proximal perforating branches. Dorsal metacarpal arteries are generally thin, but they are connected to the palmar arteries, forming a complete and uniform stereoscopic artery structure of the hand.

2.4 Fingers

Fingers are connected to the palm through the metacarpophalangeal joint, and the movement is very sensitive. The thumb is thick and short, with only two phalanxes, but the range of motion is maximal, and it can complete half of the hand functions.

2.4.1 Superficial Layer Structure

1. Skin: The skin on the palmar side of the fingers is relatively thick and rich in perspiratory glands and fingerprints, but it has no hair and sebaceous gland; thus, pain and swelling tend not to occur. At the finger pulp, the nerve endings are very rich, with especially sensitive tactile sensation, through which the shape and texture of an object can be identified. Because there are no subcutaneous tissues at the digital palmar transverse creases, the skin is directly connected to the tendon sheath; in the case of stab wounds and infection, tenosynovitis may occur. The skin at the digital dorsum is relatively thin, with few subcutaneous fats, and it has a larger range of motion than that on the palmar side. The finger skin has a very rich blood supply; it should be retained as far as possible in the case of treatment for trauma or burns.
2. Finger nail: This is a derived structure of the skin at the digital dorsum and is formed by the clumping of multiple layers of closely connected keratinized epithelial cells. It plays the role of protecting the finger tips, assisting the hands to give full play to their functions and beautifying the fingers; however, it is the most vulnerable part.
3. Subcutaneous tissues: The subcutaneous fats on the palmar side of the finger are relatively thick and become aggregated into a globular shape, in which fiber bundles are intermingled; they connect skin with the phalangeal periosteum and tendon sheath (Fig. 2.40). In the case of trauma and infection, they often become diffused toward the deep layers. The subcutaneous fats at the dorsal side of the finger are thin and loose, with a higher chance of slippage.
4. Digital arteries of the hand: In theory, each finger has two digital palmar arteries and two dorsal digital arteries for blood supply. The arteries with an apparent trunk visible to the naked eyes are the palmar digital arteries, the dorsal digital artery is generally immature (except for the thumb's arteries), and they are merely scattered fine and small branches.

2.4.1.1 Dorsal Digital Artery

There are great variations in the arteries on the dorsal side of the fingers. The dorsal digital arteries of the index, middle, and ring fingers origi-

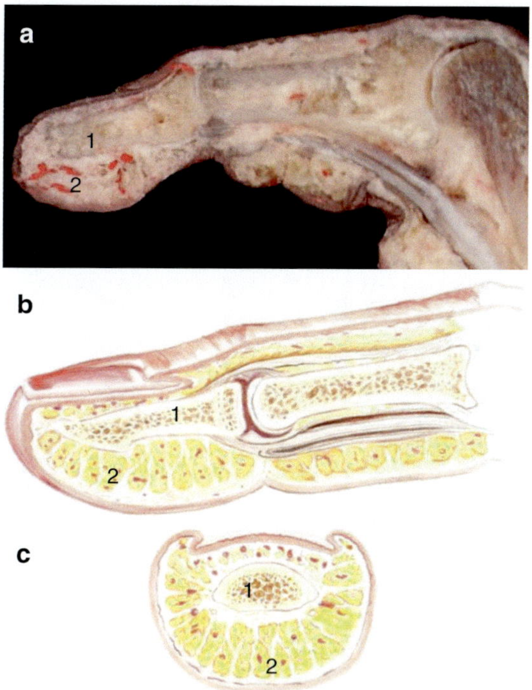

Fig. 2.40 Finger structure. (**a**) Sagittal view (specimen). (**b**) Sagittal section (schematic diagram). (**c**) Phalangette cross-section (schematic diagram). *1* Phalangette. *2* Fats

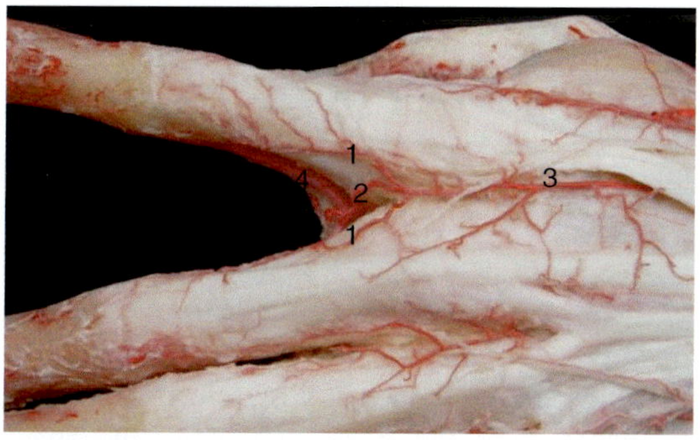

Fig. 2.41 Origin, course, and distribution of the dorsal digital artery. *1* Dorsal digital artery. *2* Second dorsal metacarpal artery. *3* Anastomotic branch. *4* Proper palmar digital artery

nate from the corresponding dorsal metacarpal arteries (Fig. 2.41). Most dorsal digital arteries are distributed to the proximal hemi-part of the proximal phalanx or the dorsal aspect of the proximal interphalangeal joints, and very few are distributed to the distal phalanx. The dorsal digital artery on the radial side of the thumb originates from the branch of the anatomist's snuff-box of the radial artery, and its outer diameter is about 0.5 mm. The dorsal digital artery on the ulnar side originates from the first dorsal metacarpal artery, and its outer diameter is about 0.8 mm. The radial side of the dorsal digital artery of the little finger originates from the fourth dorsal metacarpal artery, the ulnar side originates from the branch of the dorsal artery of the wrist, and the outer diameters range from 0.3 to 0.4 mm.

2.4.1.2 Proper Palmar Digital Artery

The common palmar digital artery is divided into two proper palmar digital arteries at the plane of head of metacarpal bone. The proper palmar digital artery runs toward the distal end along the two sides of the flexor tendon sheath, and, accompanying the digital proper nerve, it runs in a narrow and long neurovascular bundle of the Cleland's ligament. The proper palmar digital artery is located at the outer dorsal side of the proper palmar digital nerve, with a smaller outer diameter than the nerve, and the proper palmar digital nerve is located at the inner palmar side of the proper palmar digital artery. During the replantation of an amputated finger, the arteries and nerves can be successfully found through this anatomical relationship. The proper palmar digital artery sends branches to the palmar side and becomes anastomosed with the corresponding contralateral branches to form the digital palmar arch, it sends several perforating arteries and articular branches toward the dorsal side, and it is distributed at the digital dorsum and the interphalangeal joints (Fig. 2.42).

At the distal phalanx, the trunk of the proper palmar digital artery gradually runs toward the medial side and becomes anastomosed with the contralateral artery, forming the vascular net of the fingertip. The middle point between the nail bed and the distal interphalangeal joint constantly sends a transverse anastomotic branch with a diameter of about 0.5 mm. This transverse anastomotic branch becomes anastomosed with the

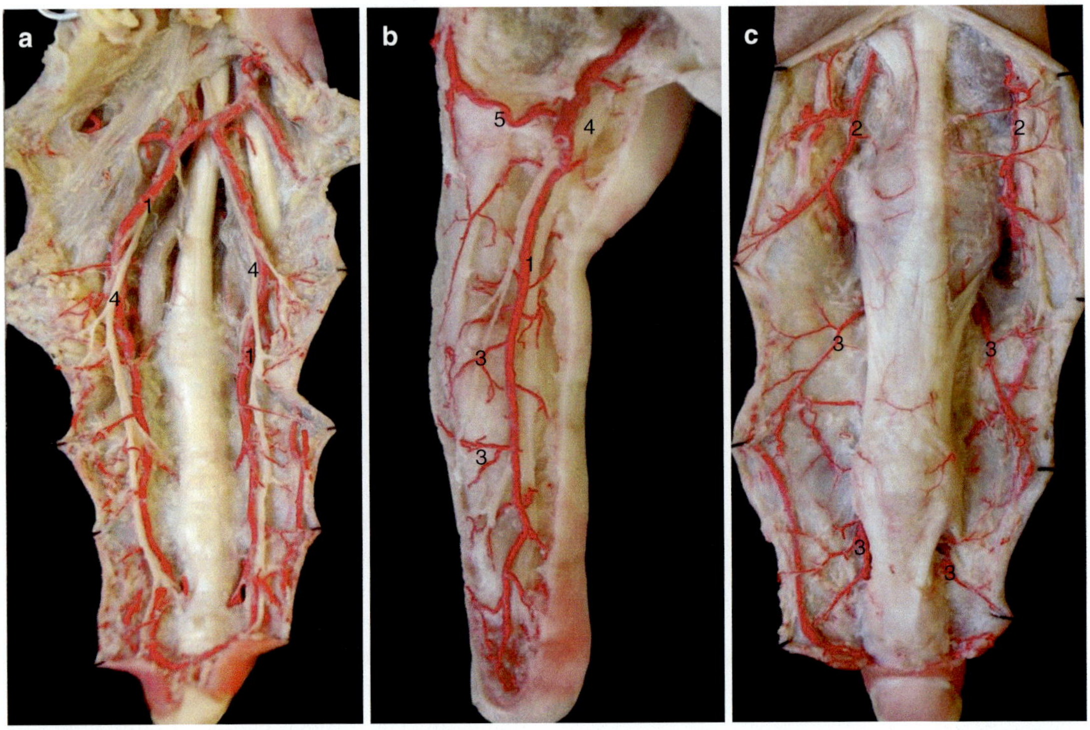

Fig. 2.42 Course, branches, and distribution of the digital arteries. (**a**) Middle finger palmar view. (**b**) Middle finger lateral view. (**c**) Middle finger dorsal view. *1* Palmar digital artery. *2* Dorsal metacarpal artery. *3* Dorsal perforating branch. *4* Proper digital nerve. *5* Anastomotic branch

contralateral branch of the same name, forming the distal dorsal arterial arch (Fig. 2.43). The digital arterial arch sends five primary branches toward the distal end, which are located on the surface of the digital flexor tendon on the palmar side; one on each side, with an outer diameter of 0.1–0.2 mm, and three are in the middle and the end branches of the finger pulp, with an outer diameter of 0.2–0.3 mm. The five trunks converge mutually, and any can provide anastomosis.

The ulnar palmar artery and the radial palmar artery of the thumb can be found at the palmar side of the thumb. The former is thicker. The starting outer diameter is 1.8 mm. It is mainly sent by the principal artery of the thumb, and then passes through the ulnar side of the long flexor muscle tendon of the thumb and passes the thumb adductor insertion and the ulnar inter-sesamoid region to become distributed toward the distal end of the thumb. The latter is thinner. The starting outer diameter is 1.1 mm. It is mainly sent by the principal artery of the thumb (85%) and the superficial palmar branch of the radial artery (15%). After being sent, it reaches the radial side of the deep surface of the long flexor muscle tendon of the thumb, and skips the free margin of the deep head of the short flexor muscle of the thumb. It runs toward the distal end along the space between the radial sesamoid bone and the long flexor muscle tendon of the thumb. The ulnar and radial palmar arteries of the thumb run toward the distal end and send branches, which are distributed in the skin and soft tissues of the palmar and lateral sides of the thumb, and at the same time, the two arteries communicate through the constant digital palmar arch and neural arch (Fig. 2.44).

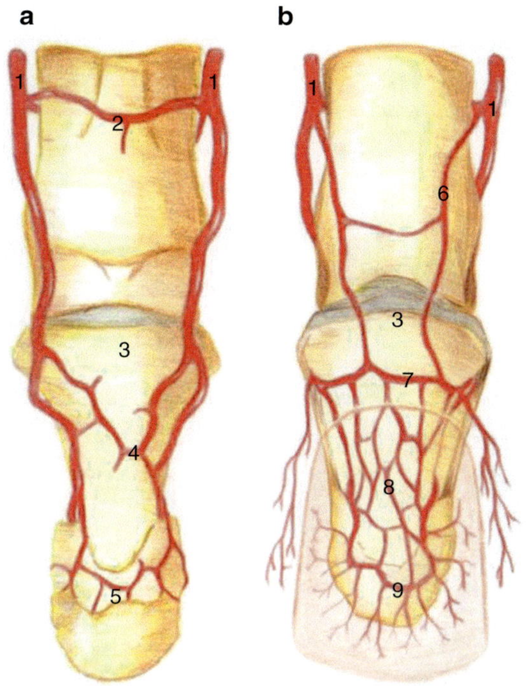

Fig. 2.43 Vascular net of the fingertip. (**a**) Palmar view. (**b**) Dorsal view. *1* Proper palmar digital artery. *2* Digital palmar arch. *3* Phalangette. *4* Proximal palmar arterial arch. *5* Distal palmar arterial arch. *6* Digital middle phalangeal dorsal ramus. *7* Proximal dorsal arterial arch. *8* Nail arterial rete. *9* Distal phalangeal dorsal arterial arch

2.4.1.3 Digital Veins

The digital veins are classified into superficial veins and deep veins. The superficial digital veins on the palmar side are closely attached to the subcutaneous regions. Thin-walled, they originate from the venous network of finger pulp and become mutually anastomosed into three to four large veins, which run toward the proximal side. During the course, they mutually anastomose into a net, and the branches run toward the digital dorsum along the two sides. The adjacent superficial veins at the finger web converge onto small veins, which flow into the dorsal digital veins.

The superficial dorsal digital veins are relatively thick and large, and are the main route for digital venous return. There is a certain law in its course, and it runs between the subcutaneous region and the digital extensor tendon. The small veins at the two sides of the nail converge onto one or two small veins in the middle of the region from the nail base to the dorsal side of the distal interphalangeal joint, with an outer diameter ranging from 0.5 to 0.6 mm, and they aggregate like a net toward the proximal end. These small veins, generated through the convergence, form several veins, with an outer diameter ranging from 0.8 to 1.0 mm on the dorsal side of the proximal interphalangeal joint; they tend to be centralized like a network structure on the dorsal side of the proximal phalanx, subsequently causing venous arches in one to three layers (Fig. 2.45). At the digital root, the venous arch feet of the mutually adjacent fingers converge onto the palmar dorsal veins or cephalic veins. The superficial dorsal digital veins are distributed based on the following law: (1) mainly at the 10 to 2 o'clock directions; (2) deviation from the midline: when the midline of the middle finger is treated as the central line, the superficial dorsal digital veins of the thumb and index finger deviate toward the radial side, and the diameters are thicker; the superficial dorsal digital veins of the ring and little fingers deviate toward the ulnar side, and the ulnar veins have thicker diameters. The deviation from the midline is most apparent in the index and little fingers.

The deep digital veins of the hand are generally accompanied by the proper palmar digital artery and dorsal digital artery, but the accompanying veins have a thinner diameter and are not located at a fixed position; the veins run tortuously by surrounding the arteries, and the distance from the arteries is sometimes long and sometimes short.

Valve distribution can also be found in the digital veins. A pair of venous valves can be found approximately every 2 cm of the dorsal veins of the hand. The valve is open from the distal end to the proximal end, and from the palmar side to the dorsal side, to guarantee that the venous blood flows from the distal end to the proximal end, and from the palmar side to the dorsal side (Figs. 2.46, 2.47, 2.48, and 2.49).

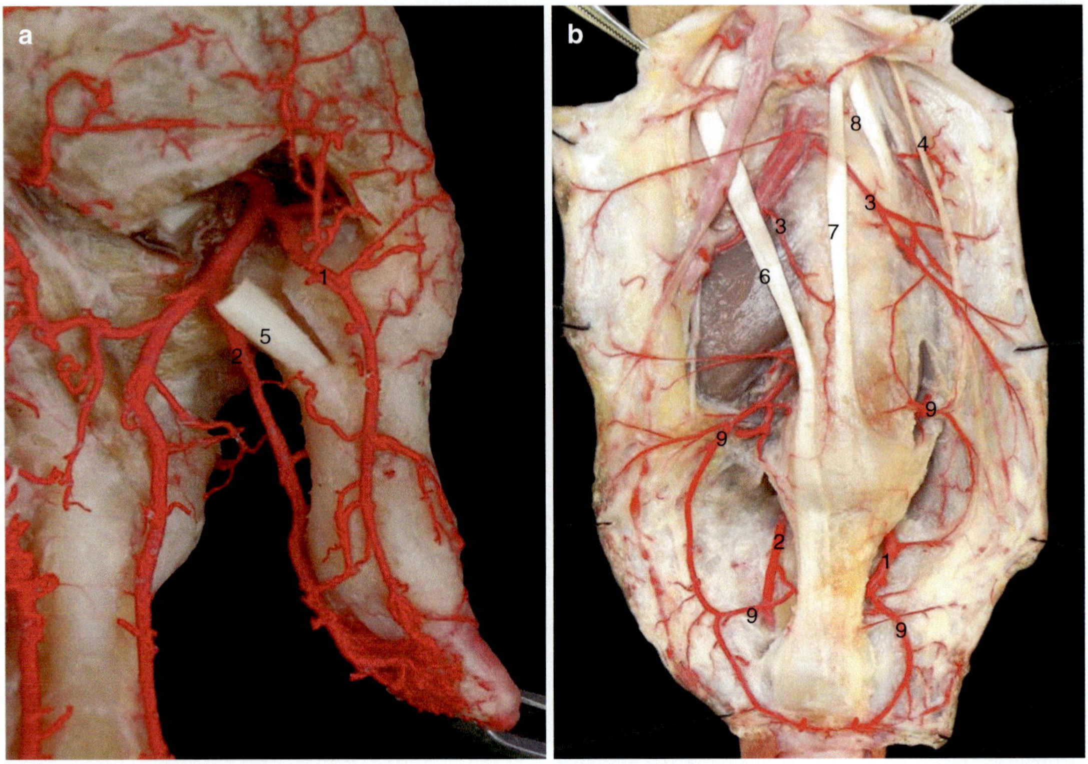

Fig. 2.44 Course and distribution of the thumb arteries. (**a**) Radial and palmar view of the thumb. (**b**) Dorsal view of the thumb. *1* Radial and palmar arteries of the thumb. *2* Ulnar palmar artery of the thumb. *3* Dorsal digital artery of the thumb. *4* Radial digital dorsal cutaneous nerves of the thumb. *5* Long extensor tendon of the thumb. *6* Long extensor tendon of the thumb. *7* Short extensor tendon of the thumb. *8* Long extensor tendon of the thumb. *9* Dorsal perforating branch

2.4.2 Deep Layer Structure

2.4.2.1 Finger Flexor Tendon

Morphological and Structural Characteristics of the Digital Flexion Tendon

The digital flexor tendons are divided into superficial and deep flexor tendons. The thumb has one flexor tendon, and the remaining fingers have a digital superficial flexor tendon and a digital deep flexor tendon, which run into the digital tendon sheaths. At the proximal phalanx, the digital superficial flexor tendon is located on the palmar side of the digital deep flexor tendon and surrounds the digital deep flexor tendon along the two sides; then it runs toward the distal end and divides into two segments, which are attached to the two margins of the middle phalanxes, a hiatus tendineus, and the digital deep flexor tendon is allowed to pass it (Fig. 2.50a). After leaving the hiatus tendineus, the digital deep flexor tendon inserts onto the base of the distal phalanx. The digital superficial flexor tendon mainly flexes the proximal interphalangeal joint, metacarpophalangeal joint, and the carpal joint, and the digital deep flexor tendon mainly flexes the distal interphalangeal joint and can also flex the fingers and wrist completely.

As a synovial fold located in the digital flexor tendon sheath, the vincula tendinum is classified

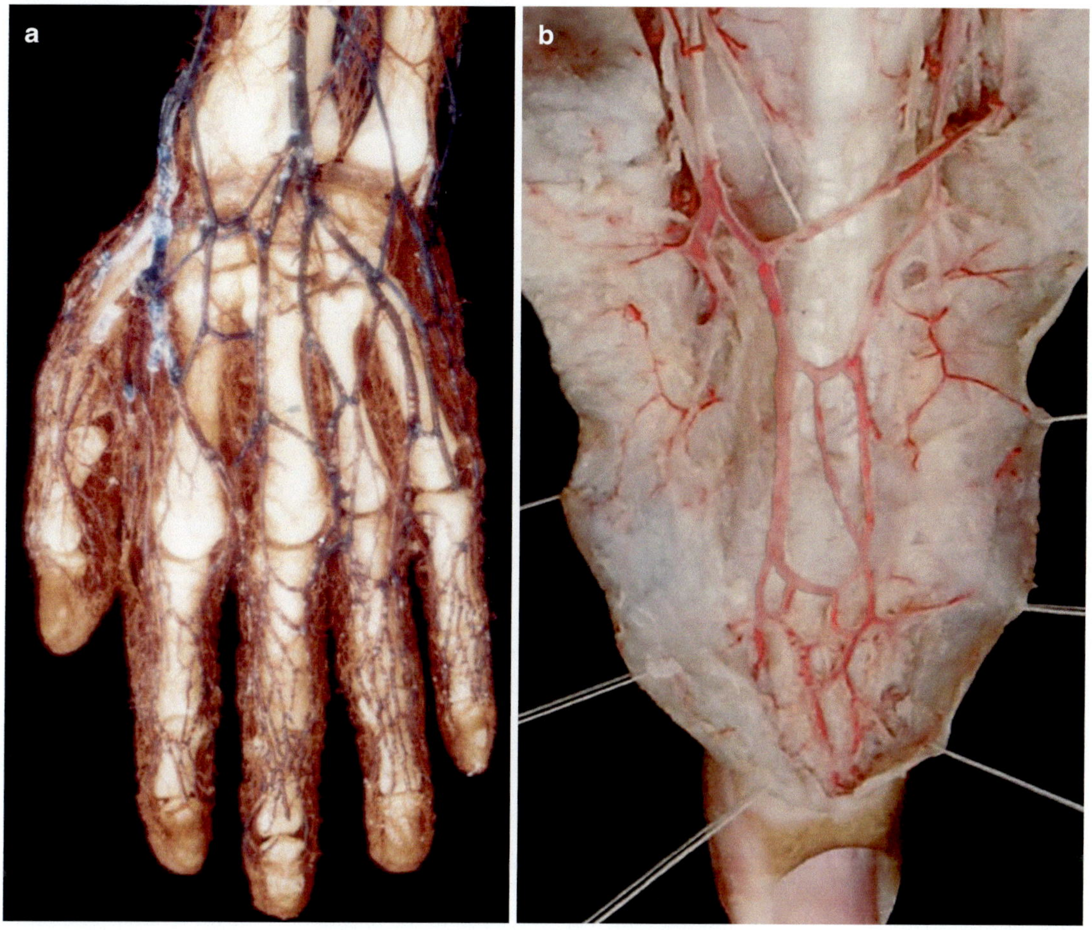

Fig. 2.45 Digital veins. (**a**) Cast specimen. (**b**) Specimen of the real object

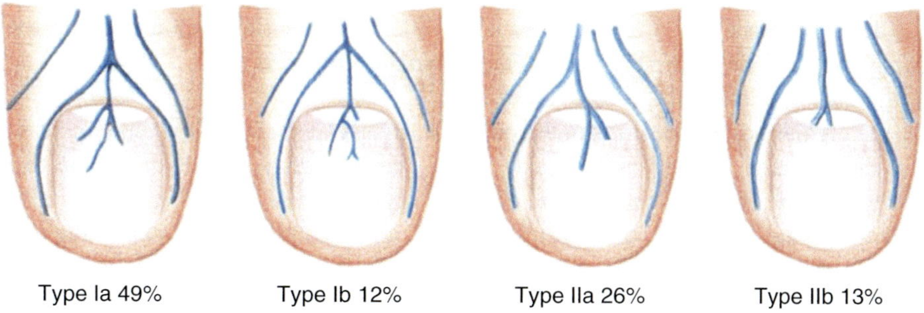

Fig. 2.46 Distribution type of the superficial veins at the dorsal surface of the phalangette. Type Ia 49%, type Ib 12%, type IIa 26%, and type IIb 13%

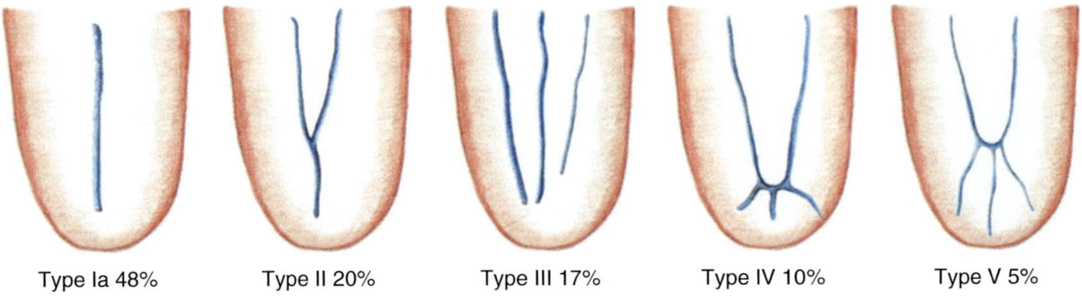

Fig. 2.47 Distribution type of superficial veins at the palmar surface of the phalangette. Type Ia 48%, type II 20%, type III 17%, type IV 10%, and type V 5%

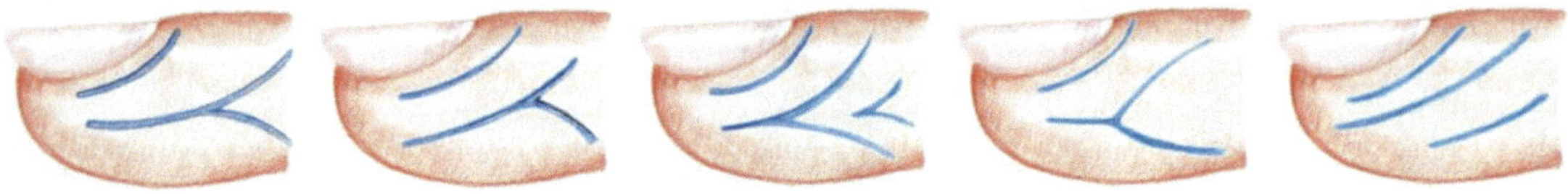

Fig. 2.48 Type of superficial veins of the phalangette

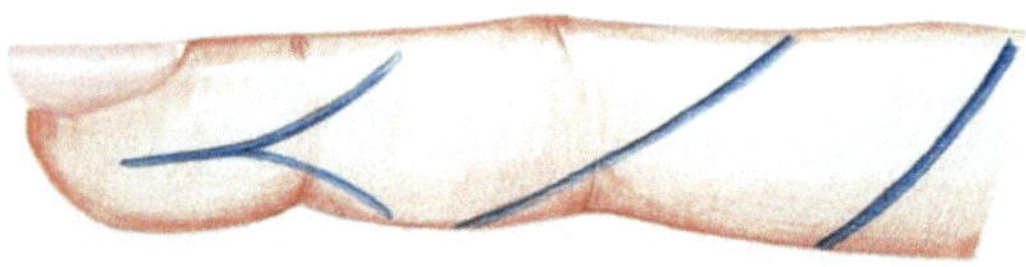

Fig. 2.49 Distribution of superficial veins at the digital lateral aspect

into the short vincula tendinum and the long vincula tendinum according to its morphology, and each flexor tendon has two kinds of vincula tendina (Fig. 2.50b).

Short vincula tendinum: This is triangular. There are two vincula tendina, which lie at the proximal side of the insertion of the superficial digital flexor and the deep digital flexor. The proximal margins are free, the dorsal side is attached to the median sagittal position at the palmar side of the phalange, and the palmar side is attached to the dorsal aspect of the tendon. The blood supply originates from the small periosteal vessels at the branches and insertions of palmar digital arterial arches, and the vessels are mutually anastomosed, forming a vascular net.

Long vincula tendinum: This is a fine and long cord-shaped structure, and its shape, position, and number are not as constant as those of the short vincula tendinum. The long vincula tendinum of the digital deep flexor tendon mostly originates directly or indirectly from the short vincula tendinum of the digital superficial flexor tendon, and the short vincula tendinum of the digital superficial flexor tendon is sent from the insertion, penetrating the center of the digital superficial flexor tendon to the digital deep flexor tendon. The number is 1–3, and its vessels supply blood to the middle segment of the digital deep flexor tendon.

The digital tendon sheath surrounds the digital superficial flexor tendon and the digital deep flexor tendon, consisting of two parts: the synovial sheath of the tendon and the tendon fiber bundle (Fig. 2.51).

1. Synovial sheath of the tendon: This is a cystic tubular structure formed by the two layers of synovia that surround the digital flexor tendon, the synovial sheaths of the tendon of the index, middle, and ring fingers extend from the proximal side to the distal side of the metacarpophalangeal joint, striding over three joints and finally reaching the base of the distal phalanx. The synovial sheaths of the ten-

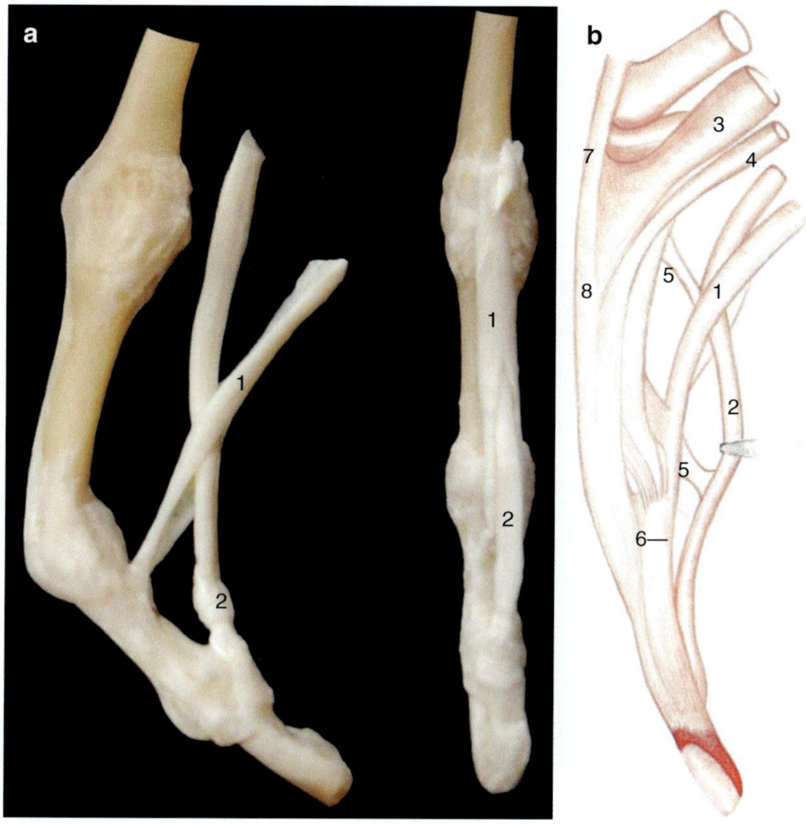

Fig. 2.50 Shape of the insertions of the digital flexor tendons. (**a**) Specimen of a real object. (**b**) Schematic diagram. *1* Digital superficial flexor tendon. *2* Digital deep flexor tendon. *3* Interosseous muscle. *4* Lumbrical muscle. *5* Vincula tendinum. *6* Vincula tendinum. *7* Digital extensor tendon. *8* Dorsal aponeurosis

don of the thumb and little finger continue to the radial and ulnar synovial sheaths of the tendon. The synovial sheaths of the tendon are divided into the visceral layer and the parietal layer, which surround the tendons, and the parietal layer is closely attached to the medial surface of the tendon fibrous sheath. The two ends of the synovial sheath of tendon are enclosed, the part of the two-layer synovia between the dorsal side of the tendon and the phalange is called the mesotendon, with the vessels, nerves, and lymphatic vessels that come in and out of the tendons.

2. Tendon fibrous sheath: This is the osseofibrous canal formed by being surrounded by the periosteum on the palmar side of phalange, the volar plate anterior to the articular capsule, and the tough connective tissues, and it can assist the fingers to give full play to their functions. To prevent the appearance of an "arch-shaped finger" caused by the tendon traction, the distal segment of the digital flexor tendon is constrained in the sheathing canal.

Different positions of the sheathing canal cater for the different functions, and the fibrous layers become thickened to form a series of trochlear systems with important biomechanical characteristics. The trochlear systems of the index, middle, ring, and little fingers consist of five annular trochleas (A, which are A1, A2, A3, A4, and A5 respectively); four chiasmatic trochleas (C, which are C0, C1, C2, and C3 trochleas), and one palmar aponeurosis trochlea (consisting of palmar aponeurosis). The sequence of the trochleae from the proximal to the distal is: PA, A1, C0, A2, C1, A3, C2, A2, C3, and A5.

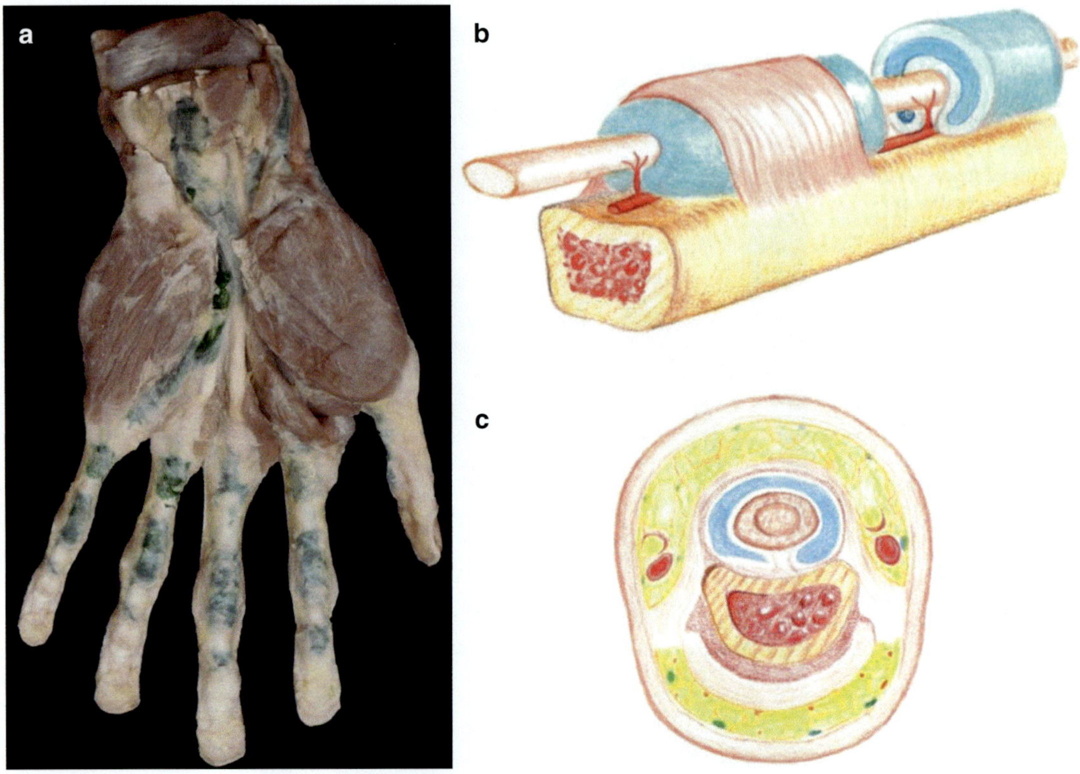

Fig. 2.51 Hand flexor tendon and sheath. (**a**) Specimen of a real object. (**b**) Schematic diagram. *1* Synovial tendon sheath of digital flexor. *2* Tendon fiber sheath. *3* Visceral layer of the synovial tendon sheath. *4* Parietal layer of the synovial tendon sheath. *5* Mesotendon. *6* Phalange. *7* Proper vessels and nerves on the palmar side of the finger

The thumb's trochlear system consists of two annular trochleae (TA1 and TA2) and one oblique trochlea (T0).

The tendinous fiber tendon trochlear system has the function of providing mechanical insertion to tendon sliding, changing the force direction, and facilitating the tendon to give full play to the tendon function of sliding.

Differentiation of the Digital Flexor Tendon

The digital flexor tendons pass through different positions and the peri-musculotendinous adjacent structures vary. Clinically, the tendon injuries at different sites are treated based on different treatment principles and result in different functional prognoses. Therefore, it is clinically significant to differentiate the positions of the digital flexor tendons. The digital flexor tendons are often divided into five regions (Fig. 2.52).

Tendon terminal region (region I or region TI): This region is the middle part of the range from the insertion of the distal phalangeal tendon to the middle phalanx (the thumb is the middle part of the proximal phalanx), and the proximal phalanx is about 1.5 cm long. In this region, there is only one digital deep flexor tendon or long flexor muscle tendon of the thumb, which is partially wrapped into the tendon sheath. There is a constant short vincula tendinum at the site where the proximal phalanx is attached, and the proximal phalanx has a good blood supply. The tendon has a small range of motion, and the early repair effect is relatively good after its rupture.

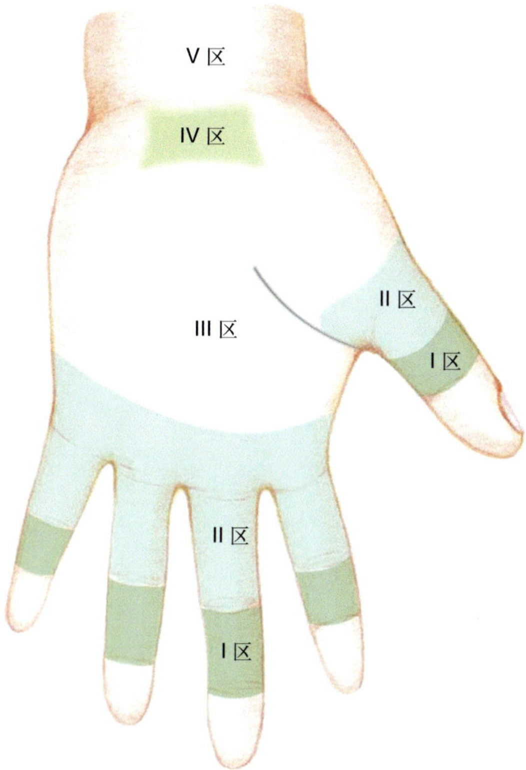

Fig. 2.52 Flexor tendon division

Sheathing canal region (region II or region TII): This is also called "no man's land." This region is the plane ranging from the middle part of the middle phalanx to the distal palmar transverse crease. There are two flexor tendons (superficial and deep) in this region. Tendons are located in the digital flexor tendon sheath, with a poor blood supply. Therefore, there is a great difficulty in surgically treating the tendon injuries, and the efficacy is also poor. In the "region TII" of the thumb, two sesamoid bones are retained at both sides of the metacarpophalangeal joint of the thumb, forming a narrow canal, in spite of there being only one long flexor muscle tendon of the thumb, which is very simple. Under pathological conditions, it is prone to becoming adhered to the long flexor muscle tendon of the thumb.

Palm region (region III or region TIII): This region ranges from the distal palmar transverse crease to the distal margin of the flexor retinaculum. In this segment, the flexor tendons of the thumb and little finger are wrapped by separate radial and ulnar synovial bursae; the flexor tendons of the index, middle, and ring fingers are located in the space of loose connective tissues and coated in paratenons outside, and the lumbrical muscles originate from the digital deep flexor tendon.

Carpal canal region (region IV): This is located in the carpal canal and in a narrow canal. In this region, nine flexor tendons and the median nerve are squeezed together, and this is the site where entrapment syndrome can be easily induced.

Forearm region (region V): This is located in the tendon region above the flexor retinaculum. There are many loose connective tissues between the structures in this segment. It is relatively easy to perform the tendon repair, the postoperative adhesion is mild, and the impact on the tendon's sliding function is small.

2.4.2.2 Digital Extensor Tendon

Morphological and Structural Characteristics of the Digital Extensor Tendon

The digital extensor tendon strides over the head of the metacarpal bone and the dorsal surface of the proximal phalanx, and becomes dilated to form the dorsal aponeurosis; it is also called the tendon hood (Fig. 2.53). The dorsal aponeurosis is distally divided into three longitudinal tendon bundles; the middle bundle runs forwards, receives the participation of some of the fibers of the bilateral bundle, and inserts on the base of the middle phalanx and articular capsule. On the two sides of the proximal phalanx, two lateral tendon bundles are added to the interosseous muscle tendons and lumbrical muscle tendons that circle from the palmar side to the dorsal side. After convergence on the dorsal side of the middle phalanx, the two lateral bundles insert on the dorsal side of the distal phalanx base and the articular capsule. The main function of the dorsal aponeurosis is to

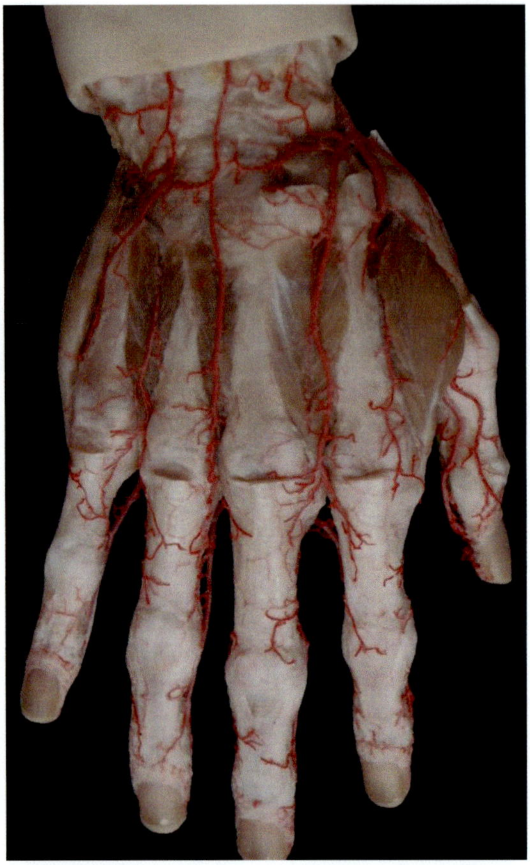

Fig. 2.53 Shape of dorsal aponeurosis

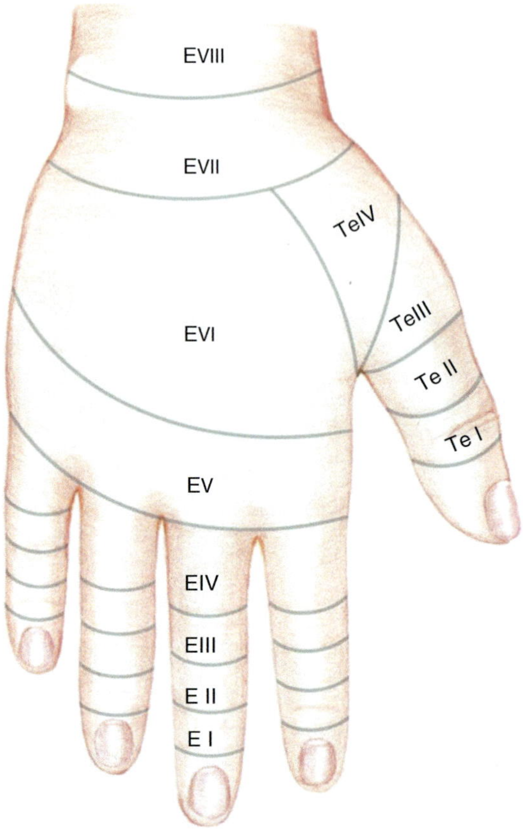

Fig. 2.54 Differentiation of digital extensor tendons

stabilize the metacarpophalangeal joint and extend the interphalangeal joint, which is the foundation for the hand's intrinsic muscles to exert their functions. After digital extensor tendon ruptures, all joints have the status of flexion. After the middle bundle ruptures, the proximal interphalangeal joint cannot extend. After the two bundles rupture, the distal interphalangeal joint cannot extend.

Differentiation of Extensor Tendon

The digital extensor tendon is divided into eight regions (Fig. 2.54) according to Verdan's method. Arranged from distal to proximal: distal interphalangeal joint region (EI), middle phalanx region (EII), proximal interphalangeal joint region (EIII), proximal phalanx region (EIV), metacarpophalangeal joint region (EV), metacarpal region (EVI), carpal region (EVII), and forearm region (EVIII).

The thumb is divided into four regions, i.e., the thumb's interphalangeal joint region (TEI), proximal phalanx region (TE II), metacarpophalangeal joint region (TEIII), and metacarpal region (TEIV). The odd number region corresponds to the joint, and the even number region corresponds to the phalangeal shaft. Injury to the digital extensor tendon at different sites cause different functional disorders of the bones and joints, deformity generation, and therapeutic measures; therefore, to differentiate the digital extensor tendons is of clinical significance.

2.5 Hand Bones and Joint

2.5.1 Hand Bones

Hand bones are divided into three types: carpal bone, metacarpal bone, and phalange Fig. 2.55.

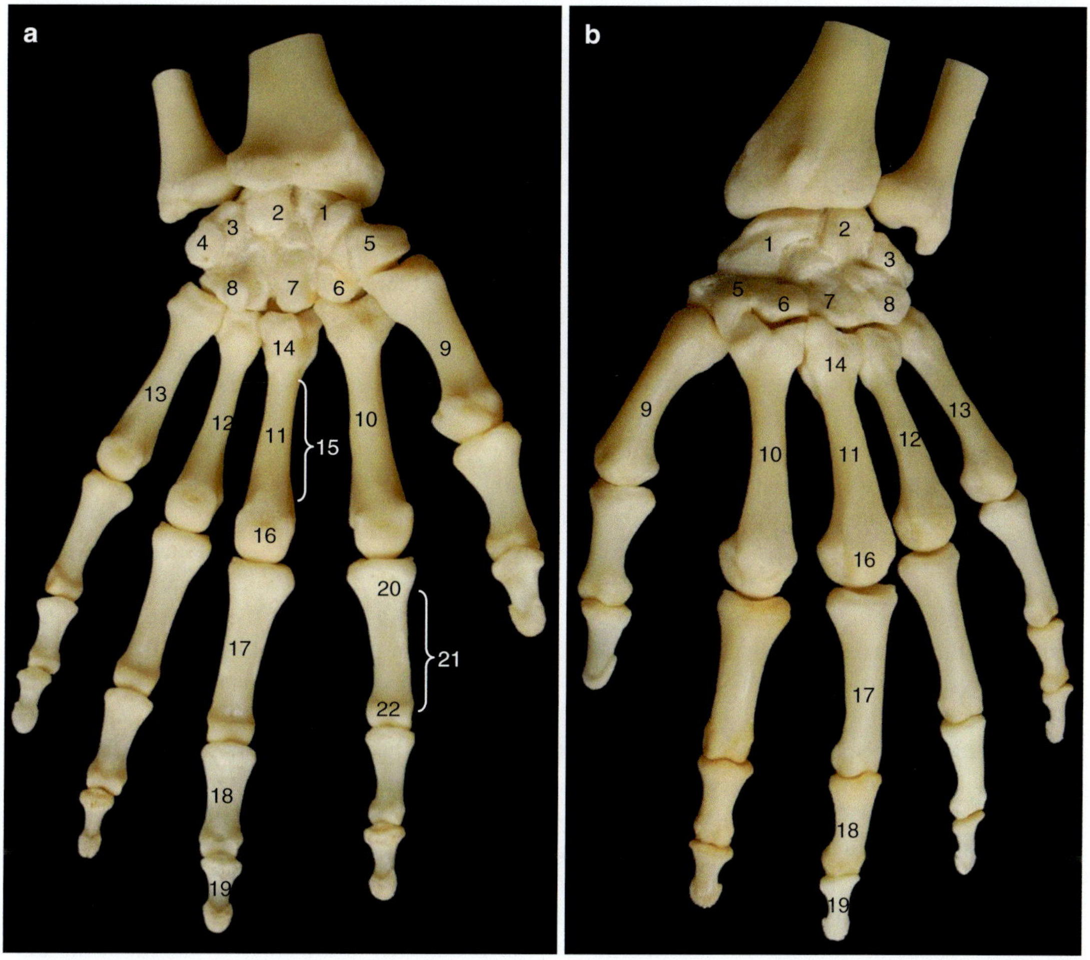

Fig. 2.55 Hand bones. (**a**) Palmar surface. (**b**) Dorsal surface. *1* Navicular bone. *2* Lunar bone. *3* Triangular bone. *4* Lentiform bone. *5* Trapezium bone. *6* Trapezoid bone. *7* Capitate bone. *8* Hamate bone. *9* First metacarpal bone. *10* Second metacarpal bone. *11* Third metacarpal bone. *12* Fourth metacarpal bone. *13* Fifth metacarpal bone. *14* Base of metacarpal bone. *15* Body of metacarpal bone. *16* Caput ossis metacarpalis. *17* Proximal phalanx. *18* Middle phalanx. *19* Distal phalanx. *20* Base of phalanx. *21* Body of phalanx. *22* Head of phalanx

2.5.1.1 Carpal Bones

The carpal bones are located at the wrist, consist of eight small bones, and are arranged in two regions at the proximal and distal rows respectively. The carpal bones at the proximal row are the navicular bone, the lunar bone, the triangular bone, and the lentiform bone, from the outer to the interior. The carpal bones at the distal row are the trapezium bone, the trapezoid bone, the capitate bone, and the hamate bone, from the outer to the interior.

The carpal bones are short bones, covered by a layer of compact substances outside and are filled with spongiosa inside. They are generally cubical and a hexahedron. Ligaments are attached to the palmar and dorsal surfaces; thus, they appear rough, and the other four planes are mutually connected, forming joints. Lunar bone has a wide palmar surface and a narrow dorsal surface whereas the remaining bones have a wide dorsal surface and a narrow palmar surface.

The capitate bones at the proximal row form an elliptically shaped convex surface on the proximal side and are articulated with the distal end and articular discs of the radius. They form a concave surface at the distal end, holding the capitate bones on the distal side, especially the capitate bone and hamate bone. The lunar bone is relatively wide and connected to the trapezium bone and the trapezoid bone; the lunar bone and the triangular bone are relatively small. The lentiform bone is located anterior to the triangular bone, and is not involved in the formation of the radiocarpal joint.

The capitate bone in the carpal bone at the distal row is located in the middle and is the strongest. The capitate bone head, in association with the navicular bone and lunar bone, forms a saddle-shaped connection. In the case of shock to the hands, the external force can be transferred to the radial bone without passing through the capitate bone head. The distal articular surface is relatively flat and forms a plane articulation together with the base of the metacarpal bone.

The dorsal aspect of all carpal bones is convex-shaped, ranging from the interior to the exterior, and the palmar surface forms a deep groove, which is also called the carpal groove; an eminence is formed at the internal and external margins of the groove, which is the carpal radial eminence and the ulnar eminence of the wrist. The radial bulge of the wrist consists of the tubercle of the navicular bone and the tubercle of the trapezium bone. The tubercle of the navicular bone is a small and circular eminence, to which the short abductor muscle of the thumb is attached; this tubercle, located in the subcutaneous region of the carpal distal crease, is palpable. The tubercle of the trapezium bone is a circular crest and shaped like an inward hook. Located at the distal side of the tubercle of the navicular bone, it is also palpable subcutaneously. The ulnar eminence of the wrist consists of lentiform bone and the hook of hamate bone. The lentiform bone is proximally located on the deep surface of the carpal distal crease, on which the ulnar flexor muscle of the wrist and little finger abductor. The hook of the hamate bone is located at the site 1 cm away from the distal radial side of the lentiform bone, and numerous structures attach to it, including the breviflexor and opposing muscle of the little finger; in case of the use of the finger for deep compression, the rolling of the superficial branch of the ulnar nerve is palpable on the hook.

2.5.1.2 Metacarpal Bones

Metacarpal bones are five small tubular bones, each of which consists of a base, body, and head.

Base: This is a bulge of the proximal end, its proximal surface articulates with the carpal bones on the proximal side, forming the carpometacarpal joint, but the articular surfaces are inconsistent; the first, third, and fifth metacarpal bones are only connected to a carpal bone, the second metacarpal bone is connected to the trapezium bone, trapezoid bone, and capitate bone, and the fourth metacarpal bone is connected to the capitate bone and hamate bone. Therefore, the capitate bone has two to four articular surfaces connected to the second to fourth metacarpal bones. The base of the first metacarpal is saddle-shaped, and forms the carpometacarpal joint of the thumb together with the trapezium bone. The two sides of the base of the metacarpal bone are connected to the adjacent base of the metacarpal bone, forming the intermetacarpal joint, but the first metacarpal bone is ruled out.

Body: The transverse head is triangular, the anterior margin is divided into an anterior medial surface and an anterior lateral surface, the anterior margins of the second, to fourth and fifth metacarpal bones are attached to the palmar interosseous muscles. The transverse head of the thumb adductor is attached to the anterior margin of the third metacarpal bone, and the dorsal interosseous muscles attached to the adjacent margins of the five bodies of the metacarpal bone. The body of the metacarpal bone is relatively thin, fracture may sometimes arise in the case of the intense shock, and the ruptured pieces are often angulated toward the dorsal side because of the large flexor force.

Head: This is circular, and its spherical joint surface is connected to the base of the proximal phalanx, forming the metacarpophalangeal joint. Most of the articular surface is located on the palmar side, the smallest proportion of the articular surface is located on the dorsal side, and the convexity in the anterior and posterior direction of the articular surface is higher than that in the transverse direction. In the case of the flexion of the metacarpophalangeal joint, the base of the proximal phalanx slides to the anterior side, and the head of the metacarpal bone is exposed at the inferior region and palpable at the body surface.

The five metacarpal bones differ slightly in terms of their shape and size. The first metacarpal bone is the shortest and thickest, concave on the palmar surface, and it is divided into the internal and external surfaces by a crest. The lateral surface is relatively large, the opposing muscle is attached to the thumb, and the medial surface is relatively small, on which nutrient foramens are visible. The dorsal surface is wide and smooth. The base is a saddle-shaped articular surface; on the lateral side, lesser tubercles are found, and to it is attached the long abductor of the thumb. The medial side is rough and the short flexor of the thumb is attached to it. The head has a lower curvature than that of other metacarpal bones, but its transverse diameter is the largest; one bulging articular surface is found on the two sides of the palmar surface of the head, and it is connected to the two sesamoid bones of the thumb.

The second metacarpal bone is the largest, and the three articular surfaces lie at the three bases, which are connected to the trapezium, trapezoid, and capitate bones. The dorsal surface of the base is rough, to which are attached the long and short radial extensors of the wrist; a nodule or crest is found at the palmar surface, to which is attached the radial flexor of the wrist. The body is shaped like a triangular prism, and it becomes slightly bent toward the dorsal side.

The third metacarpal bone is slightly shorter than the second metacarpal bone, and the base is connected to the capitate bone; the palmar surface is rough, to which the oblique head of the thumb adductor and the radial flexor of the wrist are attached. The dorsal surface is attached to the radial short adductor of the wrist.

The fourth metacarpal bone is relatively short and thin, its base is relatively narrow, and two articular surfaces are connected by the capitate bone and the hamate bone. Its body is relatively thin, three interosseous muscles are attached to it, and nutrient foramens can be found at the lateral surface.

The fifth metacarpal bone is thin and short, and the base articular surface is saddle-shaped and connected to the hamate bone. The palmar surface is rough, to which is attached the piso-metacarpal ligament. There is a nodule at the medial surface of the base, to which is attached the ulnar extensor muscle of the wrist.

For the hand's activities (such as pinching and beating), gravity is mostly imposed on the first to third metacarpal bones, the force of the second metacarpal bone can be transferred to the radial bone via the trapezium and navicular bones, the force of the third metacarpal bone can be transferred to the radial bone via the capitate and navicular bones, and the force of the fourth and fifth metacarpal bones can be indirectly transferred to the radial bone only through the tip of the capitate bone via the navicular bone. The development of the metacarpal bone is associated with the above-mentioned functions.

2.5.2 Phalanges

There are 14 phalanges; the thumbs have two phalanges whereas the other digits have three phalanges, i.e., the proximal phalange, middle phalange, and distal phalange. Each phalange consists of three parts: the base, body, and head. The base is wide, with an oval and sunken articular surface; the body is relatively thin and part of the bone fibrous tube, and its palmar surface is flat and sunk. Its dorsal surface is an excavation and is covered by the dorsal aponeurosis. The head is relatively narrow and trochlear shaped, and there are two small condyles on the articular surface, with a groove in the middle.

The proximal phalanx is the longest, the base and the head of the metacarpal bone grow into the metacarpophalangeal joint, the cross-section of the body is half-moon-shaped, the palmar surface is flat, to its margins are attached the digital superficial flexor tendon, and the head and the base of middle phalanx form the proximal interphalangeal joint. The middle phalanx is relatively short and thin, and two sunk articular surfaces at the base are separated by a small crest and connected with the head of the proximal phalanx. The palmar surface of the body is slightly concave on its two sides, and it attaches to the digital superficial flexor tendon. The head is smaller than the proximal phalanx and connected to the distal phalanx. The distal phalanx is the smallest and its base is articulated with the head of the middle phalanx. The palmar surface of its base is slightly concave, to which is attached the deep superficial flexor; the palmar surface of its head has a heel-iron-shaped tuberosity, which is called the tuberosity of the distal phalanx.

Sesamoid bones are a small round bone blocks, contained in the tendon and ligament, and five sesamoid bones are found in a hand, two of which constantly appear on the palmar surface of the thumb's metacarpophalangeal joint.

2.5.3 Hand Joints and Ligaments

Hand joints include the radiocarpal joint, intercarpal joint, middle wrist joint, metacarpophalangeal joint, intermetacarpal joints, metacarpophalangeal joint, and phalangeal joint Fig. 2.56.

2.5.3.1 Radiocarpal Joint

The radiocarpal joint is a biaxial ellipsoidal joint, consisting of the carpal articular surface of the radius, the inferior surface of the articular disc, navicular bone, lunar bone, and triangular bone. Its joint capsule is thin and flaccid, peripheral to which the carpal palmar ligament of the radius, the carpal dorsal ligament of the radius, the radial collateral ligament of the wrist, and the ulnar collateral ligament of the wrist for reinforcement. The articular surface and articular head are covered by thin-layered cartilage. The articular cavity is wide. The radiocarpal joint functions as a whole during movement. During the pronation and supination (actually generated by the radioulnar distal joint), the simultaneous movement of the radiocarpal joint and intercarpal joints can result in an anteflexion of 60–70°,

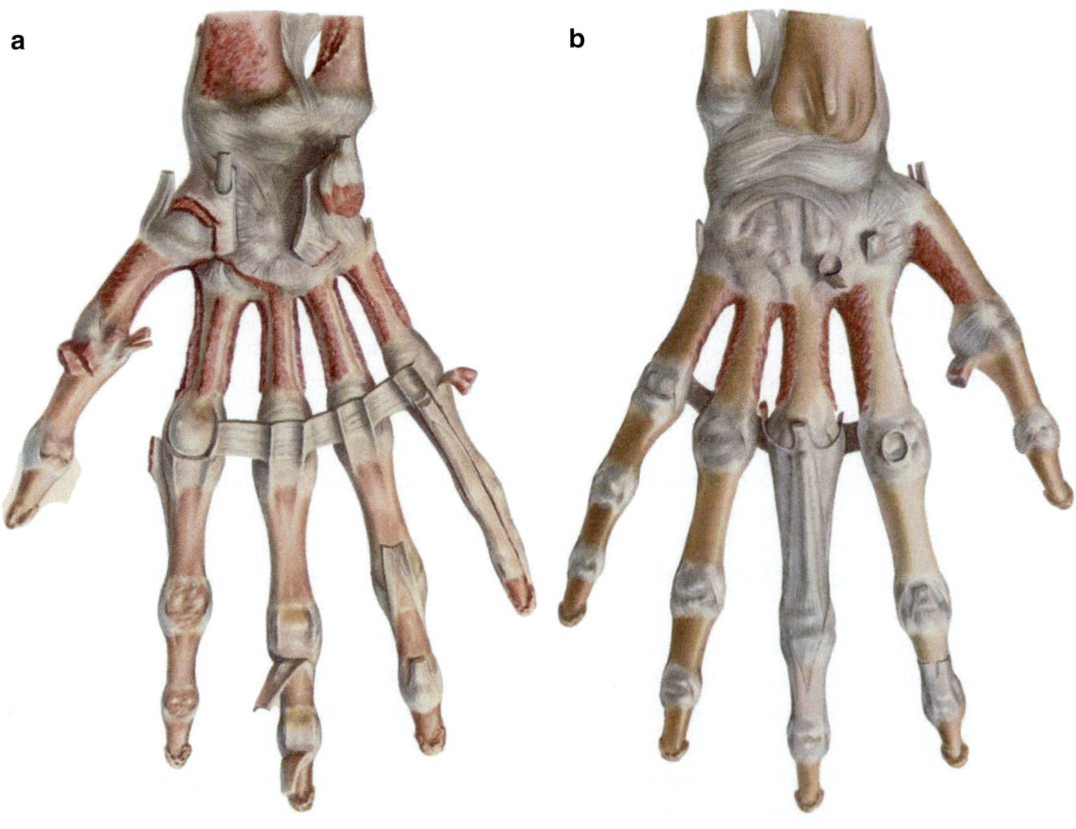

Fig. 2.56 Hand joints. *1* Radiocarpal joint. *2* Intercarpal joint. *3* Middle wrist joint. *4* Carpometacarpal joint. *5* Intermetacarpal joints. *6* Metacarpophalangeal joint. *7* Proximal interphalangeal joint. *8* Distal interphalangeal joint

a posterior extension of about 45°, an adduction of 35–40°, and an abduction of about 20°.

2.5.3.2 Intercarpal Joint

The intercarpal joint at the proximal row consists of navicular bone, lunar bone and triangular bone, and it is amphiarthrodial. It is reinforced by the palmar intercarpal ligament, dorsal intercarpal ligament, and interosseous intercarpal ligament. In addition, a lentiform bone joint is formed between the lentiform bone and the triangular bone; it has an independent articular capsule and articular cavity, and is reinforced by the pisometacarpal ligament and the pisohamate ligament.

The intercarpal joint at the distal row consists of the trapezium bone, trapezoid bone, capitate bone, and hamate bone; being amphiarthrodial, it is reinforced by the palmar intercarpal ligament, dorsal intercarpal ligament, and interosseous intercarpal ligament.

2.5.3.3 Middle Carpal Joint

Located between the two rows of carpal bones, it is a deformed plane joint and an ellipsoidal joint, in fact. The shape of the articular surface is bent like the symbol "~", the trapezium bone and the trapezoid bone on its lateral side form a concave side, which is connected to the navicular bone, and the capitate bone and hamate bone at its medial side form a convex side, which is connected to the navicular bone, lunar bone, and triangular bone. Its articular cavity is very large and can communicate completely transversely, and it can still communicate with the intercarpal joint cavity at the proximal row and the intercarpal joint cavity at the distal row. The joint capsule is reinforced by the radiate carpal ligament and the dorsal intercarpal ligament.

The joint cavity is tortuous; on the proximal side, it can communicate with the intermetacarpal joint at the distal end, and on the distal side, it can communicate with the cavities of the second to fifth intermetacarpal joints. The joint capsule is reinforced by the palmar metacarpal ligament of the wrist and the dorsal metacarpal ligament of the wrist, which lie peripherally.

2.5.3.4 Intermetacarpal Joint

There are three intermetacarpal joints, which are located ranging from the second to the fifth base of the metacarpal bones. Being amphiarthrodial, they have their own joint capsules, and the joint cavity can communicate with the carpometacarpal joint. The joint capsule is reinforced by the palmar metacarpal ligament, dorsal metacarpal ligament, and interosseous metacarpal ligament.

2.5.3.5 Metacarpophalangeal Joint

Metacarpophalangeal joint is a ball-and-socket joint consisting of the capitellum of metacarpal bone and the proximal phalanx. It can perform the movements of flexion and extension, adduction and abduction, and rotation, but the thumb metacarpophalangeal joint is a hinge joint and can only perform flexion and extension movements. The joint capsule is reinforced by the palmar ligament (volar plate) and accessory collateral ligament. The second to fifth heads of the metacarpal bones are connected via the deep palmar transverse ligaments.

2.5.3.6 Interphalangeal Joint

There are nine interphalangeal joints consisting of the head of the proximal phalanx, the base of the middle phalanx, the head of the middle phalanx, and the base of the distal phalanx. It belongs to the axial hinge joint. Being flaccid and thin, the joint capsule is reinforced by the palmar ligament (volar plate), accessory ligament, and accessory collateral ligament.

3 Replantation with Commonly Used Instruments, Equipment, and Materials

Finger replantation is an important part of microsurgery, and the key to success is fine blood vessels and nerve anastomosis. Finger blood vessels and nerves are very small; thus, it is very difficult to distinguish them with the naked eye. All surgical protocols must be performed with a microscope, micro-instruments and various special repair materials. The development of the replantation of amputated fingers is closely connected to the development of surgical equipment and materials. It is the continuous development of surgical equipment and materials that promotes the development of replantation of amputated fingers. Below, some of the commonly used equipment and materials for finger replantation are described (Fig. 3.1).

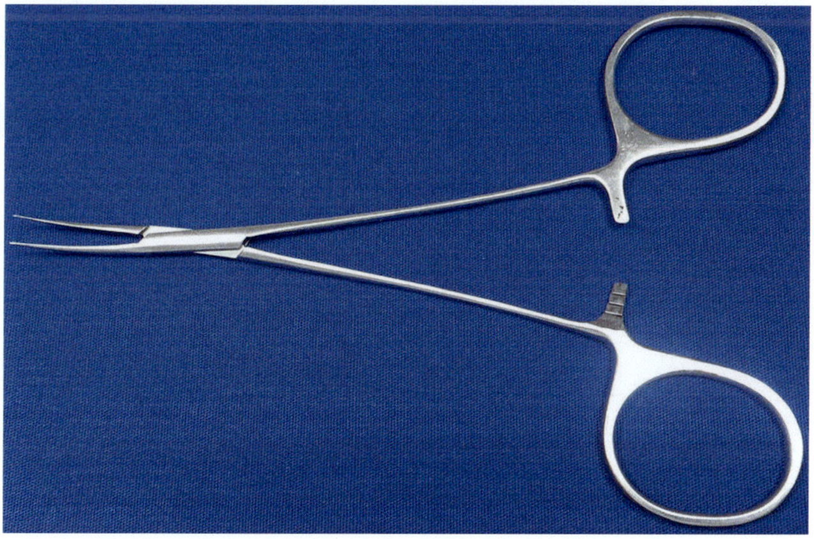

Fig. 3.1 Commonly used equipment and apparatus for replantation

J. Lin et al., *Special Type of Finger Replantation*, https://doi.org/10.1007/978-981-10-6229-2_3

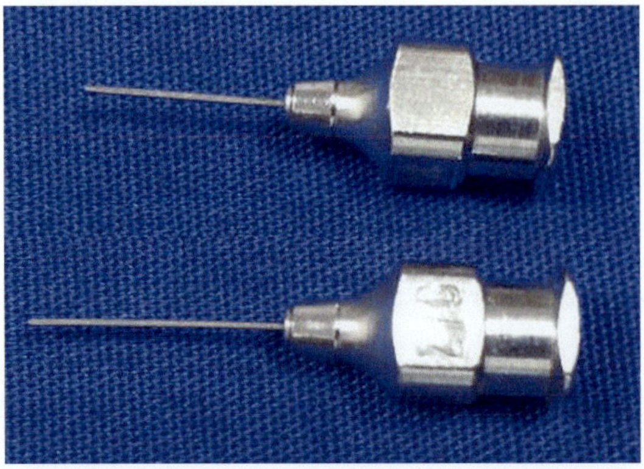

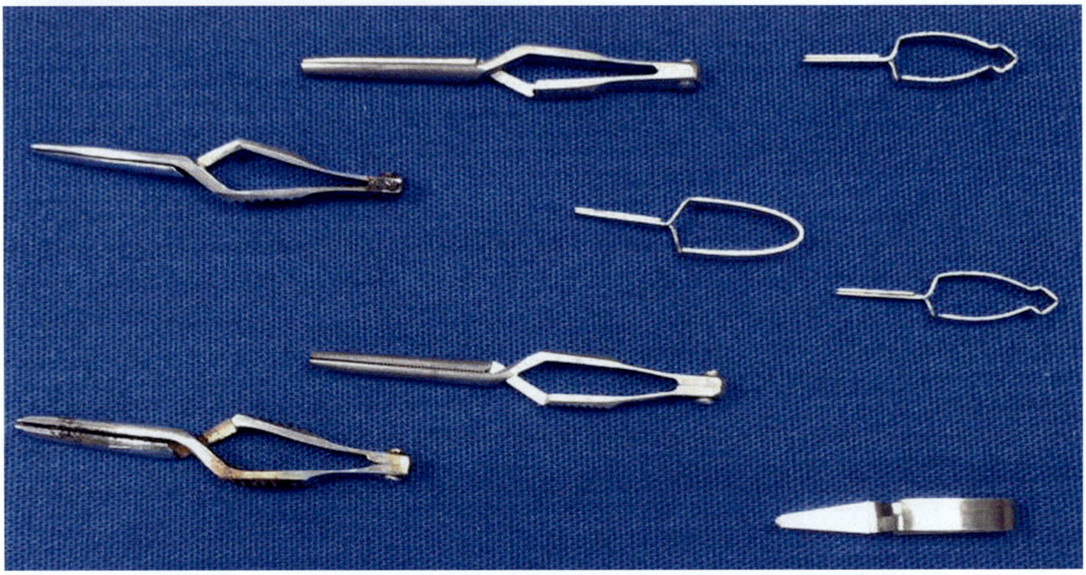

Fig. 3.1 (continued)

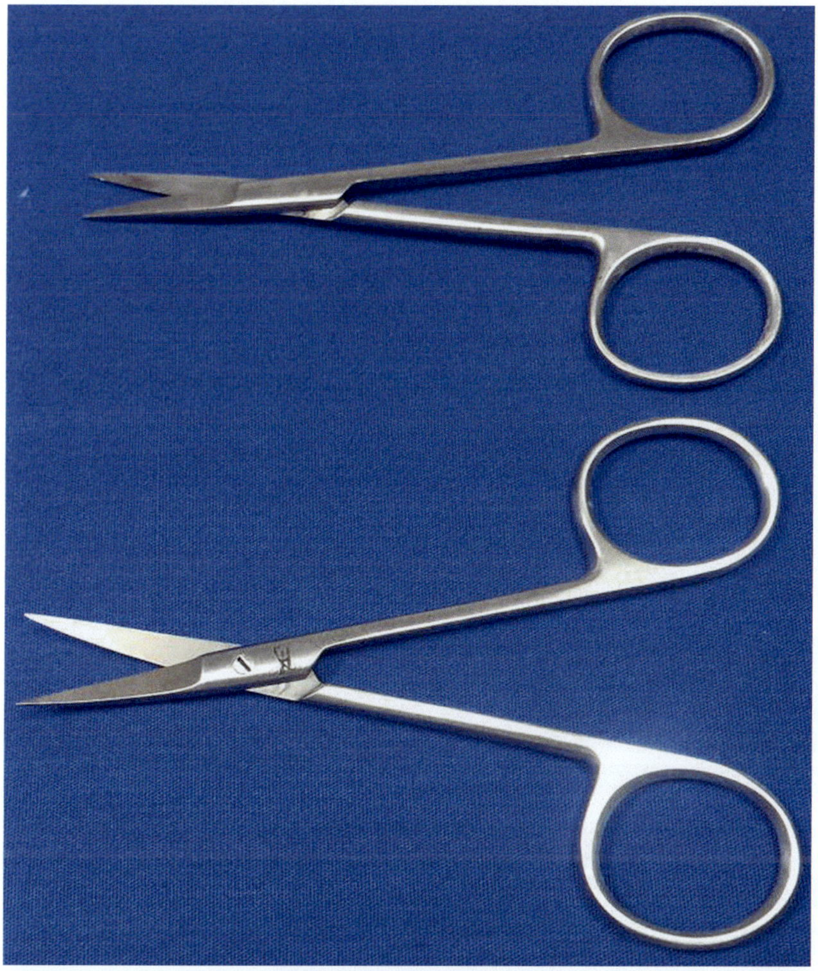

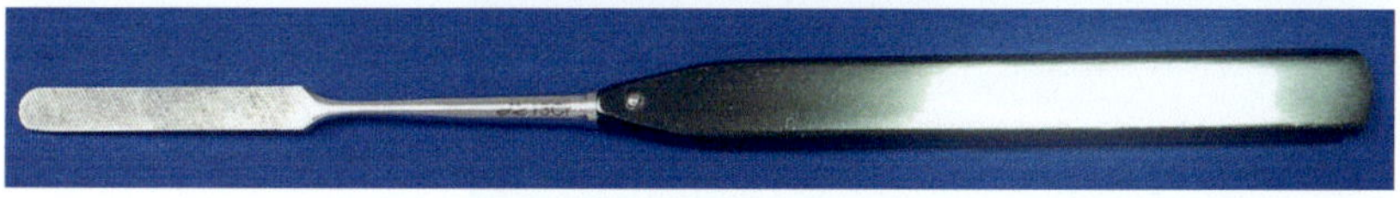

Fig. 3.1 (continued)

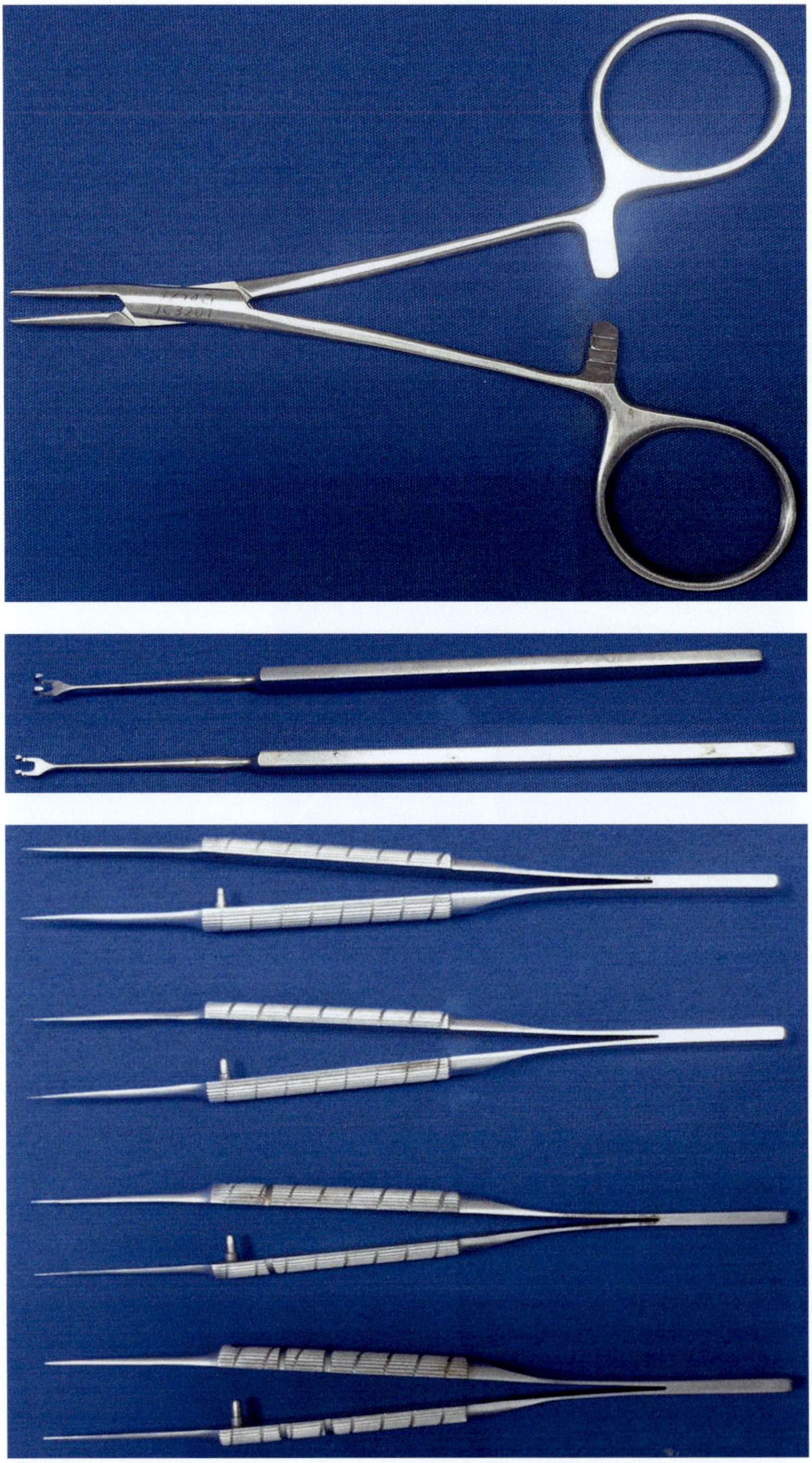

Fig. 3.1 (continued)

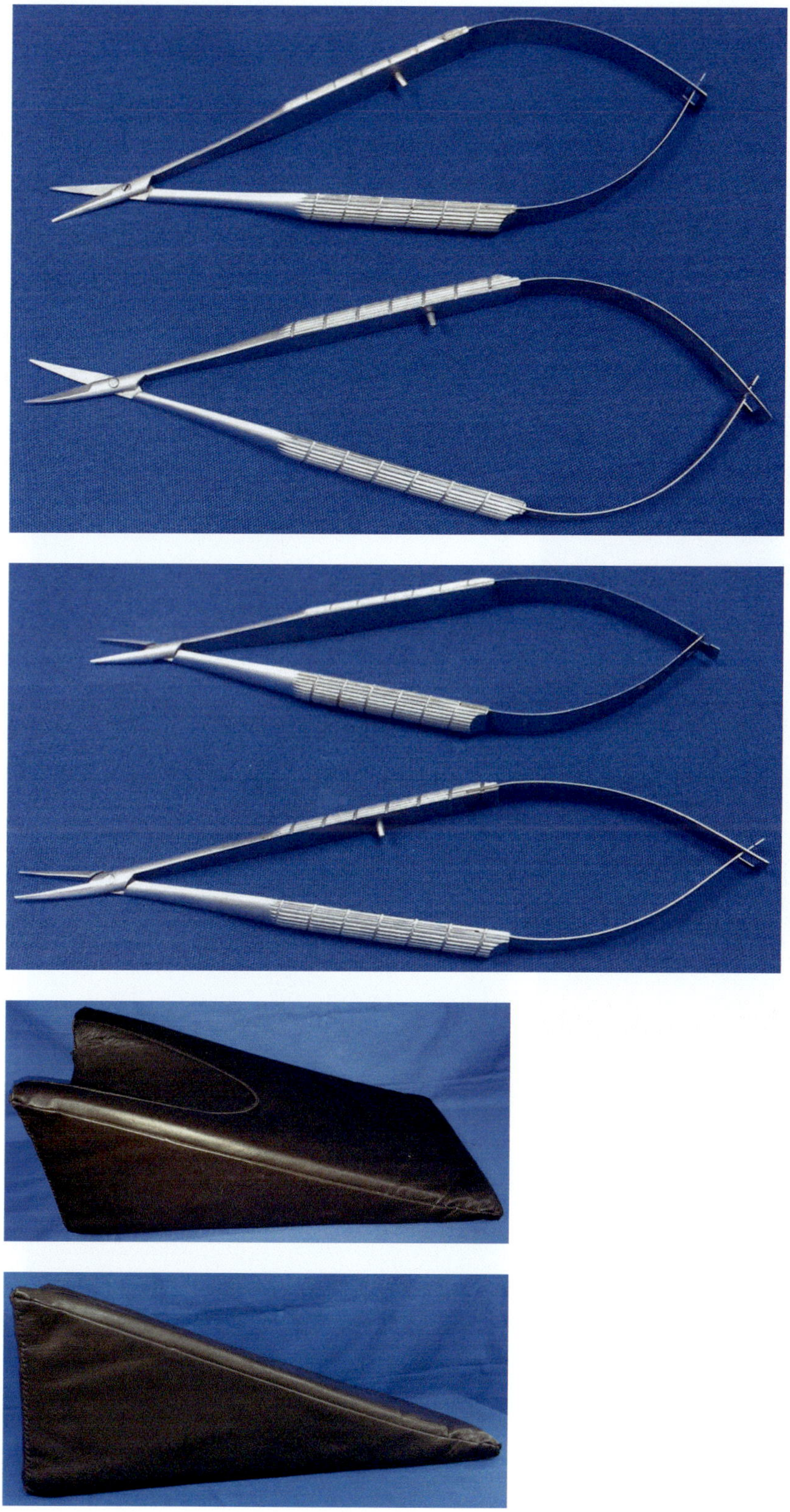

Fig. 3.1 (continued)

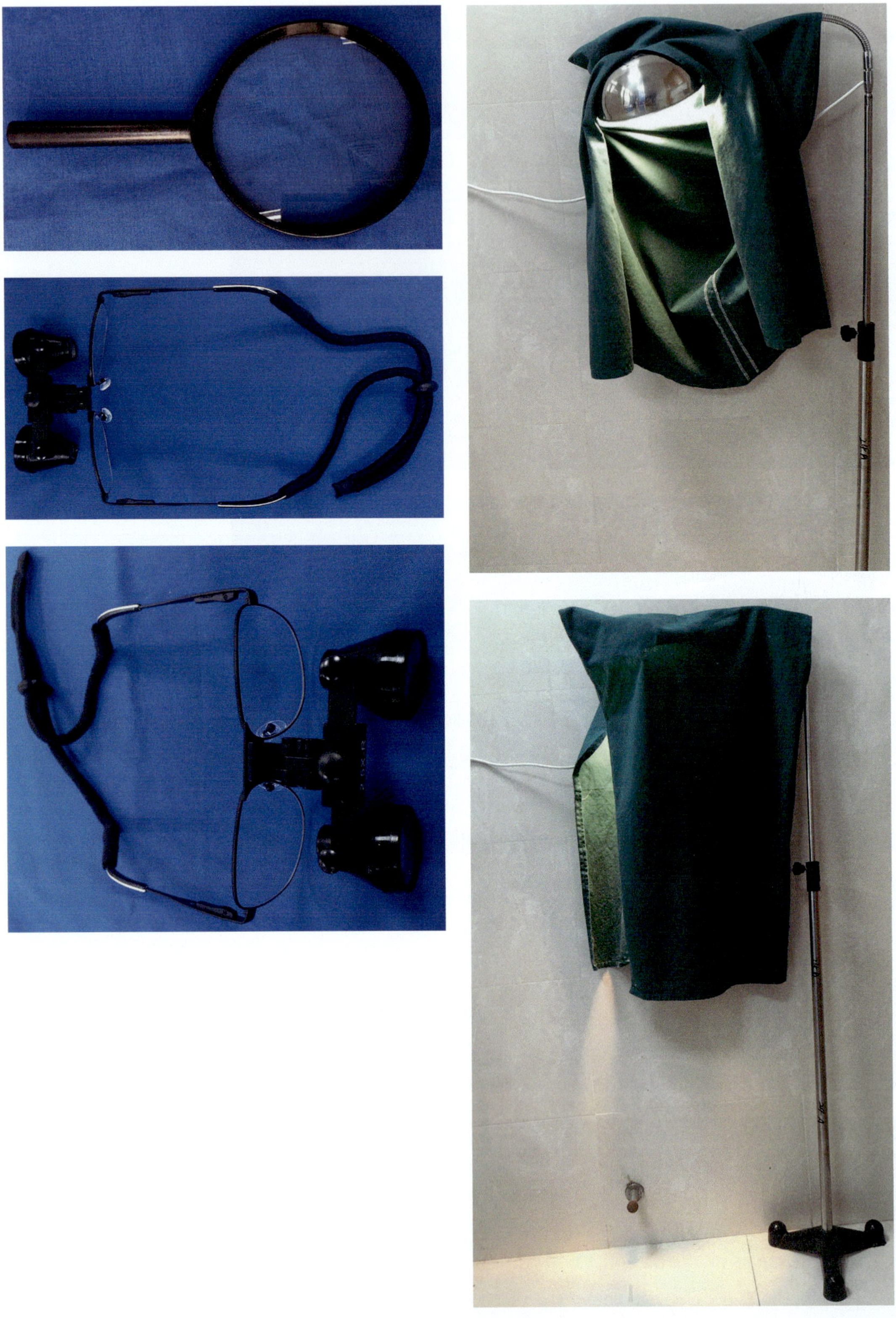

Fig. 3.1 (continued)

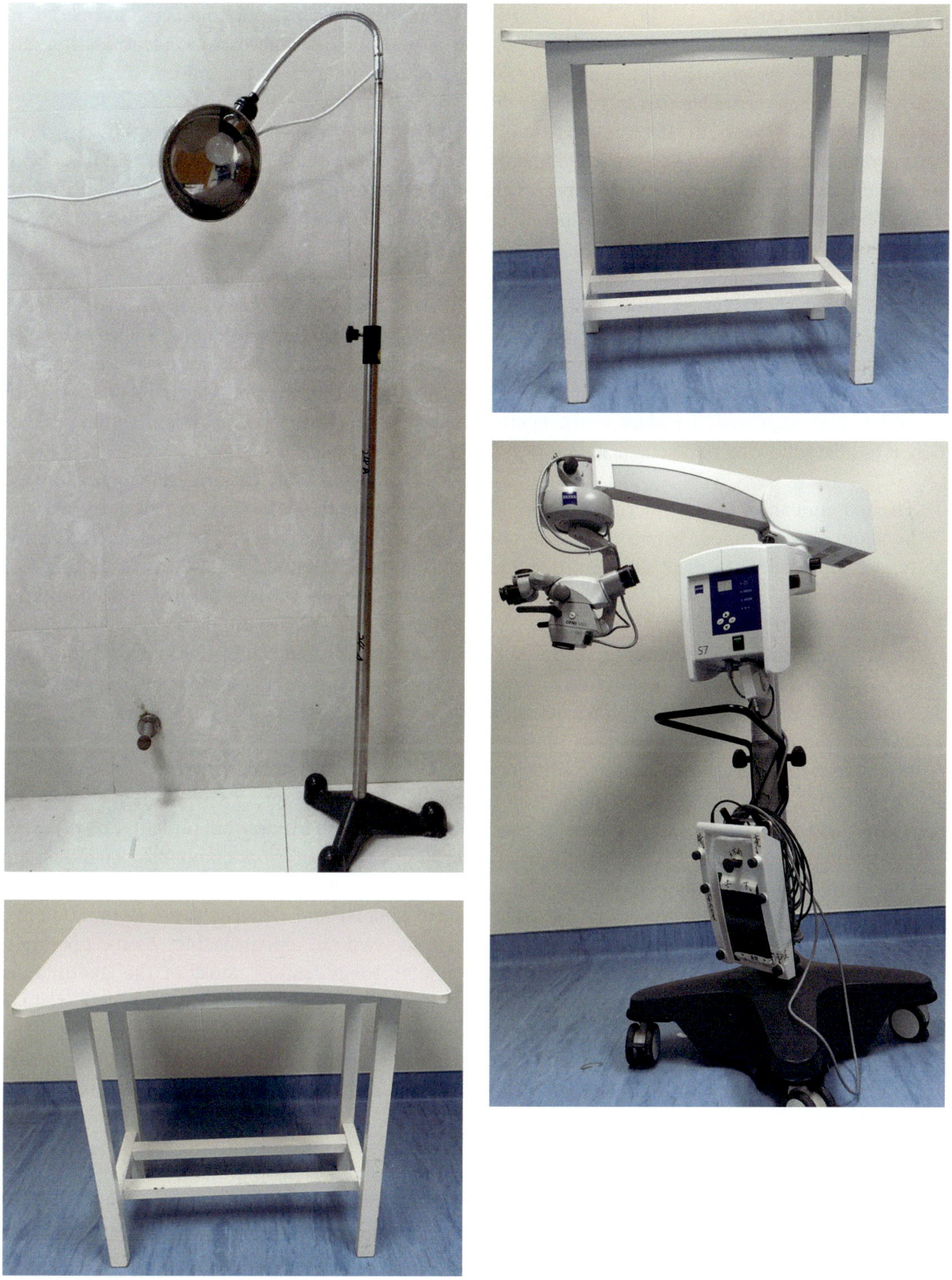

Fig. 3.1 (continued)

3.1 Microscope

The invention of the microscope has a history of nearly 400 years, its application in surgery, only 90 years. In the past 90 years, the microscope has also been updated. The first microscope used in microsurgery consisted of biological microscopes, with a small field of view and inconvenient operation. Later, there were a variety of surgical magnifying glasses. These were cheap, but the focal length cannot be fixed, there was an intraoperative need to focus repeatedly, and surgery was very inconvenient. In recent years, with the development of microsurgery, the functional design of the microscope has also improved. To adapt to the operation, it has the following basic characteristics:

1. The magnification of the microscope should be about ×10, changing between ×6 and ×40 times, and be able to meet different demand amplifications.
2. The working distance of the microscope can be adjusted randomly according to the surgeon's needs, usually at 200–400 mm.
3. Ensuring that the light source can cover the entire operation field, providing enough brightness; the light source needs to filter out infrared rays, prevent long-time radiation burn tissues, and a cold light source should be used as a priority.
4. The microscope has more than two sets of binocular tubes for the surgeon's and the assistants' use, the eyepiece should focus on the same field of view, and with visual adjustment and two pupil focal length adjustment function, to adapt to different surgeries. Notes: as each eye has a different diopter, the eyepiece should be adjusted before the surgery. After adjustment in the distance between the eyepieces, to make it consistent with patients with IPD. It may be necessary to adjust the microscope at any time during the operation. All operations should be performed under aseptic conditions. During the operation, the magnification of the image cannot be blindly chosen, so that the brightness of the imaging becomes weaker, and the depth of field becomes smaller, which is not conducive to operation. Therefore, the microscopic identification rate is the primary reference index.

First generation: Five-head magnifying glass: early application, the advantage is that it is cheap and easy to use, but the use of instability, the amplification effect is poor, and the surgery is fatiguing.

Second generation: The domestic optical microscope was a head-mounted magnifying glass. At ×16, the magnification improved, more stable, has a better effect, but for the fine operation of paratelum replantation, this does still not meet the requirements, for the operation personnel or with regard to fatigue.

Third generation: The imported optical microscope magnification. To further improve the image more clearly, it can be connected to a TV or computer interface, be used for teaching and research, the electric foot controller is helpful for adjusting the focal length and magnification. However, the price is high, and the operation and maintenance are more complicated.

3.1.1 Micro-Instruments

It is not enough to carry out replantation of a severed finger, and it is not enough to depend on the microscopic equipment of the operation. We also need special and delicate surgical instruments, and the two are indispensable. As the operation time is long- lasting, most of the instruments have spring-type handles, which can reduce hand fatigue, and when the spring is relaxed, the hand maintains the resting position. The spring is not too tight, otherwise there is adductor pollicis and dorsal interosseous muscle fatigue, causing shaking during surgery, which is not conducive to the operation; on the contrary, if the spring is too loose it will fall off the devices, and it must have a certain elasticity. Retractable hand instruments should not bounce or vibrate. The slight vibration has a significant effect on surgical microscope, the mismatch phenomenon, forceps tip scissors blade, uneven needle holder locking teeth during the operation are caused by vibration and have an impact on the quality of the operation. To make the fingers turn, it can complete all kinds of actions. The handle part of the instrument is usually made into a circle, so that the operating instrument can rotate along its longitudinal axis. The handle has different thickness knurling, so as to increase the friction force and make the grip more stable. The type and practicability of micro-instruments are keeping pace with the times. Traditional micro-instruments mainly include micro-forceps, scissors, needle holder, blood vessel clamp, irrigator, etc. They are relatively simple, meets the basic demands of the operation, the price is low, but the function is poor. Modern micro-instruments mainly include micro-closure devices, micro-hemostatic forceps, microvascular hook, micro-vascular fork, microvascular hemostatic forceps, micro-wire clip, micro-needle-holding forceps, micro-scissors, irrigator, etc. The operation is more convenient, more accurate, and even a single person can complete vascular anastomosis. However, the price is high, and maintenance is relatively troublesome. The characteristics of the current commonly used micro-instruments are introduced as follows.

3.1.2 Micro-Tweezers

The width of the forceps is 0.15 mm, the tweezers tip is well closed, and the positioning pin for protecting the tip is incorrect. It is suitable for the suturing of small vessels and lymph vessels of less than 0.5 mm in diameter.

3.1.3 Micro-Needle Holder

The narrow 0.2 mm needle holder head has certain advantages for the needle clamp 12-0, avoids the head being too wide and using the needle clamp. When tying the knot, the needle holder can be used to grip the thread accurately. The handle spring is of moderate hardness and less laborious when holding the needle.

3.1.4 Micro-Scissors

The length of the scissors is generally 12–15 cm, there are two kinds of scissors, bent and straight, for the separation of blood vessels and nerves. Scissors should be used if trimming or if trimming of the vessel is necessary.

3.1.5 Hemostatic Clamp

The normal pressure is 2.5 g/mm^2, and the small vessels with a diameter of less than 0.5 mm are enough to block the blood flow, and suture the 1–1.5-H vessel wall without pressure marks. a larger caliber of blood vessels can be used to adjust the pressure of the mini-fold.

3.1.6 External Diameter Measuring Ruler of the Blood Vessels

The outer diameter of the blood vessel can be accurately measured so as to record the diameter of the vessel accurately during the operation.

3.1.7 Micro-Irrigator

This is mainly used to flush the lumen of the vessels.

3.1.8 Notes on the Application of Microsurgical Instruments

The application of microsurgical instruments to the rotation of the operation of most fingers only needs to perform a variety of actions; i.e., the multipurpose gripping device for writing, eating food between the thumb and middle finger, clamp handle, and end devices should be able to increase its stability. Micro-scissors are thin; thus, they can only be used to cut blood vessel, nerve tissue, and the micro-suture line. All micro-instruments should be placed in the tip to avoid collision and dropping, to prevent damage to the sophisticated tip of the instrument. Clean the tip of blood at any time during the use of the instrument so as not to adhere to the suture and influence the operation. The blood on the instrument should also be carefully cleaned and dried.

3.1.9 Other Related Equipment

Operating table, surgical basic instruments, portable Doppler, baking lamp, etc.

3.2 Commonly Used Materials

3.2.1 Fracture Fixation Materials

Traditional methods: traditional fracture reduction internal fixation with Kirschner wire and cross steel wire based, easy to operate, fast, low price, and low cost. However, the fixation is not strong enough, it is easy to fracture displacement after the operation, and often needs to be fixed across the joint. Early functional exercises cannot be performed.

Modern methods: mini plates and screws are widely used in hand surgery, but are also applied to finger replantation. The method of fracture fixation is firm, early postoperative functional exercises can be performed, and the function is adequately restored. However, the mini-plate and screw internal fixation has some deficiencies and complications, such as it cannot be used for finger replantation, operation, and cross Kirschner wire as it is simple and prolongs the time needed to perform replantation, and the price of the materials price is higher. In addition, there may be a need for repeat internal fixation surgery.

Intramedullary nailing for the removal of the proximal phalanx is another new method that has been developed in recent years. It has the advantages of fixation, the reliability and time-saving, and it minimizes the destruction of soft tissue. However, this technique lacks a large amount of long-term follow-up data, its clinical application has been limited, and it is still in the exploratory stage.

With regard to general parallel longitudinal Kirschner wire fixation for middle transverse fracture of the bone fixation, cross-wire fixation is relatively reliable, and is especially suitable for near-periarticular fractures, but can also be used for arthrodesis. Screw fixation is suitable for short oblique fractures, whereas small plate fixation has the advantage of good stability, but it is offset by the deterioration of soft tissue. To avoid bone fracture, it is important to keep in mind the principle of screw fixation: the length of the broken end of the fixed point should be at least three times the diameter of the screw. The risk of complications after standard small plate fixation is relatively high, and the "H"-shaped plate designed for replantation of the severed finger can be chosen.

In summary, replantation should be based on fixed methods and choosing the specific circumstances, such as a combination of traditional methods and modern methods, and even other innovations, as long as it is conducive to the survival and function of the reconstructed finger.

3.2.2 Nerve Repair Materials

Traditional methods: If a nerve defect occurs, autologous nerve graft or nerve transposition method are usually used, and another nerve needs to be sacrificed.

Modern methods: With the development of modern materials for nerve repair, for replantation treatment of the nerve defect, artificial nerve conduit repair, or nerve allograft to repair, can be chosen, without sacrificing the autologous nerve, but the prices of materials are higher.

3.2.3 Tendon Repair Materials

Traditional methods: If a tendon defect occurs during replantation of the finger, traditional tendon autograft or autograft should be sacrificed, and other tendons should be sacrificed.

Modern method: If a tendon defect occurs during replantation of an amputated finger, allograft tendon repair can now be used, but the material price is higher, and a rejection reaction may occur.

3.2.4 Vascular Repair Materials

Replantation surgery has been successfully implemented for decades, using artificial vascular anastomosis suture needles. In recent years, anastomotic devices have been widely used for relatively coarse microvascular anastomosis, such as the ulnar radial artery and the cephalic vein. This has achieved a good clinical effect, a simple method of anastomosis, and satisfactory anastomotic effect. With the development of science and technology, the microvascular anastomosis device will be applied to the anastomosis of finger blood vessels. At the same time, finger replantation will be easier to perform, and the survival rate will be greatly improved.

Bibliography

Chen X, Gao W, Jian H. Study on the application of cryopreserved allogeneic tendon. J Chin J Surg. 2001;17(4):223–4.

Freeland AE. Open screw fixation. In: Freeland AE, editor. Hand fractures repair reconstruction and rehabilitation. Philadelphia: Churchill-Livingstone; 2000. p. 46–51.

Grewal AS, Emvic B, Strumas N, et al. The utility of the microvascular, anastomotic, coupler, transfer in free tissue. Can J Plast Surg. 2012;20(2):98–102.

Gu L, Qingtang Z, Wang Overseas Chinese. Expert opinion on symposium on microsurgical vascular anastomosis technique. Chin J Microsurg. 2014;37(2):105.

Guoliang C. Development and improvement of digital replantation. Chin J Hand Surg. 2003;19:129–31.

Guoliang C. Review and prospect of limb (finger) replantation in China. Chin J Microsurg. 2007;30:253–6.

Huang J, Mintao T, Xueyuan L. Medicon mini titanium plate in replantation of amputated fingers. Chin J Hand Surg. 2010;26(5):303.

Kayikcioglu A, Karamursel S, Mavili E, et al. Ann Plast Surg. 2000;45(3):258–63.

Minami A, Usui M, Ishii S, et al. The in vivo effects of vatic US immunoreactive treatments on allogenic tendon grafts. J Hand Surg (Am). 1983;8:888–93.

Qingtang Z, Canbin Z, Xiaolin L. Clinical adaptation of peripheral nerve defect repair materials. The consideration of syndrome. Chin J Microsurg. 2013;36:417–21.

Reddy C, Pennington D, Stem H. Microvascular anastomosis using the vascular closure device in free flap reconstructive surgery: a 13-year experience. J Plast Reconstr Aesthet Surg. 2012;65(2):195–200.

Rovak JM, Bishop DK, Boxer LK, et al. Peripheral, nerve transplantation: the, role, of, chemical, acellularization, in, eliminating, allograft antigenicity. J Reconstr Microsurg. 2005;21:207–13.

Shu W. Atlas hand surgery. Beijing: People's Medical Publishing House; 2011. p. 12.

Sun T, Peng W, Jianrong F, et al. Analysis of the effect of microvascular stapler on repair of vascular injuries in extremities. Chin J Microsurg. 2014;37(2):123–5.

Tang J, Fang Y, Panfeng W. Acellular allograft nerve repair for radial nerve and digital nerve defect. Chin J Microsurg. 2014;37(5):449–52.

Tao Z, Jun Z, Baozhan I. Mini titanium plate in multi finger replantation. Appl Pract Hand Surg. 2013;04:356–7.

Teng X, Hong C, Sihong L. Application of microvascular stapler in free flap repair of upper limb tissue defects. Chin J Chin Surg. 2015;38(4):385–7.

Xi ZX, Linquan Y, Hong M. Glutaraldehyde and deep hypothermia treatment of tendon transplantation for the repair of hand tendon defect. J Hepatopancreatobiliary Surg. 2003;26(4):305–6.

Yu F, Meng XZ. Macro observation of tendon allograft for repairing tendon defect of hand effect. J Zhongshan Univ. 2004;25(z1):285–6.

Yudong G. Basic concept and treatment principle of peripheral nerve defect. Chin J Hand Surg. 2002;18:129–30.

Yudong G, Shuhuan W, Li D. Hand surgery. Shanghai: Fudan University Press; 2010. p. 6.

Yun SL, Yuhui C, Fangliang Z, et al. Internal fixation with mini phalanx steel plate for finger replantation applications. J Pract Hand Surg. 2004;18:52–3.

Yun SL, Fangliang Z, Tao X. Clinical comparison of three different internal fixation methods in finger replantation. Chin J Surg. 2005;21(4):205–6.

Common Medicines Used after the Replantation of Amputated Fingers

4

The successful replantation of amputated fingers is based on not only the microsurgery technique, but also the medicines used postoperatively. Three kinds of medicines are generally used after an operation, which are antibiotics, antispasmodics, and anticoagulant drugs. Antibiotics must be used intraoperatively and postoperatively because of complex injuries, the long duration, and prolonged exposure of the wound. The common reasons why the antispasmodic drugs and anticoagulant drugs should be used after an operation are:

1. Blood coagulability is increased after injury and operation, which is the body's protective physiological response
2. Adrenaline is released after the injury and operation; thus, patients are prone to experiencing vasospasm, an increase in platelets and an increase in blood coagulation, which easily leads to thrombosis
3. Spasticity and thrombosis can be easily induced because of the small diameter, which is commonly 1–3 mm (a minimum of 0.2–0.5 mm), and easy susceptibility to physicochemical factors
4. There is a higher chance of thrombosis because of the small scouring force to anastomotic stoma caused by the small diameter and low blood flow. It is necessary to use antispasmodic drugs and anticoagulant drugs because experiments have proved that the smaller diameter of the vessel, the more likely it is that thrombosis will occur, because the 1-mm vessel has a platelet absorption density twice as high as the 2-mm vessel. In Table 4.1, the commonly used drugs are shown.

Characteristics, indications, adverse reactions, and precautions for these drugs are described as follows.

Table 4.1 Commonly used drugs

Antibiotic drugs	Penicillin, cephalosporins, macrolide, et al., used alone or in combination
Anticoagulant drugs	6% dextran 40 iv drip (500–1000 ml/day); or aspirin (3 times/day, each 0.5–1 g); or 5% glucose injection 1000 ml + low molecular heparin 1500 IU (for children: 11–150 U/kg + 5% glucose injection 500 ml), maintained for 24 h
Antispasmodic drugs	Benzazoline 25 mg or papaverine 30 mg/6–8 h, intramuscular injection, used alone or in combination

J. Lin et al., *Special Type of Finger Replantation*, https://doi.org/10.1007/978-981-10-6229-2_4

4.1 Dextran 40

Dextran is clinically used to decrease blood viscosity, improve microcirculation, and expand blood volume. With a high molecular weight and not prone to exuding from vessels, Dextrose 40 can improve plasma colloid osmotic pressure, and further expand blood volume and maintain blood pressure. It also has the effects of inhibiting platelet aggregation and reducing erythrocyte aggregation to decrease blood viscosity, in addition to the effects of inhibiting blood coagulation factor II to prevent thrombosis and improve microcirculation. The general dose is 1000 ml/day, for 7–10 days and the dose can be reduced gradually according to the severity of the disease.

4.1.1 Adverse Reactions

(1) Anaphylaxis: Skin pruritus and even refractory skin pruritus may occur, and in some cases, it will last for 6 months; these are the most prominent characteristics. This pruritus is characterized by long duration, the fact that there are no effective mitigating methods, and its insufferability. Red papules, urticaria, and asthma, etc., may occur. There is a small chance of anaphylactic shock; thus, the first drip should be observed for 5–10 min and the drug should be withdrawn immediately if there are any symptoms. (2) Febrile response occasionally occurs, manifesting as shivering and high fever. The fever may be periodic or persistent low heat and there is a small chance of enlarged lymph nodes and joint pain. (3) Excessively large doses may cause bleeding such as nosebleed, skin and mucous membrane bleeding, gingival bleeding, wound blood oozing, and hematuria. The daily dose should be no more than 1500 ml.

4.1.2 Precautions

(1) It is contraindicated in patients with congestive heart failure and hemorrhagic disease. (2) Great caution should be exercised in patients with liver and kidney diseases.

4.2 Papaverine

Papaverine is one of the opioid alkaloids, but has no obvious anesthetic effect. It is a nonspecific vasodilator that can cause a direct nonspecific relaxation effect on the blood vessels, heart or other smooth muscles. It has the obvious effects of relieving vasospasm and improving circulation of the replanted finger. Intermittent and repeated intramuscular injection or intravenous administration after dilution is commonly used clinically. There are reports that local application at a small dose can relax the vessels completely so that the vasospasm can be mitigated; papaverine injection at a low dose near the anastomotic stoma can used if an arterial crisis occurs during or after the operation.

4.2.1 Adverse Reactions

(1) As papaverine is a strong irritant, the long-term intramuscular injection of the drug at the hip causes local edema and histiocyte metabolism disorder; thus, the drug cannot be absorbed and becomes stagnated locally, causing further chemical stimulation to local sites. The mechanical stimulation of the injection also induces the chemical and traumatic damage to muscle fiber. As the injection frequency increases, the muscle fiber gradually atrophies and is replaced by connective tissues. Collagenous fibers become gradually proliferative gradually, forming induration. (2) Jaundice will occur, and eyes and skin are clearly stained yellow after administration, indicating the liver damage. (3) An excessive dose may cause blurred vision, double vision, drowsiness, and/or weakness. (4) A large intake can inhibit mitochondrial oxidation reactions, serious lactic acidosis, an increase in blood ketone, and mild hyperglycemia and hypokalemia. (5) It can cause exaggerated respiration and thrombocytopenia.

4.2.2 Precautions

(1) Interference with diagnosis: During administration, blood acidocytes, alanine aminotransferase, alkaline phosphatase, aspartate amino transferase, and bilirubin may increase, indicating liver function impairment. (2) Glaucoma patients should have their intraocular pressure checked regularly. (3) The liver function should be examined regularly, especially when gastrointestinal symptoms or jaundice occur. The drug should be withdrawn in the case of liver function insufficiency.

4.3 Heparin

As an intense anticoagulant and a kind of heterogenous mucous polysaccharide, heparin has the mechanism of action of providing negatively charged matrix to the endothelial cells, providing compounds to AT-III, providing necessary conditions for the repair of endothelial cells, blocking the vasospasm substances, and further inhibiting the prothrombin from being converted into thrombin. The characteristics of action: rapid anticoagulation, short duration, and no accumulative effects. Currently, large-dose heparin is not clinically available, and small-dose heparin is used to prevent postoperative vasospasm and thrombosis. The general usage is 500 ml of normal saline + heparin sodium 6250 U daily, maintained with an intravenous drip for 24 h. The drip speed is adjusted to be within the range of 5–10 gtt/min according to the blood oozing from the lateral incisions. The speed of blood oozing is generally maintained to be within the range 3–5 gtt/min as appropriate, to guarantee capillary engorgement; the heparin is used for 3–7 days continuously.

4.3.1 Adverse Reactions

(1) The most common and important complication is bleeding, with an incidence rate of 8–33%; it is associated with an excessively high dose, age, heart failure, liver function insufficiency, and trauma. (2) Thrombocytopenia: This is divided into the transient type and the persistent type. Transient thrombocytopenia may be caused by the aggregation of heparin-induced transient platelets and stagnation in these regions, and the patient may recover several hours after the intravenous infusion. Persistent thrombocytopenia (subdivided into the moderate type and severe type, potentially with thrombosis) may be caused by the in-vivo antibody damage of platelets and endothelial cells, and the patient may recover after drug withdrawal. (3) Decrease in plasma AT: This leads to gradual failure of heparin anticoagulation, and low-molecular-weight heparin will not cause the decrease in the AT-III level. (4) Allergic reactions: These may be caused by the impurity of the drugs used, manifesting as mild bronchospasm, lacrimation, rhinitis, urticaria, etc.. The incidence rate is less than 1% in the case of pure drugs.

4.3.2 Precautions

(1) People with an allergy to heparin, spontaneous hemorrhagic tendency, slow blood coagulation, canker, postpartum hemorrhage, and serious liver function insufficiency are contraindicated. (2) Coagulation time should be tested regularly during administration. In children, heparin should be administered according to body weight. For patients aged over 60, especially women, a dose reduction is necessary. (3) Low-molecular-weight heparin, i.e., heparin with a relative molecular weight of less than 6.5 kDa, is clinically recommended and it can be obtained from the direct separation of the unfractionated heparin or the re-separation after degradation of unfractionated heparin. It is active on the selective anticoagulin X and has little impact on other coagulation factors; it is characterized by intense anti-FZa effects, weak anti-Flla effects, high bioavailability, long plasma half-life, and low hemorrhagic tendency, etc., when compared with heparin.

4.4 Benzazoline

This is an α receptor blocking agent, which can directly expand the smooth muscles. Adrenergic blockers have direct effects on smooth muscles, can dilate the peripheral vessels, and relieve vasospasm. It is used alternately with papaverine, 25 mg po or im every day, three to four times per day.

Adverse reactions and precautions: (1) It can induce central nerve excitation, thus causing nausea, vomiting, dysphoria, aversion to cold, flushing, palpitation, and postural hypotension. It is contraindicated in patients with canker and coronary arterial blood supply inadequacy. (2) A high dose can induce orthostatic hypotension. At this time, the patient should be asked to lie in the horizontal position with the head down, and electrolyte solution should be supplemented and ephedrine given. Adrenaline should not be used because it aggravates the hypotension.

4.5 Aspirin

The pharmacological action of aspirin can be summarized as: (1) Inhibiting platelet aggregation and expanding blood vessels; (2) prolonging bleeding and coagulation time; (3) analgesia; (4) relieving fever and pain, mitigating inflammation and swelling, and inhibiting acute inflammatory exudation. General usage: enteric type in adults 150 mg per day, three times a day, po. Some people take aspirin to prevent and treat the blood crisis after the replantation of an amputated finger: 0.6 g aspirin administered at 30–60 min after the operation, 0.45 g in the morning, at noon, and in the evening after the operation; an additional 0.6 g at 2:00 am to resist the low peak of the in-vivo hormone level that occurs in the morning. After maintaining therapy according to the above usage for 7 days, the dose is changed to 0.6 g to be taken every early morning for 7 days.

4.5.1 Adverse Reactions

(1) Gastrointestinal symptoms: These are the most common adverse reactions, and common symptoms include nausea, vomiting, and discomfort or pain in the abdomen. (2) Allergic reactions: Allergic reactions such as skin rash, angioneurotic edema, and asthma are induced after idiosyncratic patients take aspirin and they are common in middle-aged people or patients with rhinitis and nasal polyps. (3) Central nervous system: The nervous symptoms occur after a large dose administration, and are called salicylism, manifesting as headache, vertigo, tinnitus, loss of hearing and vision, and even mental disorder, convulsions, and coma; they recover after 2- to 3-day drug withdrawal. (4) Hepatic function impairment: This often occurs in the case of a high dose; this impairment is not an acute action and is characterized by the occurrence several months later after large-dose treatment; it is usually asymptomatic or accompanied by discomfort in the right abdomen, tenderness, increased aminotransferases, etc., but obvious jaundice is uncommon. This impairment is reversible after withdrawal. (5) Renal function impairment: Interstitial nephritis, necrosis of the renal papillae, and renal hypofunction may occur during the long-term administration of aspirin. Long-term administration at a high dose may lead to potassium deficiency, and excessive discharge of urine acid, and the relative damage is the appearance of protein, cells, and casts in the urine. (6). Impact on blood: the long-term administration can cause iron deficiency anemia. (7) Cardiotoxicity: aspirin at the treatment dose has no significant direct cardiovascular effects, and administration at a high dose can directly act on the vascular smooth vessels, leading to the peripheral vasodilation. (8) Reye's syndrome: Treatment in pediatric influenza or chicken pox can induce Reye's syndrome, which is an acute encephalopathy and liver fatty infiltration syndrome and often occurs after some acute viral infectious diseases. (9) Cross-allergic reaction: This means that the patient who is allergic to this drug is also allergic to another salicylic acid drug.

4.5.2 Precautions

It should be taken with food or water to reduce gastrointestinal irritation and it should not be taken with wine; otherwise, this will aggravate generalized pain and cause liver damage.

4.6 Dipyridamole

Dipyridamole can inhibit adenosine diphosphate, reduce platelet aggregation and platelet factor IV release, dilate blood vessels, and relax smooth muscles. The combination of aspirin enhances anticoagulation. Usage: Three to four times a day, 25 mg per dose, po.

4.6.1 Adverse Reactions

(1) Adverse reactions are associated with dosage. About 25% of patients have adverse reactions if more than 400 mg is taken per day; (2) Dizziness is relatively common, and discomfort in the abdomen, headache, and skin rash, etc., are relatively rare; (3) Diarrhea, vomiting, blushing, pruritus, angina pectoris, etc., are rare; (4) Liver function abnormality occurs occasionally.

4.6.2 Precautions

(1) It is contraindicated in people with hypotension and hemorrhagic tendency, and in pregnant and breastfeeding women. (2) It may not be injected together with other drugs except for dextrose solution. (3) In the treatment of embolism, the daily dose should not be less than 400 mg, in four doses po; otherwise, the anti-platelet effects will not be obvious. (4) Hypotension caused by overdose can be corrected by vasoconstrictor. (5) The dose should be reduced if dipyridamole is used with aspirin; if the daily oral dose of aspirin is 1 g, the dose of dipyridamole should be not more than 100 mg.

In addition to the above anticoagulation and antispasmodic drugs, there are many Chinese patent medicines available with significant blood flow-promoting effects and anticoagulation effects, such as urokinase, salvia miltiorrhiza, danhong, shuxuetong, and xuesaitong. Combined application with the above common drugs will be more effective during the actual clinical application. No drug is a panacea without adverse reactions, and different patients have different conditions. Microsurgeons should keep up to date to choose the more suitable medicines for obtaining better surgical results.

Bibliography

Chengqi W, Zhongwei C, Shengxiu Z. Practical microsurgery. 1st ed. Beijing: People's Military Medical People's Press; 1992. p. 103.

Guoliang C. Finger replantation and reconstruction. 2nd ed. Beijing: People's Medical Publishing House; 2005. p. 113.

Haibo D, Liping T. Serious anaphylactic shock induced by Dextran-40: an analysis on 59 cases. Drug Clin. 2002;17:52–3.

Huilong L. Adverse reactions induced by Dextran-40: a retrospective analysis of 696 reports. Chin J Hosp Pharm. 2006;26(8):1049–50.

Jinfang C, Chengqi W, Bin C, et al. Study and clinical application of replantation of amputated finger through approaches of arteriovenous reversal. Chin J Microsurg. 2000;23:65–8.

Lingfeng H, Xueyuan L, Xin W, et al. Clinical case control study on different medication regimens after the replantation of amputated finger. Chin J Hand Surg. 2014;30(3):230–1.

Lisheng G, Jianhua G, Ling Y, et al. Study on microcirculation of transplanted flap. Chin J Microsurg. 1997;20:207.

Mingtong H, Guangrong F. Application of anticoagulant drugs after replantation of amputated finger. Chin J Microsurg. 2012;35:347. 123.

Pharmacology and pharmacotherapeutics. 1st ed. Beijing: People's Medical Publishing House; 2000. p. 977–80.

Tao W, Yudong G, Jifeng L, et al. The influence of heparin on proliferation of endothelial cell and release of contractile factors. Chin J Microsurg. 1999;22(3):195–7.

Weizhi M. Serious adverse reactions induced by Dextran-40: an analysis on 46 cases. China Pharm. 2010;13:138–9.

Xigui P, Wancheng T, Quanzhong L, et al. Clinical application of moderate dose heparin in replantation of amputated fingertip. Chin J Pract Hand Surg. 2003;17(1):17–8.

5 Preoperative Treatment for Replantation of Amputated Fingers

Amputated fingers are not uncommon today because of mechanical accidents, traffic accidents, and other hazards. Replantation is the best method of recovery for amputated fingers. At present, the survival rate of replantation-receiving patients is more than 90%, no matter whether they have an amputation of one finger or all ten fingers, and the postoperative appearance and function are good. To achieve successful replantation does not just depend on the simple replantation and postoperative treatment, and preoperative preparation is also a prerequisite; thus, surgeons should spare enough time to carry out proper preoperative preparations. Routine preoperative preparation includes:

(a) Drying and refrigeration are the main methods of storage for amputated fingers, which cannot be soaked in water or disinfectant and can be placed among ice blocks in summer.
(b) The wound should be pressurized and bandaged with clean gauze in the case of emergency treatment.
(c) Psychological preparation is needed for postoperative recovery.
(d) General assessments should be performed by a doctor before the operation to rule out life-threatening risks, determine the indications, and rule out any contraindications.
(e) Preoperative preparations for surgical fields and surgical instruments and materials.

The details are as follows.

5.1 Preoperative Emergency Resuscitation

1. The preservation and perioperative treatment of amputated fingers is vital to the success of the operation. Replantation of amputated fingers is time-limited. The prime time to close the wound is 6–8 h after the finger amputation in summer and 10–12 h in winter. The injured should be taken to a hospital nearby after simple treatment and tetanus antitoxin should be conventionally injected to reduce the risk of postoperative bleeding and infection.
2. If the amputation is associated with limb fractures, the fractures should be fixed temporarily using materials nearby, such as a board, iron bar, and hardback books or magazines, before the patient is moved to avoid secondary injury.
3. The amputated finger should be wrapped in a plastic bag and put in a low-temperature barrel and taken to the hospital with the injured. Storage at room temperature or above is not

J. Lin et al., *Special Type of Finger Replantation*, https://doi.org/10.1007/978-981-10-6229-2_5

permitted. The best storage temperature is 4 °C (as shown in following figure).

Schematic diagram

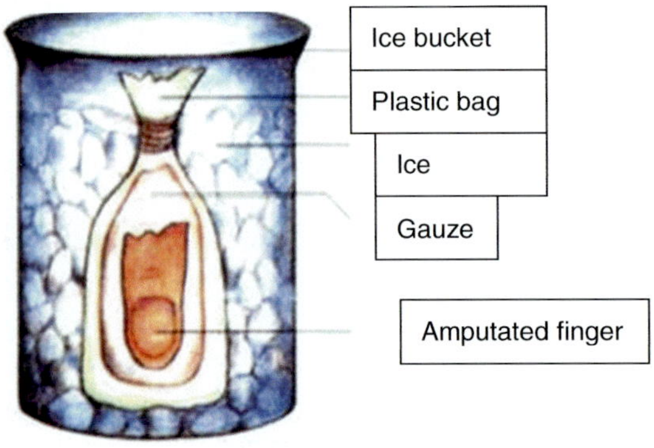

Schematic diagram

The methods of amputated finger preservation are:

(a) Ice bucket preservation: putting the amputated finger into a dry sealed plastic bag, then transferring the bag into an ice bucket, padded with ice cubes around the bag, and finally covering the bucket with a lid.
(b) Ice plastic bag preservation: putting the amputated finger bag into another plastic bag, which is full of ice and should be sealed.
(c) Packing method: the amputated finger is packed with a towel or gauze and taken to the hospital with the injured (the cold storage method may not be necessary in winter or during transfer within a short distance).

At the hospital, the amputated finger should be wrapped with aseptic gauze before the operation and put in a refrigerator at 4 °C after it is debrided and disinfected by the medical staff. In the case of multiple amputated fingers, the fingers should be properly marked and wrapped separately. The amputated finger can also be preserved in a holeless plastic bag, which is then put into an ice bucket if there is no refrigerator. The finger should be wrapped with an 8-to-10-layer aseptic gauze and put into a holeless plastic bag, which is then sealed and placed into an ice bucket if the injured must be transferred to a remote place for replantation. Ice cubes can be placed close to the bags, and ice cream or ice block will also do if there are no ice cubes. The doctor should replant the fingers one by one and the remaining finger(s) should be preserved in a refrigerator and properly marked. Cryopreservation means preserving the amputated finger with liquid nitrogen at −196 °C.

5.2 Assessment of General Conditions

The general state and medical condition of the injured should be assessed to rule out any life-threatening risks and underlying diseases.

5.3 Evaluation of the Injury

It is very important to evaluate the condition of the injured because the structure of the hand is very delicate and complex. In hand trauma, the tissue that is first affected is the skin, followed by muscles, tendons, nerves, vessels, bones, and joints.

(a) Evaluation of skin conditions: The rupture of the skin is very visible, but the prognosis varies in different types of skin ruptures. Skin scratches caused by a sharp instrument is relatively easily treated, but they can still be easily infected if the sharp instrument is polluted with heterogeneous immune substances such as meat, and healing will be difficult, especially wounds caused by human or animal bites. A cotton opener will cut skin into pieces that are hard to suture and repair. It is worth noting that it is hard to judge the blood supply of a serious degloving injury, which is preferably observed under a microscope.
(b) Evaluation of nervous injuries: There should be a high degree of suspicion of whether nerves have been damaged in the case of sensory degeneration, disappearance, and (or) movement in the area distal to the wound, and the wound should be repaired as early as possible to achieve beneficial effects.

(c) Evaluation of vascular injuries: Bleeding is unavoidable in an open injury. However, pressure should be applied to the wound or a tourniquet should be used at the proximal part to stop the bleeding promptly when pulsating bleeding is seen in the wound; otherwise, this may cause arterial injury. In addition, paleness, absence of a pulse, and a reduction in skin temperature in the area distal to the wound indicate a poor blood supply in the area; in the case of no vascular anastomosis and blood circulation, the finger will not survive.
(d) Evaluation of muscle and tendon injuries: When disruption of movement occurs in one or more fingers, but it is not accompanied by sensory degeneration, the disorder may be caused by muscle and tendon injuries.
(e) Evaluation of bone and joint injuries: The occurrence of deformity and abnormal movement of bones and joints or local obvious swelling and tenderness indicates bone and joint injury. At this time, an X-ray should be performed to discover the severity of the injuries. Anteroposterior and oblique radiography films of not only the whole hand, but also the specific fingers or joint should be observed.

5.4 Preparation for Surgical Fields

(a) Psychological preparations for medical staff and the injured: As it is an important factor for success in the replantation of amputated fingers, the medical staff should be confidentially devoted to the rescue of the amputated finger based on the fact that every decision is made in the interest of the injured party. With kindness and patience, they should educate the injured to ease their tension and strengthen their confidence in surgery, which will make the injured cooperate closely intraoperatively and postoperatively.
(b) When the injured is taken to the emergency room, medical history should be requested and a physical examination must be carried out: Rapid treatment should be given in the case of severe bleeding and shock. Amputated fingers should be put in a refrigerator at 2–4 °C and surgeons should be called for further immediate processing. Relevant departments such as the clinical laboratory, the radiology department, the blood bank, the anesthesiology department, and the operating room, should be prepared to conduct the necessary examinations and preparations, and the injured should be taken to the operation room as soon as possible.
(c) Preparation of the surgical equipment: In addition to the equipment used in the department of traumatology, the equipment for small blood vessel suture should also be prepared. For non-invasive suture needle lines, injury-free small vessel suture needles are required, which are connected at the two ends of the nylon monofilament. Currently, 7-0, 8-0, 9-0, 10-0, 11-0, 12-0 are available. Non-invasive suture lines of the corresponding model should be selected according to differences in vascular diameters. The following types of needle holder should be available: vessel forceps type, pen type or spring piece type. Small vascular forceps and vascular clamp are required: toothed and nontoothed. With regard to small scissors, we provide special microscopic surgical scissors that can be replaced by ophthalmological small scissors. Flat and sharp needle tips for flushing the blood vessels can be made by all kinds of needles whose tips have been made round, blunt, and smooth. A surgical microscope with a simple 2- or 2.5-fold magnifying glass with glasses is needed. A complex, accurately structured surgical microscope may be a vertical type or a suspending type, which can be magnified by 6, 10, and 16 times and can be used by two or three people; it is also equipped with devices for lighting, automatic control of zooming, ascending and descending, photography, filming, and video-making, etc.

5.5 Indications and Contraindications

Indications:

(a) The general conditions are stable, with no life-threatening risk, and the patient can tolerate the surgery.
(b) The patient and his/her family desire replantation very eagerly.
(c) The structure of amputated fingers should be comparatively complete, postoperative complications few, and the appearance and function have a good recovery.
(d) The replantation should be performed according to the time limit and the patient's age. The tolerance of amputated fingers to ischemia would be reduced. A higher environmental temperature means a more active metabolism of histiocytes and a shorter duration of the tolerance of the amputated finger to the ischemia. Generally, there is no absolute limit for replantation time and age currently, and the right judgment should be made according to the specific conditions and after various factors have been taken into consideration.
(e) Replantation can only be performed under necessary device conditions by skilled surgeons who have professional training.

Contraindications:

(a) Replantation is not indicated in people with systemic disease, poor constitution or concomitant serious organ injuries. The aim of replantation is to recover the function of the amputated fingers, not purely for survival; thus, maintaining the finger's integrity is essential.
(b) Amputated fingers associated with multiple fractures or severe soft-tissue defects result in poor appearance and function.
(c) (c) Severe damage to the integrity of the finger's vascular bed, such as in squeezing-induced finger amputation, manifest as subcutaneous blood stasis at the two sides of fingers; even if the vessels are connected, the replanted finger cannot survive easily because of the extensive blood oozing in the soft tissues and thrombosis.
(d) Replantation is not suitable if the time-limit has been excessively exceeded and the tissues have become deformed. Amputated fingers can be replanted and survive within 24 h of the amputation without refrigeration, and the limit time for replantation can be prolonged to 30 h. The shorter the ischemic time, the higher the survival rate. Replantation is not indicated for the finger if the finger nerves, vessels, bones, and muscles have been damaged because the effect of nerve repair will be relatively poor and post-survival functions will not be as good as expected.

5.6 Selection of Anesthesia

Hand injury draws less attention in most comprehensive hospitals, and surgery is usually performed under local anesthesia in the emergency room. However, local anesthesia often generates poor efficacy, and the anesthesia range is too narrow. This is very unfavorable to complete debridement and comprehensive injury exploration, and is very likely to lead to incomplete debridement or missed diagnosis and treatment. Generally speaking, brachial plexus block anesthesia is recommended for hand surgery because this covers the entire upper limb, during which the pneumatic tourniquet can be easily used. This practice not only reduces intraoperative bleeding, but also makes the surgical fields cleaner, thus increasing the efficiency of surgery. Currently, the most popular finger root anesthesia is tendon intrathecal injection of anesthetics. This anesthesia mode is characterized by the speed at achieving the anesthetic effect with only one injection, involving little pain for the patients and a positive anesthetic effect. General anesthesia can be considered if multiple injuries are involved, or the skin flap or tissue flap transposition at other sites are scheduled, or combined anesthesia is not an option because the patient is a child.

6 Selection of Anesthesia for Replantation of an Amputated Finger

Replantation of an amputated finger refers to a surgery on the complete or incomplete amputated finger(s) during which the vessels, nerves, tendons, bones, and skin are re-anastomosed and repaired to make the amputated fingers recover certain functions. It is characterized by a complex surgical process, accurate operation, long duration, and the need for complete immobilization. The requirements for anesthesia are a simple operation, a small impact on the patient's physiological functions, complete immobilization, painlessness during the operation, easy monitoring, perfect postoperative analgesia, maintenance of dilation of local small vessels, and reduction of vasospasm. This chapter focuses on the common anesthesia modes for replantation of amputated fingers.

6.1 Nerve Block Anesthesia

6.1.1 Brachial Plexus Block

Brachial plexus block anesthesia is the commonest anesthesia mode for hand trauma surgery, especially the replantation of severed limbs.

Brachial plexus mainly consists of $C_{5–8}$ and T_1 anterior branches of the spinal nerve, mainly dominating the sensation and movement of the entire hands and arms. These nerves are located at the supraclavicular regions after efference from the intervertebral foramens and are further divided into superior, middle, and inferior trunks via the intramuscular groove between the anterior and middle scalene muscles. The superior trunk consists of $C_{5–6}$ anterior branches, the middle trunk consists of C_7 anterior branches, and the inferior trunk consists of C_8 and $T_{1,2}$ anterior branches. The three nerve trunks pass through the lower margin of the space between the anterior scalene muscle and the middle scalene muscle, the accompanying subclavian arteries extend toward, outward, and downward, each nerve trunk is divided into the anterior section and the posterior section when they reach the middle exterior margin of the post-clavicular first costal cartilage, then they pass the first costal cartilage and the clavicular median point and finally enter the armpit through its apex. All the sections of nerves become re-combined into bundles at the armpit, the three sections become combined into bundles posterior to the axillary artery, and then they become extended into axillary nerves and radial nerves; the anterior sections of the superior trunk and the middle trunk become combined into lateral bundles at the lateral side of the axillary artery, and then extend into the lateral roots of the musculocutaneous nerves and the median nerves; the anterior section of the inferior trunk becomes extended into the medial trunk, and finally into the medial roots of the ulnar nerves, the medial cutaneous nerves of the forearm, the medial cutaneous nerve of the arm, and the median nerves.

J. Lin et al., *Special Type of Finger Replantation*, https://doi.org/10.1007/978-981-10-6229-2_6

Brachial plexus block can be achieved through four routes: the intramuscular groove, the supraclavicular region, the infraclavicular region, and the armpit. The brachial plexus block via different routes is selected according to the degree of hand trauma and the site of the amputated limb.

6.1.1.1 Intramuscular Groove Brachial Plexus Block Method

This is the commonest brachial plexus block method. Oblique angle intramuscular groove is located at the apex of the lung, above the subclavian artery and between the anterior and middle scalene muscles. The patient is asked to lie in a recumbent position without a pillow, the head slightly turned toward the contralateral side, the arm is closely attached to the body, the hands should be dropped as far as possible, and the patient is first asked to actively lift the head to show the sternomastoid muscle. First, the anesthetist's index finger and the middle finger are placed behind the posterior margin of the clavicular head of the sternocleidomastoid muscle, and then the patient is asked to relax the head. At this point, the fingers of the anesthetist are above the anterior scalene muscle. The index finger and the middle finger are gently moved toward the posterior and lateral directions, and then the intra-scalene-muscular groove can be found. The needle is inserted between the anesthetist's index finger and the middle finger at the level of the cricoid cartilage, namely, the level of the transverse process of the sixth cervical vertebra. The direction of needle insertion is vertical to the lateral surface of the neck, and then the tip is slightly directed to the lower region. The needle is inserted slowly until paresthesia is felt, when the drug should be injected, or the tip is first pushed against the transverse process of the cervical vertebrae, then the tip is moved from the anterior to the posterior to find the paresthesia, and once it is found, the drug is injected. The ulnar nerves may not be anesthetized completely. During anesthesia, if the paresthesia that radiates to the shoulder is found, then the anesthetic effect will be more satisfying.

Block anesthesia at the intramuscular groove has the advantage of being simple operation, especially for obese patients. Good anesthetic effects at the upper arm and shoulder can be achieved only with a relatively small quantity of anesthetic drugs. The blocking effect at the shoulder, upper arm, and radial side is relatively good, and the blocking effect at the forearm and the ulnar side is slightly poor. The salvage method means increasing the volume of anesthetic drugs or including the ulnar nerves at the elbow. As needle insertion is performed in a high position, pneumothorax can be avoided. For patients with an upper limb infection or malignant tumor, the higher position of the needle insertion can avoid the spread of infection or tumor. The main complications are injection of the drug into the subarachnoid cavity, epidural cavity, and vertebral arteries; thus, the tip is directed slightly downward during needle insertion. At this time, the phrenic nerve block induced by injection of the drug to the front of the anterior scalene muscle or toward the head so that the dispersive block of C_3–C_5 occurs. As the unilateral phrenic nerve block reduces lung function, this method of anesthesia is not recommended for patients with contralateral diaphragmatic paralysis.

6.1.1.2 Supraclavicular Brachial Plexus Block Method

The patient is asked to in at a horizontal position, a thin pillow provides padding on the affected side, with the head turning toward the contralateral side, and the affected upper limb is closely attached to the body. The needle is inserted through the site 1–1.5 cm above the clavicular median point, the tip is pushed inward, backward, and downward to find the first rib, and the tip is moved along the first rib from the outer margin of the anterior scalene muscle to the anterior margin of the middle scalene muscle. In the case of paresthesia, the tip is fixed, and if there is no blood and gas during the pump-back, the local anesthesia drug liquid is injected. This method is characterized by a good anesthetic effect, speed at achieving efficacy, fewer adverse reactions, and fewer complications; however, it can also result in complications, such as pneumothorax, phrenic nerve block, and Horner's syndrome.

6.1.1.3 Infraclavicular Brachial Plexus Block Method

The patient is asked to lie in the same body position as for the intramuscular groove method. After the intrascalene muscular groove is found, the finger is moved downward; after the subclavian arterial pulsation is palpated, the needle is inserted from the posterior margin of the subclavian artery, and the tip faces the caudal side. If the subclavian arterial pulsation is not palpable, the needle is inserted along the front of the middle scalene muscle. The brachial plexus is located in front of the middle scalene muscle, and touching the brachial plexus with the tip induces paresthesia. In most cases, the middle trunk of the brachial plexus is encountered first. If the brachial plexus is not encountered, the tip will be against the first rib; attempts are then made to find paresthesia along the first rib. In the case of paresthesia, then 20–30 ml of local drug liquid is injected. This method is characterized by simple operation, low consumption of anesthetic drugs, and rapidness in achieving efficacy. There are no complications induced by injecting the drug into the subarachnoid space, epidural space, and vertebral artery. However, it does result in complications such as phrenic nerve block, recurrent laryngeal nerve block, and pneumothorax.

6.1.1.4 Axillary Brachial Plexus Method

As the axillary arteries and veins and brachial plexus are located in a superficial position, the operation is relatively simple, and this method is also the commonest anesthesia method in hand surgery. During axillary brachial plexus block anesthesia, the patient is asked to lie in the supine position, with the head turned toward the contralateral side, the upper arm is abducted by 90°, the elbow is bent by 90°, the forearm is externally rotated, and the back of hand is close to the bed or the face is resting on the palm of the affected limb. During the operation, palpation is performed at the apex of the axillary fossa to judge the relative position between the nerves and the arteries. The main operation methods include the axillary arterial puncture method, seeking paresthesia peripheral to the axillary artery, and the peri-axillary arterial wide infiltration method. Signs indicating the success of axillary brachial plexus block are: (1) the puncture needle tip is fixed and vibrates along the arterial pulsation; (2) there is no blood during pump-back; (3) fusiform diffusion after the drug injection; (4) the patient complains of numbness of the upper limb; (5) inability to lift the upper arm, especially the forearm; (6) vasodilation of the skin surface.

Axillary brachial plexus block anesthesia has the advantage of being simple and safe and hardly ever results in the complications of pneumothorax, diaphragmatic paralysis, stellate block, and mis-injection of the anesthetic drug into the subarachnoid space, epidural space, and vertebral artery. It has a wide range of indications, including patients with bilateral brachial plexus block or with emphysema, pediatric patients, uncooperative patients, and outpatients. Its disadvantage is the inapplicability of the method in the case of the failure of the passive abduction of the shoulder.

6.1.1.5 Brachial Plexus Block Location Technique

The development of nerve block is closely associated with the development of anatomy, local anesthetics, puncture devices, and the nerve location technique. As the development of anatomy, local anesthetics, and puncture devices is fully fledged, the current main limitation that has an impact on the effects of nerve block is whether the nerves can be accurately located. The nerve location technique goes through three stages: (a) Blind detection for the location of paresthesia, (b) nerve stimulation for location, and (c) location using ultrasound.

(a) Blind detection for the location of paresthesia: This method means using body surface marks and anatomy to determine the general position and needle insertion point to find the target nerves and then seek paresthesia by direct use of the needle. However, owing to the anatomical variation, it has unavoidable disadvantages such as unclear body surface marks and non-obvious paresthesia: (1) The success rate of complete block is not satisfying, and even experienced anesthetists may have a failure rate of 4–20%; (2) multiple detection and intense electrical sensation can easily induce patient discomfort, anxiety, and panic; (3) the incidence rate of complications such as nerve injury, hematoma, accidental injection of local anesthetic drug into the vessels, and pneumothorax; (4) nerve block is very difficult and cannot be carried out for some patients who are extremely obese.

(b) Nerve stimulation localization method: This technique has been applied to nerve block for more than 30 years. A nerve stimulator helps to accurately locate the nerves by stimulating the nerve fibers using a specially made nerve puncture needle, discharging the electricity to generate single stimulus waves to stimulate the peripheral nerve trunks and then inducing the contraction of the muscle fibers dominated by the motor branch of this nerve. As it is close to the nerves instead of touching them, the nerves are less frequently injured; thus, the location is relatively accurate. For obese patients or patients with unclear anatomical structures, the success rate of the operation is significantly improved.

The nerve-stimulator-guided nerve block, like the conventional nerve block, is performed based on the following procedures: asking the patient to lie in the specified body position, locating, disinfecting, and inserting the needle and the nerve stimulator. First, charge at the current of 1–2 mA to determine whether it is close to nerves, and then adjust the direction and depth of the puncture needle and the current of the stimulator until the minimal electric current (0.3–0.5 mA) produces the maximal muscular contraction or skin paresthesia to determine the nerve position; stop the needle insertion when the puncture needle has been close to the nerve, and the local anesthetic drug is injected if there is no blood and liquid during the pump-back of the syringe.

Increasing emphasis has been placed on the role of nerve stimulators in improving the nerve block technique. Stimulation has been more widely applied clinically, and the quality of nerve block anesthesia has been further improved through accurate location and accurate operation. However, the nerve stimulation technique has some limitations, including individual differences in patients' reactions to nerve stimulation, the impacts of injected liquid or peripheral nerve regions on the conduction of electricity, and anatomical variation or abnormality. It is difficult or impossible to observe the muscular contractions. Generally speaking, the nerve stimulation technique has the disadvantages of blind puncture and failure of using it to guide the puncture direction, and the proper position can be found by judging the position of the tip.

(c) Location using ultrasound: The development of high-frequency ultrasound technology during recent years has significantly improved the resolution of superficial tissues; during the location, the nerve structures can be clearly displayed, providing the conditions for its application in nerve block. Ultrasound can realize the real-time observation of the local structures of target nerves, the insertion route of the puncture needle, and diffusion of the local anesthetic drug, making the nerve block visible, so that the success rate of the nerve block reaches 100% and there is no need for the patient to express paresthesia, making it possible to perform the anesthesia when the patient is under sedation.

The current method of nerve location under the guidance of ultrasound in combination with the nerve stimulation puncture needle can visualize the nerve structures under ultrasound and make the muscles contract using the nerve stimulator. The combination can improve the quality and effect of nerve block; thus, it is worth clinical application and study.

6.1.1.6 Common Complications of Brachial Plexus Block

(a) Pneumothorax: This occurs with the supraclavicular or infraclavicular block method in most cases. Owing to the incorrect puncture directions and the excessively deep puncture, or the cough during the puncture, the lungs may have hyperdistention, and the pleurae and the pulmonary apex can be punctured so that the intrapulmonary gas can enter the pleural cavity. The patient should be diagnosed and treated in good time, and in severe cases, air extraction or closed drainage of the thoracic cavity can be performed.

(b) Bleeding or hematoma: During the puncture, the internal and external jugular veins, subclavian artery, axillary artery or axillary vein can be punctured, inducing bleeding. If there is a need for blood pump-back during the puncture, the puncture needle should be withdrawn and local compression should be performed to arrest the bleeding so that the continuous bleeding or hematoma formation can be avoided.

(c) Toxic reactions induced by local anesthetic drugs: The reactions are mostly induced by an overdose of local anesthetic drugs or misinjection into the vessels.

(d) Diaphragmatic paralysis: This occurs when the intramuscular groove method or supraclavicular puncture method are adopted, during which chest distress, shortness of breath, and decreased ventilatory capacity can occur; oxygen inhalation or assisted respiration can be given if necessary.

(e) Hoarseness of voice: This occurs when the intramuscular groove method or supraclavicular puncture method is adopted, and it is often induced by the recurrent laryngeal nerve block. During drug injection, neither the pressure nor the dose should be excessively high, which helps to avoid complications.

(f) High epidural block or total spinal anesthesia: This is induced by the infusion of the local anesthetic drug into the epidural space or subarachnoid space owing to the excessively deep entrance of the needle into the epidural space or subarachnoid space when the intramuscular groove method is adopted. If this occurs, it should be treated as total spinal anesthesia that results from epidural block anesthesia.

(g) Horner's syndrome: This occurs when the intramuscular groove block method is adopted; it is induced by stellate block and can subside per se without any treatment.

6.1.1.7 Advantages and Disadvantages of Brachial Plexus Block Anesthesia

(a) Advantages: (1) This has little impact on the function of the heart, lungs, liver, and kidneys and it is indicated for patients with disorders in the cardiovascular system, respiratory system, and liver and renal functions. (2) Nerve block anesthesia blocks the nerve impulses in the position at surgery from entering the central nervous system and additionally blocks the vessel-contracting nerve impulses from the central nervous system from being sent to the vascular walls of the surgical fields, thus relieving the patient's postoperative pain, making the small local vessels relax, improving the blood circulation, and reducing the vascular crisis of vasospasm. It is very important for the postoperative recovery of patients undergoing amputated limb replantation. (3) Patients can have a clear mind, and various kinds of protective reflexes are present; compared with general anesthesia, it can result in a few complications such as nausea, vomiting, atelectasis, amnesia, somnolence, and dysphoria. (4) Less postoperative care is needed; most patients can directly go back to the ward without having to go to the anesthesia recovery room. (5) As for the patients with concomitant cervical vertebral fractures or with serious airway problems, nerve block anesthesia can avoid the movement of the patient's neck and tracheal intubation; otherwise, the patient's conditions can be avoided.

(b) Disadvantages: (1) The reasons why patients refuse to receive nerve block anesthesia is fear of the pain, the puncture, the paresthesia induced by the insertion of the needle tip on the nerves, hearing sounds in the operation room. (2) The time needed for the nerve block anesthesia to take effect is relatively long, and the incidence of anesthesia insufficiency is relatively high. It is often necessary to add intravenous anesthetic drugs and analgesic drugs during the operation. (3) Although the incidence of anesthesia insufficiency or failure is very low, it should be transformed into general anesthesia during the operation. (4) The duration of replantation of amputated limbs is relatively long, the patient should maintain a position, which often causes discomfort in the lumbar region or the back and the lower limb, and the subconscious activities of the lower limbs interfere with the surgery.

Before the operation, the patients should be interviewed and communication should be carried out with them about the advantages and disadvantages of the anesthesia methods and the precautions to be followed by the patients during the operation. The anesthesia method that is satisfactory to the patient is selected to guarantee that the surgery proceeds safely and smoothly.

6.1.2 Other Nerve Block Anesthesia Methods

Elbow, wrist, and finger nerve block can be selected for the patients who receive simple finger replantation.

6.1.2.1 Elbow Nerve Block Anesthesia

Behind the humeral bone, the radial nerve runs downward along the radial nerve groove; above the extensor condyle of the humerus. It passes through the lateral intermuscular septum, and runs to the lateral side of the elbow between the biceps muscle of the arm and the brachioradial muscle. The median nerve runs downward to the elbow along the medial side of the biceps muscle of the arm. At the lateral side of the elbow median nerve is the brachial artery and biceps muscle of the arm, and at the medial side is the brachial muscle. At the middle segment level of the humeral bone, the ulnar nerve starts to deviate from the brachial artery and run toward the inner and posterior direction, and it enters the ulnar nerve groove at the outer margin of the elbow; on the medial side of the ulnar nerve groove is the internal epicondyle of the humerus, and on the lateral side is the medial wall of the humeral trochlea. Nerve block anesthesia is performed on the ulnar nerve, median nerve, radial nerve, forearm median, and lateral cutaneous nerves at the elbow, according to the surgical needs.

6.1.2.2 Wrist Nerve Block Anesthesia

The ulnar nerve, median nerve, and radial nerve run on the medial side, central part, and lateral side of the wrist. The ulnar nerve and ulnar artery alternatively run between the tendon of the wrist ulnar flexor muscle and the tendon of the finger's superficial flexor, the ulnar nerve is on the ulnar side of the ulnar artery and its endings dominate the skin sensation of the hypothenar eminence, 1.5 fingers on the volar side (little finger and ring finger) and 2.5 fingers on the dorsal side (little finger, ring finger, and middle finger). The median nerve of the wrist runs between the tendon of the long palmar muscle and the tendon of the radial flexor muscle of the wrist, it is at a superficial position, and its endings dominate the sensation of the palm radial skin and the 3.5 fingers (thumb, index finger, and ring finger) on the volar side. The superficial branch of the radial nerve passes through the spinal lateral side of the wrist, and its endings dominate the skin sensation of 2.5 fingers (thumb, index finger, and ring finger) on the dorsal side and the dorsal side of the palm.

6.1.2.3 Finger Nerve Block Anesthesia

Finger nerve block anesthesia is divided into three categories: (1) Trans-sheathing canal injection, (2) trans-metacarpal injection, (3) subcutaneous injection. As for finger root anesthesia, annular injection is not recommended to prevent the finger mortification induced by excessive pressure. Trans-sheathing canal injection starts from the flexor tendon sheath, where the needle is inserted into the bone surface at the level of the finger root transverse striation, and the local anesthetic drug is easily pushed in when the needle is withdrawn slowly to the area between the periosteum and the flexor tendon (the volume of the injected local anesthetic drug is 2 ml). The advantage of this method is the need for only one injection and its speed at taking effect. During trans-metacarpal injection, the point for inserting the needle is often located at the site 1 cm away from the proximal end of the volar metacarpophalangeal joint, and some tend to insert the needle toward the dorsal side because the patient has few subcutaneous tissues at the dorsal side. After the needle is inserted, 2 ml of local anesthetic drug is injected at the level of the neck of the metacarpal bone. Subcutaneous finger nerve block is often performed at the distal end of finger transverse striation, the needle is inserted vertically on the two sides of the flexor tendon sheath, and 2 ml of a local anesthetic drug is injected. During finger nerve block anesthesia, it is forbidden to add adrenaline to the local anesthetic drug because it causes vasospasm due to the vasoconstrictive action and compromises the surgical effects. In addition, it carries the risk of increasing the blood crisis after the operation.

6.2 General Anesthesia

General anesthesia is rarely selected for patients with a good general condition who undergo simple replantation of a severed limb. General anesthesia is mainly applicable to children, surgery involving multiple sites, surgery with a long duration, uncooperative patients, patients who refuse nerve block anesthesia, patients with serious multiple injuries, and patients with functional insufficiency in the heart and lungs.

The previous common use of an endotracheal tube for general anesthesia can effectively maintain the smooth respiratory tract, benefit the clearance of secretions in the trachea and bronchi. Assisted respiration or controlled respiration can be performed for patients with respiratory insufficiency or defective laryngeal reflex; various positive pressure ventilations are allowed; the surgeons are allowed to place the patient in any position that does not cause excessive ventilation dysfunction; the anesthetist is permitted to be away from the patient to continue effective anesthesia control and ventilation.

In 1981, a British anesthetist named Brain designed and made the laryngeal mask airway. The emergence of the laryngeal mask airway undoubtedly marks a major breakthrough in airway management, especially patients with a difficult airway. In the case of a difficulty in endotracheal intubation, a laryngeal mask plays an important role, and can even save a patient's life. After the application to large quantities of clinical patients for more than 30 years and the constant updates and improvements in laryngeal mask models, laryngeal mask general anesthesia has distinguished itself from other methods by means of the following universally recognized advantages: (1) The placement of a laryngeal mask results in fewer injuries, less stimulation, and mild stress. Anesthesia induction and hemodynamics have a high stability during the recovery period, and bucking and secretions decrease during recovery from anesthesia. (2) Ventilation can be easily maintained during airway processing, which can effectively lower the incidence of difficult airways. (3) The operation is simple, first learners can master the technique after training several times, and the success rate is higher. (4) It can be easily used, insertion is rapid, and airway maintenance is simpler. (5) It can be placed without the need to use a laryngoscope and muscle relaxants, and cervical vertebrae have a smaller range of motion. (6) Patients can tolerate it easily, and need fewer anesthetic drugs for tracheal intubation. (7) The incidence of postoperative complications is low, and the incidence of sore throat and a hoarse voice is relatively low. Laryngeal mask general anesthesia can be applied to the surgery of the four limbs, especially to the replantation of amputated limbs.

Midazolam, propofol, and sufentanil with or without muscle relaxant are placed in the laryngeal mask to induce general anesthesia; inhalation of sevoflurane and intravenous pumping of remifentanil are mainly performed for anesthesia maintenance. The continuous pumping of analgesic drugs is performed for postoperative analgesia.

To sum up, attention should be paid to the following points, no matter what anesthesia mode is adopted: (1) Anesthesia effects should be consolidated to avoid pain-induced vasospasm, and for patients who are too nervous, adjuvant analgesic and sedative drugs are intravenously administered to guarantee that the patient is quiet without body movement. (2) Good vasodilation benefits accurate suturing to improve the success rate. (3) As for patients with excessive intraoperative bleeding, a colloid solution and blood should be supplemented to improve the ending circulation, and vasoconstrictive drugs should be used with great caution if blood pressure needs to be increased. (4) All parameters of physiological functions are closely monitored during the operation, and their normal range should be maintained. (5) The continuous postoperative analgesia benefits vasodilation and wound recovery.

Bibliography

Alemanno F, Capozzoli G, Egarter-Vigl E, et al. The middle interscalene block: cadaver study and clinical assessment. Reg Anesth Pain Med. 2006;31(6):563–8.

Arbona FL, Khabiri B, Norton JA. Ultrasound-guided regional anesthesia. New York: Cambridge University Press; 2011. p. 31–191.

Farquhar-Thomson DR, Baker AK, Satapathy AR, et al. Minimum volume of local anaesthetic required for an axillary brachial plexus block. Br J Anaesth. 2010;105(3):382–3.

Fuchun Y, Jinmin Z, Zhi Y, et al. Investigation of reasons of delayed vascular crisis caused by replantation of amputated finger and the prevention. Chin J Microsurg. 2006;29(4):305–6.

Ge H, Yu B, Guanxian T. Impact of continuous brachial plexus block for analgesia after the replantation of an amputated finger on the survival of the replanted fingers. Chin J Microsurg. 2005;28(3):273–4.

Hadzic A. Peripheral nerve blocks and anatomy for ultrasound-guided regional anesthesia. 2nd ed. Beijing: Peking University Medical Press; 2014. p. 107–36.

Jeng CL, Torrillo TM, Rosenblatt MA. Complications of peripheral nerve blocks. Br J Anaesth. 2010;105(1):97–107.

Kapral S, Greher M, Huber G, et al. Ultrasonographic guidance improves the success rate of interscalene brachial plexus block. Reg Anesth Pain Med. 2008;33(3):253–8.

Lecamwasam H, Mayfield J, Rosow L, et al. Stimulation of the posterior cord predicts successful infraclavicular block. Anesth Analg. 2006;102(5):1564–8.

Mahmoud KM, Ammar AS. Ultrasound-guided continuous infraclavicular brachial plexus block using bupivacaine alone or combined with adenosine for pain control in upper limb surgery. Saudi J Anaesth. 2011;5(2):132–7.

Minville V, Fourcade O, Bourdet B, et al. The optimal motor response for infraclavicular brachial plexus block. Anesth Analg. 2007;104(2):448–51.

Peng L, Bing C, Meiting L. Comparison of the anesthetic effects between two approaches of infraclavicular brachial plexus block assisted by ultrasound and never stimulator. J Clin Anesth. 2015;31(7):644–7.

Shiqiang J. Evaluation of intramuscular groove and axillary combined brachial plexus block in replantation of amputated finger. China Med Eng. 2013;12(1):51–2.

Xi L, Aizhong W, Daqiang Z, et al. Clinical study on the brachial plexus approach of the ultrasound-guided complete upper limb nerve block. Shanghai Med J. 2014;37(6):496–73.

Xian MW, Mingrui Z, Shaocheng Z, et al. Intra-tendon sheath anesthesia for replanted distal phalanx after the amputation: a study on 21 cases. Chin J Pract Hand Surg. 2005;19(2):126.

Xiaofang L. Analysis and treatment policies of the reasons for the vascular crisis after the replantation of amputated finger. Chin J Microsurg. 2005;28(3):274–6.

Xiaoming D, Shanglong Y, Buwei Y, Yuguang H, editors. Modern anesthesiology. 4th ed. Beijing: People's Medical Publishing House; 2014. p. 1115–41.

Yang X, Yongzhu C, Junzhen W. Impact of ultrasound-guided elbow continuous target nerve block after the replantation of severed limb on the skin temperature and survival rate of replanted fingers. Shanghai Med J. 2015;38(4):272–5.

Youcun Y, Yong F, Keyan F, Yan H, et al. Comparison between one-point and two-point combined method in the application to brachial plexus block. J Pract Hand Surg. 2007;21(2):127.

Yuanxin Z, Shujian H, Jurong W, Xuejun Y, et al. Clinical study on the effects of papaverine on brachial plexus block. Chin J Hand Surg. 2000;14(2):43–5.

7 Routine Surgical Procedures for the Replantation of Amputated Fingers

Replantation of amputated finger is a detailed and difficult project, requiring surgeons to perform the operation all through the course under the surgical microscope. Besides basic knowledge of orthopedics, vascular surgery, plastic surgery, it is necessary to being proficient in microsurgery technology operation, to achieve stable, accurate, skillful operating skills. According to the general principles, the order of replantation and the specific circumstances, flexible control and temporary adjustment of the surgical plan is needed to ensure that every step of the operation is correct. There are two orders of replantation of amputated fingers. One is antegrade replantation, using by most scholars conventionally, that debridement—skeletal fixation—repair of the flexor and extensor tendon—dorsal vein anastomosis-dorsal skin suture—inherent artery anastomosis—nerve anastomosis-palmar skin suture. The other one is retrograde replantation: debridement-palmar skin suture—finger nerve anastomosis—inherent arteries anastomosis—flexor tendon suture- skeletal fixation—extensor tendon suture—dorsal vein anastomosis-dorsal skin suture. The latter has the advantage of not having to turn over the hands during the surgical procedure, especially for replantation of thumb amputation, and severed fingers in children. Avoiding to pull and sprain the anastomosed blood vessels and nerves when a fracture is fixed. The specific operation are as follows (Fig. 7.1).

7.1 Effective Debridement

Emergency debridement of open wound is of vital importance, the quality of debridement directly determines whether the wound can be healed in one stage post-operation, and whether there will be infection. Debridement should include necrosis, inactivated organization, and severely contaminated tissue. Rinsing the wound with saline, hydrogen peroxide and iodophor. If necessary, debridement again until the wound is clean and fresh. In order to thoroughly debridement and prevent the secondary damage, debridement should be performed under microscope. Careful and gentle operation is needed to avoid injury to blood vessels and nerves. After a thorough debridement, the suture line marks the blood vessels and nerves. After debridement, the surgeon should further confirm the outcome of the preoperative assessment. If a new injury is found, a detailed record should be performed, and adjusting the operation plan and repairing as soon as possible in one stage (Fig. 7.2).

7.2 Reconstruction of Bony Framework

The end of the fracture is usually shortened each side by 2–3 mm at debridement. Amputation should be performed at the end of the fracture adjacent to joint. If the joint capsule is intact,

J. Lin et al., *Special Type of Finger Replantation*, https://doi.org/10.1007/978-981-10-6229-2_7

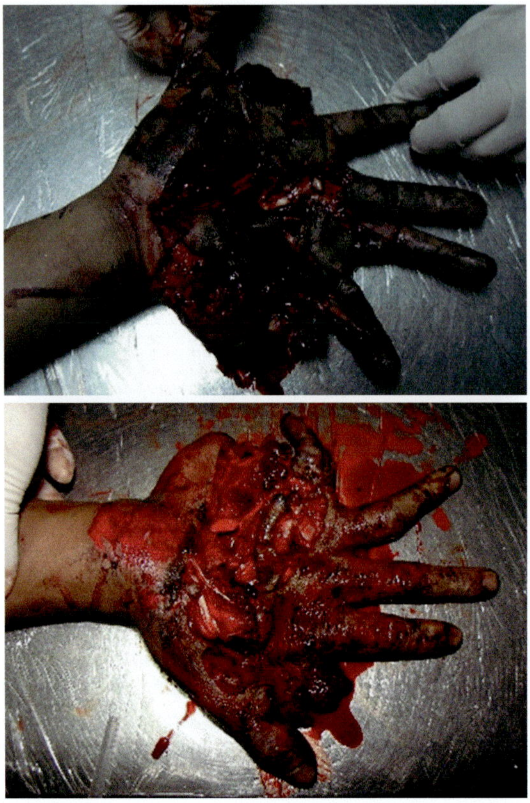

Fig. 7.1 Preoperative injury and contamination

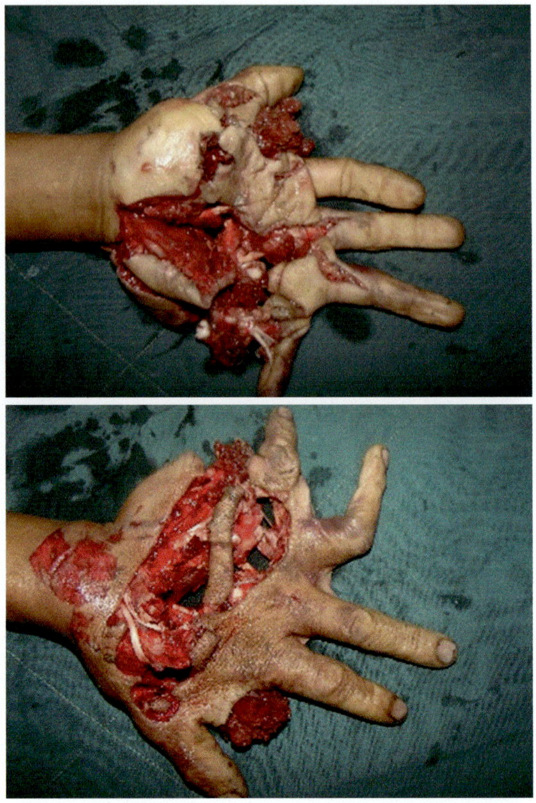

Fig. 7.2 Effective debridement

more bone is removed at the end of the fracture far from the joint, than the end adjacent to joint, to ensure the integrity of the joint. Joint fusion is applied to disarticulation of interphalangeal joints or metacarpophalangeal joints of thumb. Arthroplasty is applied to damage of metacarpophalangeal joint of the on the 2–5 finger. It was found that the bone defect was serious during the operation, kirschner needle "stenting" fixation in one stage, bone grafting treatment in two stage. The fracture end of the severed fingers of children is usually shortened each side by 1–2 mm. Bone shortening is far away from the epiphysis area and the epiphysis is preserved as much as possible, avoiding joint fusion. To part of the severed finger trans-articular or trans-epiphysis, bone can be shortened far away from the severed plane, and then replanted to preserve the function of the joint and protect the epiphysis. Internal fixation of joint could be performed with vertical or oblique Kirschner wire and cross Kirschner wire and cross steel wire cross. The reduction of the end of fracture is required to contact accurately, closely, fixed firmly, and easy to do. Most scholars use Kirschner wire to fix penetrating the medullary cavity in longitudinal direction. When the severed plane is near the proximal phalanx, to avoid injury to extensor tendon and dorsal finger vein, the Kirschner pin points should be on the middle of the middle phalanx of the middle segment. When severed plane is in the middle section of the middle phalanx, the Kirschner pin points should be selected at distal phalanx. After fixation, suturing the periosteum and the aponeurosis and fascia of the bone surface, to prevent bony separation and rotation, reduce the adhesion of tendons (Tendon adhesion is common after tendon rupture and suture, especially in the dorsal hand). Then the extensor and flexor tendons are sutured. Maximum recovery of the motor function of the affected finger should be taken into consideration after fixation (Fig. 7.3).

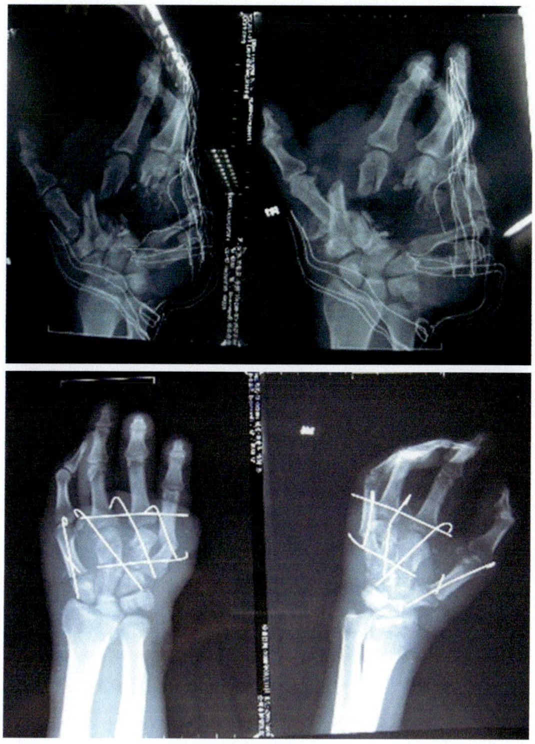

Fig. 7.3 Reconstruction of sbony scaffold

7.3 Tendon and Ligament Repair

Most scholars suture the flexor tendon followed by the extensor tendon. Intermittent suturing of extensor tendon with 3-0 nylon in figure of "8". When severed plane is in the metacarpophalangeal and proximal phalanx planes, In addition to the suture of the central tendon, the lateral tendons of vermis and interosseous muscles extending to the distal end should be repaired. It is only that extended tendons of the lateral tendons is sutured in the fracture of phalanx of middle section. When the flexor tendon is broken, it is usually to suture the tendon of the flexor digitorum. Excision of tendons of superficial flexor digitorum, greater retracting force can be obtained at the proximal end of the flexor tendon. Near the broken end 1 to 1.5 cm, a needle crosses the tendon to make it not retracted, the suture the digitorum flexor tendon with Kessler's suture. The tendon can be sutured between the ends of the tendon by 7-0 lines of

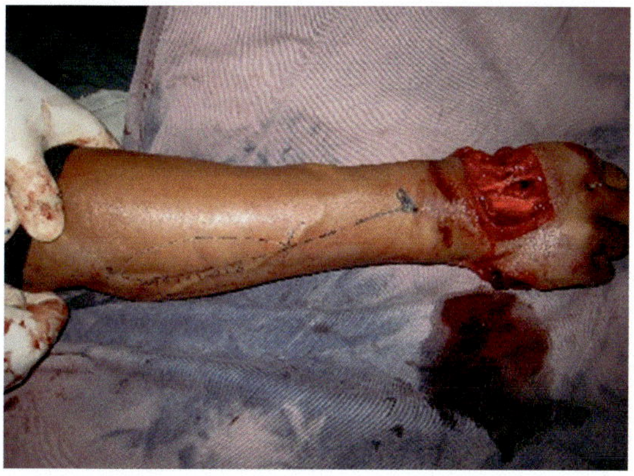

Fig. 7.4 Repair of tendon

interrupted or continuous suture, so as to increase the suture strength, eliminate the rough surface, and make the finger in rest position. Joint capsule and collateral ligament can be sutured with single needle or 3-0 nylon in figure of "8" (Fig. 7.4).

7.4 Vascular Anastomosis Repair

Fine vascular anastomosis is the key to the success of the replantation of amputated fingers, so as to anastomosed blood vessels as much as possible in principle. Anastomosis of 2 digital arteries and 2–3 dorsal digital veins, to reduce the symptoms of thin, cold, and poor blood supply after the operation, increase the chance of replantation success. However, 1 arteries and 1–2 dorsal veins of the finger can be sutured with high quality, the finger can also survive. Vascular quality must be checked before anastomosis. Flushing blood clots and attachments in the lumen of the tube with heparin salt water. If the endometrium is damaged, the blood vessel should be pruned to the normal segment, to make sure that there is no thrombosis in the cavity and spurting well of proximal arterial. Most scholars believe that the artery is first anastomosed and then anastomosing the veins. The advantage is that the artery is first anastomosed to facilitate the search of venous blood vessels. When the artery is difficult to find in the operation, the tourniquet can be loosened properly, to search the artery, according to the arterial pulse and ejection of broken end. The proximal artery of the finger is mostly retracted with less exposure, a lateral incision is needed to find the artery. Only a small amount of blood, or even no bleeding, indicates vasospasm or vascular injury in the proximal artery. According to the different reasons for correcting, the intractable vasospasm could be handle with closed treatment by papaverine, wet compression by warm salt water, exfoliation of the epicardial membrane, mechanical dilatation of vascular broken by tweezers. If the distal artery of the finger can't be found during the operation, or severe defection of distal artery, or too small diameter of the vascular lumen, with no condition of anastomosis, the proximal arteries can be anastomosed to the appropriate distal vein for venous arteriolarization. 10-0 or 9-0 noninvasive nylon lines are used for end to end anastomosis with 6–8 needles (12-0 or 11-0 noninvasive nylon lines for children). It is easy to find the dorsal digital vein after arterial anastomosis, 10-0 or 9-0 noninvasive nylon lines for venous anastomosis with 8–10 needles. Venous anastomosis of the veins in the dorsal digital vein. If the patient's venous injury is serious, it needs to be anastomosed to digital ventral vein. As the ventral vein is located in the subcutaneous, protection of tissue and fiber around the veins, and it is less hurt in the damage, therefore, the operation is easy to be anastomosed, and the curative effect is good after the operation. If the vascular defect is above 1.5 cm, vascular transplantation should be performed selecting carpal-opalmar vein, without tension. If the defect of dorsal vein is too large, it is advisable to carry out a vein graft. The anastomosis of the artery is best performed under the control of a tourniquet or a rubber band at the root of finger or with a vascular clamp (except for children's amputated Fingers).

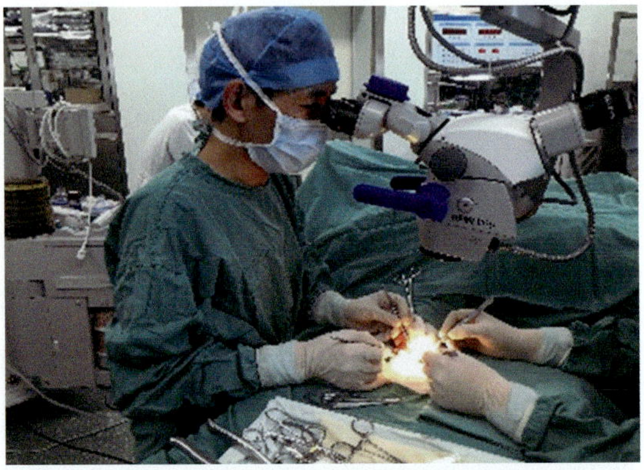

Fig. 7.5 Anastomosis of blood vessel and nerve

7.5 Nerve Repair

The nerve should be debrided and trimmed again before suturing. Suture of outer membrane or fascicular membrane is performed under a microscope with 9-0 noninvasive nylon lines. Each nerve was sutured with 3–4 needles to make the nerve fibers unexposed. Both sides of the nerve should be repaired. If there is a defect, it is needed to harvest the free nerve from the sural nerve or the dorsal cutaneous nerve of the foot and hand for transplantation. In principal, the main aim is to repair the finger nerve in the ulnar side of the thumb and the small finger, to repair nerve in the radial side of the indication, middle, and ring finger. Nerve repair requires tension-free suture of the outer membrane and the fascicular membrane of the nerve (Fig. 7.5).

7.6 Skin Suture, Wound Closure

Checking the stability of fracture fixation, the degree of tightness of tendon and nerve, circumfluence of vessel, tension of finger pulp; skin color turned to ruddy, capillary filling time is normal, the temperature of the finger becomes warm; distal section hemorrhage; small incision is bleeding in the lateral side. After flushing the wound with warm water, suture the skin and close the wound. The wound is covered with a number of small slices of Vaseline and aseptic gauze. The finger-tip should be exposed to facilitate the observation of blood transport. Flap repair skin defected. It is worth noting that, if the finger ischemia duration prolonged, severe injury or finger preservation was unsuitable, although the finger had a received blood supply, only high tension was shown. Finger-tip small incision is bleeding, but temperature and capillary fullness is not up to normal. This condition can be restored after several hours of heat preservation, antispasmodic and dilatation treatment (Fig. 7.6).

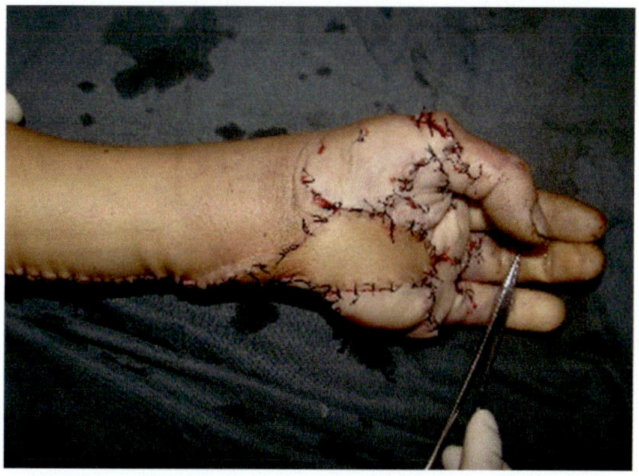

Fig. 7.6 Suture the skin and close the wound

8 Treatment and Management After the Replantation of Amputated Fingers

China's amputated finger replantation technology is in the leading position worldwide in terms of replantation techniques, the number of cases, replantation difficulty, and survival rate after development for nearly 50 years. The success of the replantation of an amputated finger is related to multiple factors such as the patient's injuries, vascular conditions, and quality of intraoperative vascular anastomosis, and is also closely associated with the postoperative treatment and management. If there is no emphasis on post-replantation treatment and management, the surgery will fail. Special attention should be paid to the vascular crisis (spasm and embolism) that occurs after the replantation of an amputated finger. Treatment and management are of great importance after the replantation of an amputated finger to improve the success rate of replantation.

8.1 Conventional Treatment After Replantation of an Amputated Finger

8.1.1 General Processing and Specialized Treatment

Gypsum can be used postoperatively to fix the affected limb, the patient is strictly confined to the bed with the affected limb raised (10–20 cm above the heart) for 1 week, and it is forbidden for the patient to engage the affected limb in both active and passive movement for 2 weeks. The replanted limb and the palm should be kept warm under the 40- to 60-W heat lamp, with a lamp distance of 40–50 cm. Hyperbaric oxygen chamber therapy can be additionally used if conditions permit, in the case of a relatively low temperature in the replanted finger, serious swelling or relatively poor circulation of the endings, and no confirmed thrombosis. Hyperbaric oxygen chamber can increase the oxygen dissolved in the blood by about 20 times, thus correcting the vicious cycle induced by anoxia, making tissue edema subside, and improving microcirculation. Hyperbaric oxygen treatment is often given in a hyperbaric chamber at an atmospheric pressure of 0.2–0.25 MPa, in which intermittent oxygen inhalation is adopted, i.e., oxygen inhalation is first given for 20 min and stopped for 10 min, then oxygen inhalation is resumed for 20 min. One to two treatments are given every day, for 7–10 consecutive days. If conditions permit, patients can inhale pure oxygen for treatment, which can be somewhat effective. The conventional treatment is the intramuscular injection of tetanus antitoxin 1500 tU, followed by "anti-inflammatory, anticoagulant, and antispasmodic" therapies, to prevent postoperative infection, thrombosis, and anastomotic vasospasm.

J. Lin et al., *Special Type of Finger Replantation*, https://doi.org/10.1007/978-981-10-6229-2_8

8.1.2 **Drug Treatment** (Table 8.1)

(a) Postoperative anesthesia: The patient is often in pain of varying intensities when the anesthetic effects disappear after the operation. The patient should be given sedative and analgesic drugs for the vasospasm induced by pain stimulation so that the patient can rest quietly and pass through the critical stage after replantation. Hibernation therapy can be given if necessary for patients with a low pain threshold and children who tend to cry because pain can trigger excitement of the patient's sympathetic nerve and central nervous system, vasoconstriction, and vasospasm as a reflex, increase the incidence rate of vascular crisis, and have an impact on the survival rate of the replanted finger. Common drugs include promethazine for sedation, and anisodamine, fentanyl, sufentanil, and pethidine for analgesia. The common drug for hibernotherapy is Lytic Cocktail 1, consisting of pethidine hydrochloride 50 mg, chlorpromazine 25 mg, promethazine 25 mg, +0.9% normal saline 500 ml, continuous intravenous pumping for 24 h (21 mL/h). On the one hand, hibernation can prevent the excessive stress of the patient's body to the pathogenic factors and improve the body's tolerance to the exteriors; on the other hand, it can lower the patient's basal metabolic rate, reduce the organs' activities and oxygen consumption, and improve the tissue's tolerance to anoxia.

Table 8.1 Common drugs in specialized departments

Anti-inflammatory drugs	Penicillin, cephalosporins, and macrolides, used separately or in combination
Anticoagulant drugs	6% Dextran-40 injection 500–1000 ml/day, intravenous drip; or Aspirin (0.5–1.0 g/time, tid); or 5% glucose injection (500 ml + heparin 6250–12,500 units, 24-h maintenance therapy at the speed of 4–5 drops/min
Antispasmodic drugs	Benzazepine 25 mg and papaverine 30 mg/6~8 h, im; red sage root injection, procaine, inositol hexanicotinate and hairy holly root, which can be used according to the specific circumstances
Nerve-nourishing drugs	Oral drugs: Methycobal 500 mg, tid, vitamin B, oryzanol etc.; injections: nerve growth factor, methycobal (cobinamide) injection, vitamin B (such as vitamin B1 100 mg, and vitamin B12 500 μg), im, qd

(b) Anticoagulant therapy: The vascular anastomosis and repair after the replantation of the amputated finger is the key to the success of the surgery. Effective postoperative anticoagulant therapy is indispensable in addition to correct anastomosis methods and exquisite operation techniques. Preventive treatment can lower the incidence rate of postoperative vascular crisis; thus, it is of vital clinical significance. Heparin normal saline (heparin 12,500 U + 0.9% NaCl 100 ml) is generally used intraoperatively to flush the vascular lumens, clear any clots, and prevent blood coagulation. After the operation, dextran-40 (500 ml intravenous drip, bid) is commonly used; if necessary, aspirin 25 mg tid can be additionally used 5–7 days continuously. Alternatively, the patient can be given 0.9% NS 500 mL+ heparin 6000–12,500 U, for 24-h of continuous intravenous pumping. Therefore, it can exert some preventive effects on thrombosis.

(c) Vasospasm-relieving and vasodilating drugs: Vasospasm-relieving drugs are used as the conventional treatment method after the replantation of an amputated finger and is of vital significance to the postoperative prevention of vascular crisis induced by vasospasm. Currently, papaverine (30 mg) and benzazepine 25 mg im q6h are alternatively or separately (in the case of the intraoperative occurrence of vasospasm, papaverine 10–30 mg should be given immediately, and locally injected into the peri-vascular region).

(d) Antibiotic application for infection prevention: Finger amputation is one of the common open injuries suffered by the human body and hand contamination is relatively serious in most cases. Although effective debridement can effectively lower the incidence of postoperative infection, it cannot prevent postoperative wound infection, which can cause replantation to fail. The scientific and reasonable postoperative application of antibiotics to prevent infection is non-negligible. The antibiotics are used according to the hospital situation, medication efficacy, and clinical route selection, and in most cases, the oral monotherapy is adopted. Intravenous administration should be considered for patients with many amputated fingers and relatively serious contamination. During medication, the changes in the body temperature, local conditions and generalized conditions should be observed closely, the antibiotic therapies should be adjusted in good time to achieve efficacy, the adverse drug reactions should be closely observed and monitored, and unnecessary damage to patients should be prevented.

(e) Nerve-nourishing drugs: Hands play an irreplaceable role in daily life. It is the patient's wish not only that the amputated fingers survive without problems after replantation, but also that the hand motor and sensory functions make a good recovery. Therefore, the postoperative recovery of nerve functions is also one of our treatment plans. The conventional treatment is to recover the sensory and muscular motor functions through the administration of nerve-nourishing drugs. The common nerve-nourishing drug is mecobalamin (0.5 mg, po, tid); patients who can afford to can additionally take nerve growth factors.

8.1.3 Symptomatic Treatment

Patients should receive timely symptomatic treatment for emotional changes such as depression and fidgeting caused by abdominal swelling, nausea, poor appetite, constipation, and generalized aching due to long-term confinement to bed, thus preventing vascular crisis. The dressings on the wound should be changed frequently; otherwise, the wound would be soaked with blood, causing infection, and the blood crusts would compress the vessels, causing a vascular crisis.

8.2 Postoperative Management of the Replantation of Amputated Fingers

8.2.1 Environmental Management

The patients should rest in a cozy and quiet ward with fresh air after replantation. A good medical environment should be created for the patients so that they feel relaxed. The environment of the ward area and the ward should be strictly managed. The indoor temperature should be controlled at 25–27 °C, especially in winter. The patient should preferably be in a room with air conditioning so that the room temperature can be adjusted at any time to be within this range. The humidity is maintained at 60–70%. Too low a temperature or a sudden decrease in temperature can cause vasospasm; too high a temperature speeds up the oxygen consumption of the tissue. Both situations are unfavorable to the patient's rehabilitation. In the meantime, the affected limb should be kept warm locally under the 60-W heat lamp for continuous radiation, with a radiation distance of 30–40 cm. The distance should be proper because too a short distance is prone to causing burns and too long a distance results in a failure to achieve the warming effects. The lamp holder is covered with a piece of sterile cloth or a long lamp case, the warming should be intensified, but the photostimulation to other sites should be reduced. Lamp heating generally lasts 7–10 days, and the its duration can be shortened according to the specific circumstances. It is forbidden for the patient and his/her family to smoke in the ward or the ward area, and fresh air should be maintained in the ward area. The cold stimulation and the nicotine in the cigarettes can result in arteriolar spasm; the nicotine in the cigarettes can also cause platelet aggregation, increase viscosity, slow blood flow, induce vascular crisis, and have an impact on the survival rate of the replantation.

8.2.2 Management of Patient's Body Position

After the operation, the patient should lie in a horizontal position, be strictly confined to bed with the affected limb raised, and it is forbidden for the affected limb to be engaged in both active and passive movement for 2 weeks. The patient's affected limb should be placed properly because an excessively high position can have an impact on the arterial blood supply and an excessively low position can be unfavorable to the venous backflow. As is appropriate, the affected limb should be slightly abducted (by about 20–30°), and the affected limb should be 10–20 cm higher than the heart. The patient should not lie in the lateral recumbent position; otherwise, the limb is compressed, affecting the arterial blood supply and venous return. In the case of improper placement of the affected limb or early off-bed activities, instable fixation of the bones and tendons or compression of the replanted limb to the vessels leads to obstructed venous return or induces vasospasm; subsequently, vascular crisis occurs, resulting in failure of the replantation.

8.2.3 Drug Treatment Management

Proper clinical medications are selected according to the patient's generalized conditions, injuries, drug category, dose, treatment course, and administration routes. Therefore, attending doctors are required to make ward rounds to learn detailed medical history, pay attention to the outcome, make reasonable treatment plans, and adjust the treatment plan at any time, from admission for surgery to discharge.

8.2.4 Special Nocturnal Management

Special management should be given because emergencies are prone to occur as the doctors and nurses, ward area environment, and patient's physiological status may change during the night.

First, the patient's physiology and emotions change. During the night, the vagus nerve becomes excited, the heart rate is lowered, the vascular flow tends to be slow, the smooth muscles have consolidated contraction, the platelets are in a state of contraction; thus, vasospasm or thrombosis is prone to occur. In addition, during the day time, the patient is often distracted, not noticing the pain, because of communication with visitor; however, during the night, he/she focuses on the pain at the affected finger, and the pain can induce the body to release vasoconstrictive substances such as prostaglandin and 5-HT, inducing a small blood vessel spasm.

Second, the nocturnal room temperature drops, and the affected limb may involuntarily move away from the heat lamp after the patient falls asleep; if not detected in a timely manner, cold stimulation is very likely to cause a vascular crisis. Therefore, the use of analgesic drugs should be increased during the night, the nursing staff are required to make more careful ward rounds and make sure that a round is made every 60 min during the night within 72 h of the operation. The affected limb should be guaranteed to be within the warming area of the heat lamp, and responses should be given in good time according to the blood supply of the replanted finger.

8.2.5 Patient's Cognition and Emotional Management

Clinically, many patients wear a cold frozen expression on the face at admission, they give a brief response or no response, they do not talk with others and seldom groan, and reactions appear to be slightly weak, but they are actually in a state of emotional shock. Patients have emotions of varying intensities for the functional and appearance recovery. The dominating harmful feelings are anxiety, depression, and self-abasement, which significantly increase the level of vasoconstrictive substances such as adrenaline and catecholamine in the blood, induce elevation of blood viscosity and initiation of the coagulating mechanism, and result in vasospasm or vascular embolism. Therefore, medical staff should give active psychological intervention and correct guidance, creating a very suitable psychological environment and atmosphere. They can play soothing music in the ward to relax patients, thus relieving them from harmful feelings, producing active emotions, and reducing the incidence of vascular crisis.

8.2.6 Diagnosis and Processing of Vascular Crisis

Vascular crisis, also called blood circulation crisis or blood circulation disorder, refers to a type of pathological phenomenon in which the spliced and anastomotic vessels have blood pathway blockade, thus compromising the survival of transplanted tissues and replanted limbs (fingers). It is the commonest and most serious complication after the replantation of an amputated finger. It is divided into arterial crisis and venous crisis according to the site of occurrence and it is divided into the vasospasm and vascular embolism, according to the pathological manifestations. It is divided into the intraoperative crisis and postoperative crisis according to the time of occurrence time. The postoperative early crisis occurs within 24 h of the operation, mainly manifesting as vascular embolism, and surgical exploration should be performed and the anastomotic stoma should be processed promptly. The postoperative late crisis occurs within 48 h of the operation, mainly manifesting as vasospasm, and active anticoagulant and spasm-relieving therapies should be given.

1. Judgment indicators for vascular crisis:
   (1) Skin temperature of the finger—normal and 1–2 °C higher than the temperature on the healthy side, and in the case of a drop of 4–5 °C, the occurrence of a blood crisis should be considered; (2) skin color of the finger—if the skin color turns light or pale, this indicates insufficiency in the digital arterial blood supply; a dark red and purplish dark skin color indicates a disorder in the arterial and venous flow; (3) finger pulp tension—if the blood circulation of the replanted finger is normal, the finger pulp should have a some elasticity, and swelling, the disappearance of cleavage lines or the appearance of blisters indicates a venous blood regurgitation disorder, and the presence of wrinkles at the digital dorsum indicates arterial crisis; (4) filling time of the nail bed blood capillary—the normal time is 1–2 s; a delay or disappearance indicates insufficiency or discontinuity in the arterial blood supply (the decrease in time indicates the disorder of venous blood regurgitation); (5) finger swelling (due to inflammation, blood stasis or congestion, and an enlargement in the volume of a certain body part); (6) test of incision bleeding on the lateral side of the fingertip (observed if necessary).
2. Specific processing method of the vascular crisis (Tables 8.2 and 8.3):

(a) Arteriospasm: this mostly occurs within 3 days of the operation and it is often induced by insufficient blood volume pain, cold, smoking, and mental nervousness (nervousness refers to the intensified response, both mental and physical, to external stimulants), and a child's crying. It is most apt to occur within 24 h of the operation. The clinical manifestations of arteriospasm are the color

Table 8.2 Vascular crisis judgment and processing form: Identification of arterial and venous crises

Essentials of identification	Characteristics of arterial crisis	Characteristics of venous crisis
Skin color	Pale	Dark purple
Skin temperature	Decreased	First high then low
Capillary filling time	Prolonged	Shortened
Skin tension	Shriveling and decreased tension	Full with increased tension
Cut open at the lateral side of the fingertip	Decreased bleeding	Excessive bleeding and dark purple
Ultrasound Doppler signals	Decreased or disappear	Decreased or disappear

Table 8.3 Vascular crisis judgment and processing form: Identification and processing of vasospasm and thrombosis

Essentials of identification	Characteristics of vasospasm	Characteristics of thrombosis
Etiological factors	The vascular walls are simulated by mechanical and chemical factors and the cold	The vascular walls are rough, the blood flow is slow, and the blood viscosity is changed
Pathological changes	Luminal shrinkage or occlusion	The lumens are occluded by thrombi
Antispasmodic drugs	Effective	Ineffective
Sympathetic block	Effective	Ineffective
Massage	Possibly effective	Harmful (the embolus is squeezed to the distal vascular bed)
Local warming	Helpful	Harmful (increasing oxygen consumption)
Cut open at the lateral side of the fingertip	Possible oozing of a small amount of blood and water	No bleeding
Vasography	Intra-luminal conical shadow	Sudden discontinuity of luminal shadows
High-pressure oxygen	Effective	Ineffective
Processing methods	Conservative therapy is given and then the patient is closely observed	Surgical exploration should be performed immediately after the diagnosis is confirmed
Surgical findings	The vessels at the distal and proximal ends of the anastomotic stoma become thin and the blood ejected from the proximal end of the vessels decreases	The vessels at the proximal end of the anastomotic stoma become dilated, the vessels at the distal end do not pulse, thrombi are present in the lumens, and no blood ejection is observed after the disjunction beyond the thrombi

Antispasmodic drugs
Papaverine hydrochloride injection 30–60 mg, q6h, im

of the amputated finger changing from rosy to pale, the decrease in skin temperature, and slow or normal capillary regurgitation; it is difficult to distinguish from arterial embolism during the early stage. Processing method: (1) Change the dressings at the wound, and remove the external compression factors; (2) increase the blood volume, specifically, increase the content of blood in the tissue or organ vessels; (3) intensify the insulation measures to make the room temperature reach 25 °C as soon as possible, and maintain the warmth through use of a heat lamp or hot water bag at the affected field; (4) for a pain-induced spasm, inject an analgesic drug as a pain-relieving therapy or for a restlessness-induced spasm in a child, sub-hibernation therapy or a proper sedative drug is given to help the child to fall in asleep; (5) give intravenous papaverine 30–60 mg; (6) some patients with intractable arteriospasm can be given relief occasionally after the brachial plexus block takes effect; [1](7) if observation for 30–60 min shows that no remission has been achieved after the above processing, surgical exploration should be immediately performed, if arteriospasm is observed intra-operatively, the wound should be wrapped with warm, moist saline gauze after the injection of papaverine in the sub-adventitial region, if the arteriospasm still cannot be relieved, from the proximal segment, and strip the adventitia (in patients whose spasm is still not relieved after the above measures, and an arterial embolism is caused by continuous or repeated arterial spasm, the spasm segment should be resected, and venous grafting should be performed to repair the vessels).

[1]The author once treated two patients who experienced arteriospasm 4 h after the operation. Remission was not achieved after the above processing, surgical exploration was prepared, the amputated finger turned full, rosy, and warm at 15 min after the brachial plexus block; thus, the exploration was not done. Since then, in patients with a long replantation duration, the author has performed one brachial plexus block if the anesthetic effect is poor or the surgery has been completed.

(b) Arterial embolism: This is often induced by incomplete vascular debridement, the poor quality of the vascular anastomosis or excessive tension at the anastomotic stoma, in addition to hematoma compression, excessive swelling and compression of the finger, local infection or long-term arterial spasm. The frequent occurrence time of arterial embolism of the replanted finger is generally consistent with that of the arterial spasm; they are difficult to differentiate because of the similar clinical manifestations. Indications for the surgical exploration of arterial embolism: (1) Patients with postoperative arterial crisis who still cannot achieve improvement in blood circulation over 30–60 min after various measures have been adopted; (2) patients with relatively severe injuries in the amputated finger and with only one artery intraoperatively anastomosed; (3) children who are at the status post-replantation, and in whom surgeons have no confidence in vascular anastomosis; (4) patients with avulsion amputation, in whom the conditions for anastomosis of the fingers are poor; (5) patients who experience hematoma compression caused by postoperative bleeding.

Several situations in which exploration is not indicated after the occurrence of arterial embolism: (1) The injured finger is not properly preserved, and it is ischemic for 24 h; (2) the wound is postoperatively infected, causing secondary arterial embolism; (3) the amputated finger is soaked in various types of stimulating liquid; (4) the patient and his/her family refuse exploration; (5) venous crisis causes secondary arterial embolism.

During surgical exploration, the anastomotic stoma should be examined under the operating microscope to determine the range of the arterial embolism. When the arterial embolism occurs, the arterial anastomotic stoma and its neighboring areas are dull purple, some hardness is felt after compression, but it has no elasticity. The arterial segment of the embolism is cut until the healthy vessels are reached and then re-anastomosis is performed. If direct anastomosis is difficult because of the relatively high arterial tension, the small veins at the volar side of the ipsilateral wrist are selected, and then inverted and transplanted for the repair; the digital arteries on both sides should be repaired as simultaneously as possible to increase the chance of survival.

(c) Venous embolism: This refers to the venous obstruction caused by the excessively high viscosity of venous blood and it can often induce varicosity. The venous crisis clinically occurs mostly because of phlebothrombosis (under the conditions of slow venous blood flow, blood hypercoagulable state, and vascular intimal injuries, the vein has acute nonpurulent inflammation, causing secondary venous embolism), and the main reasons for venous crisis is poor anastomosis quality, incomplete venous vascular debridement, excessively tight skin suturing, and excessive swelling and compression of the finger. Different processing methods should be adopted for the venous embolism based on the injury reasons and the differences in amputation sites. Surgical exploration should be performed on the patients with amputation near the middle phalanx caused by a simple incised wound or a power saw injury, during which the embolism segment should be resected and re-anastomosed, or venous grafting should be performed for repair. The blood dripping method can be adopted for patients with amputation beyond the middle phalanx caused by a wringer injury, who experience local infection or embolism more than 5 days after the operation. The blood dripping method: (1) An incision about 0.5 cm long and 0.3 cm deep is made at the junction between the lateral side of the fingertip and the lunula of the nail, and a heparin saline cotton ball is applied to the surface so that blood can ooze from the wound; (2) the finger nail can be extracted, several longitudinal small incisions can be made on the nail bed, and a heparin cotton ball can be applied locally so that blood can ooze from the wound; (3) the above two methods can be combined, during which the tip can be repeatedly used to stir the wound to maintain the oozing of the blood (if the blood dripping is excessively rapid, a saline cotton ball can be used to compress the incision for several minutes).

The systemic application of an intravenous heparin drip is also an option if required. The blood dripping method is maintained until approximately 7 days after the operation, when the collateral circulation is established. At this time, despite no more blood dripping to the wound, the fingertip remains red, without obvious cyanosis and swelling.

Bibliography

Fuchun Y, Jinmin Z, Zhi Y, et al. Investigation of reasons of delayed vascular crisis caused by replantation of amputated finger and the prevention. Chin J Microsurg. 2006;29:305–6.

Jian Z, Zhongwei C. Review and forecast of replantation of amputated finger. Chin J Microsurg. 2000;23:82–3.

Jing L, Qingsheng Z, Guangyue Z, et al. The analysis on the risk factors of circulatory crisis of distal finger after replantation. J Chin Orthop. 2004;24:478–81.

Jiyuan N, Linong Y, Xude S, et al. Effect of acute hypervolemic hemodilution with hydroxyethyl starch 130/0.4 on hemorheology and microcirculation in patients with finger replantation. J Fourth Mil Med Univ. 2006;27:730–2.

Kiyoshige Y. Effect of hyperbaric oxygen therapy as a monitoring technique for digital replantation survival. J Reconstr Microsurg. 1999;15:327–30.

Kroll SS, Schusterman MA, Reece GP, et al. Timing of pedicle thrombosis and flap loss after free-tissue transfer. Plast Reconstr Surg. 1996;98:1230–3.

Leach RM, Rees PJ, Wilmshurat P. Hyperbaric oxygen therapy. BMJ. 1998;317:1140–3.

Lianchu L. Analysis of four patients with delayed vascular crisis at 32 to 50 days after the replantation of amputated finger and the treatment. Chin J Microsurg. 2012;35:39–40.

Mingtong H, Guangrong F. Application of anticoagulant drugs after replantation of amputated finger. Chin J Microsurg. 2012;35:347–9.

Qisheng F. Experiences and summary of replantation of amputated finger. Chin J Microsurg. 1999;22:32–4.

Tao W, Yudong G, Jifeng L, et al. Impact of heparin on endothelial cell proliferation and contraction. Chin J Microsurg. 1999;22:195–7.

Wancheng T, Fengyu P, Quanzhong L, et al. Experiences of clinical application of replantation of amputated finger in the retrograde way. Chin J Microsurg. 2008;3:456–8.

Xiaofang L. Analysis and treatment policies of the reasons for the vascular crisis after the replantation of amputated finger. Chin J Microsurg. 2005;28:274–6.

Xiaohua W, Tao F, Mingzhong Y. Comparison of curative effect of urokinase and heparin sodium after digital replantation. J Reg Anat Oper Surg. 2013;22:384–5.

Xu H, Shujian H, Jing Z, et al. Analysis of the risk factors of circulation crisis in digit replantation. Chin J Hand Surg. 2007;23:38–9.

9 Methods and Significance of Hand Rehabilitation for Finger Replantation

Rehabilitation refers to the comprehensive coordination and application of medical, educational, occupational, social, and other methods, making it possible for sick, injured, and disabled persons (including those with congenital disability) who have lost function to restore and reconstruct to the maximum extent as soon as possible, allowing them to recover their ability in physical, mental, social, and financial states as much as possible, bringing them back to life, back to work, back to society (WHO). Rehabilitation is not only for the disease, but also for the whole person, from physical, psychological, social, and financial abilities to comprehensive rehabilitation.

In modern life, it is not uncommon for a finger to be severed because of machinery, traffic accidents, and other causes. Replantation is an effective way of recovering the amputated finger for the best possible outcome. Replantation is merely to obtain the structural basis for restoration of hand function, owing to the physical rehabilitation treatment of swelling and pain, loss of sensation, contracture, and joint caused by brake tendon adhesion, which were carried out after replantation of the fingers for recovery of system function. At present, China's digital replantation regardless of the number or the survival rate has reached an international advanced level, from single referrals to 10-finger replantation, survival was above 90%. However, if the completed first step of replantation is successful, the ultimate goal of digital replantation is through surgery and active rehabilitation treatment, to maximize the finger function recovery. This is the ultimate pursuit of the microsurgical practitioner.

9.1 Replantation of Amputated Fingers, Functional Rehabilitation, Staged Treatment

The rehabilitation of finger replantation has special features, and the rehabilitation exercises of related organizations are carried out at different times. The task of early rehabilitation is to reduce muscular atrophy and contracture, promote tissue recovery, and maintain overall health. After 1–2 weeks of rehabilitation, physical rehabilitation measures may include rehabilitation therapy and surgical treatment of the injury of team, operation mode, operation requirements, function evaluation, and judgment about early expected functions, such as understanding tendon anastomosis, fracture fixation, finger rehabilitation needs outside other injuries and patients; an appropriate shoulder and elbow joint placement guide can prevent shoulder joint and elbow joint stiffness, psychological counseling may ease the anxiety and depression of the patients, and helping patients and their families to understand the treatment plan. This period does not require too many physical therapy interventions, and continues to emphasize

J. Lin et al., *Special Type of Finger Replantation*, https://doi.org/10.1007/978-981-10-6229-2_9

the placement of shoulder joints in a slightly extended position, with the hands slightly higher than the heart level, to facilitate venous reflux, to eliminate swelling, and to shake the head to the supine position. Three to 4 weeks after the operation, the soft tissue has basically healed. The fingers have survived, and the stitches were removed. This period was based on whether the patient had residual wounds, swelling, joint stiffness, contracture, etc. Principles of rehabilitation therapy according to the fracture and nerve injury after early rehabilitation: 6 weeks after the operation, fracture healing, external fixation after removal of persistent comprehensive rehabilitation exercise late fractures, tendon, nerve injury, the recovery of hand function is not perfect. To restore the activities of daily life, special forms of appliances, such as toothbrush, comb, and other fixed length in the palm of the hand, and exercise can be used.

9.2 Common Finger Replantation Rehabilitation Therapy

There are many functional rehabilitation therapies after finger replantation. The common methods include physical therapy, occupational therapy, traditional rehabilitation, occupational rehabilitation, prosthesis rehabilitation, psychological service, etc.

9.2.1 Physiotherapy

This is referred to as physical therapy, and is the use of electricity, light, sound, magnetism, heat and exercise, and other natural or artificial physical factors acting on the body of the rehabilitation treatment methods. Many methods can be selected according to the requirements, to achieve different treatment objectives: to promote the growth of granulation tissue and skin and soft-tissue healing, ultraviolet, infrared, and laser irradiation are usually used; to promote fracture healing, DC power, etc., and ultrashort wave therapy, is often used; inflammation. Laser and ultraviolet irradiation can be used in shallow inflammation; deep inflammation can be treated with shortwave, ultrashort wave, or microwave treatment. In the traditional Chinese medicine fumigation method, after 2–4 weeks, drug fumigation is applied to improve skin nutrition, Shujin, swelling, and pain. The audio frequency electric therapy with strip electrodes on both sides of the juxtaposition of the scar is carried out every 20–30 min, one to two times daily, to soften the scar, improve scar itching and pain symptoms. It should be ensured that the electrode is placed firmly, that the wiring is not loose, and that the patients are asked how they feel in a timely manner, to prevent electric burns (Fig. 9.1). Ultrasound therapy is carried out using a mobile method, each session 1–1.5 W/cm^2 part 5–15 min, once a day, 15–20 times for a course of treatment (Fig. 9.2). A wax disc method uses wax, which can improve the blood circulation of the hands, soften the scar, and relieve the pain, and is generally used in exercise therapy before- hand

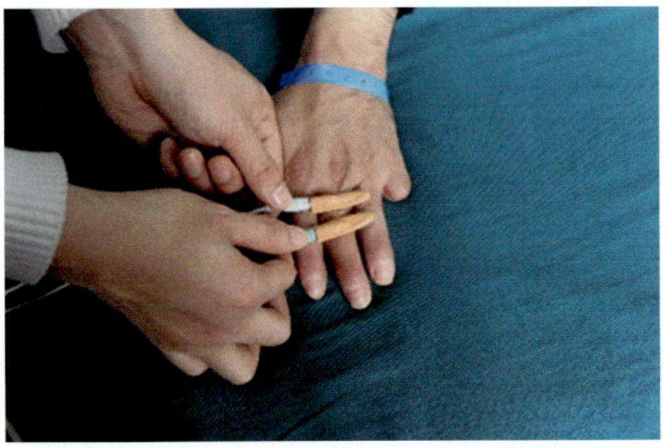

Fig. 9.1 Audio frequency electrotherapy

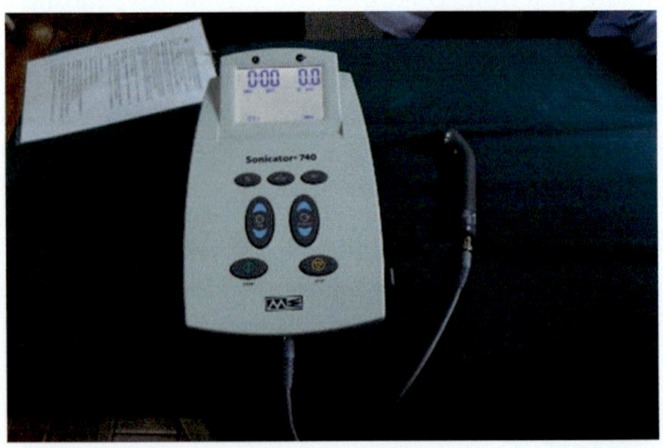

Fig. 9.2 Ultrasonic therapy

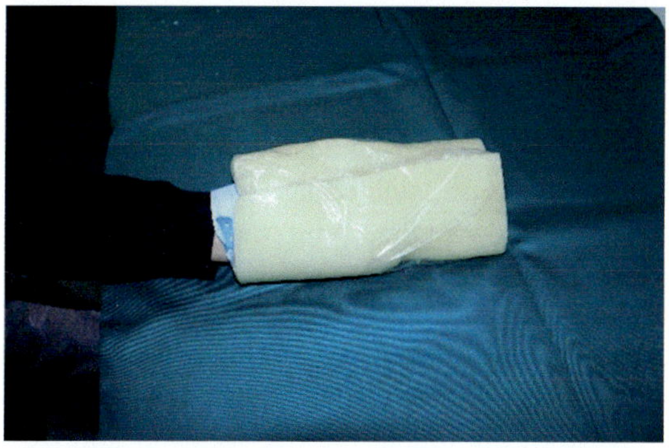

Fig. 9.3 Wax treatment

(Fig. 9.3). In addition, physical therapy can help detumescence, dilate the blood vessels, and relieve pain, softening scar tissue, stimulating muscle contraction, preventing and treating muscle atrophy, physical therapy, reasonable can achieve a multiplier effect.

9.2.2 Exercise Therapy

Exercise therapy, also known as functional exercise, is the basic rehabilitation therapy, including exercise, muscle exercises, general health care, and sensory training.

1. *Joint activity training*: Joint activity damage is the primary problem to solve. In the hand joints, because of their structure and functional characteristics, there are different rules: contracture of thumb adduction contracture is prone to lose,abduction and finger function; the metacarpophalangeal joint of finger lateral ligament in flexion relaxation, tension in the straight, and interphalangeal joints in the metacarpophalangeal joint easy contracture in extension or flexion, and interphalangeal joint in flexion contracture easy. Rehabilitation methods are: (1) Using active or passive motion, power movement or a combination of the two, in the early postoperative period (after 1 week) of fibrous tissue gradually drawing contracture adhesion, gradual recovery of the joint function; (2) the joint function of early exercise cannot be restored, late after anesthesia or release of joint implementation of practice operation, and then in the early postoperative continuous passive movement exercise (Continuous passive motion movement, CPM, is a relatively new method of treatment, in which the limb is fixed onto the special equipment, the equipment drives the passive movement of the limbs continuously, mainly for the prevention of joint adhesion and contracture caused by breaking, promoting the repair of articular cartilage, ligaments, and tendons. It can promote swelling. CPM should pay attention to the following: (a) According to the practice methods, a strong degree of contracture of joint adhesion, the early course of the passive joint motion showing greater flexibility and is easy to cause tension pain, availability of active and passive activities of the joint treatment; a longer course of disease, lack of passive elastic activities, not easy to cause the feeling of pain is often required for joint traction. The gradual recovery of joint function; (b) After 2–3 days should begin joint activity training or continuous passive motion of arthrolysis, continued fixation should be discontinued; (c) New pain should be avoided, so as not to cause new damage or muscle spasm, thereby affecting the curative effect).
2. *Muscle exercise*: In addition to the damage of the muscle or its innervation, immobilization of the injured muscle and its adjacent joints can lead to disuse atrophy. Disuse atrophy of muscle is usually reversible, but it is characterized by degeneration of muscle during long and severe muscle atrophy, the disappearance of fine fibers, phagocytosis, and disappearance. Finally, muscle fibrosis is irreversible. The median nerve and ulnar nerve injury of the hand muscle usually cannot be recovered, and these are problems that still need to be solved. Usually a grading of muscle contraction and isometric contraction in two ways are necessary for daily life, but also with access to prevention and treatment of muscle atrophy. In recent years, isokinetic exercises and hand muscle exercises have been practiced with specialized instruments. Isotonic exercises are muscle exercises with isotonic

contractions using a pulley system, such as an isotonic con- traction exercise tension arm assembly. Isometric exercises consist of muscle exercises with isometric contractions, such as the use of walls and strength training apparatus, and the further use of equipment for multiangle isometric exercises has reached the hands of many aspects of exercise. Constant speed exercise involves the use of special isokinetic exercise apparatus. During exercise, the lever of the exerciser is wound around the axis of the motion of the joint, which is consistent with the mechanical axis. The movement speed of the mechanical axis is preset, and when the body starts to reach the set speed, it can only be carried round at a constant speed; thus, it is called isokinetic exercise. Exercises of hand muscles entail fewer manual muscle strength exercises and resistance exercise methods are used, and the ball and rubber net are used as the representative exercises for the fingers, flexors, and all the internal muscles of the hand. Regarding muscle function exercise, according to the selection of patients with muscle strength exercise and equipment conditions, methods, and make the corresponding change according to the progress of the right; grasp the rhythm exercise, each exercise should be moderate muscle.

3. *General health care movement*: From a biological point of view, human beings are a type of advanced animal that depends highly on the movement of muscles during their race and individual development. Lack of exercise, especially because the injury bed muscles are greatly reduced, can cause a series of adverse reactions, such as a change in the heart and lung function, muscle atrophy, loss of appetite, immunity, and decreased ability to adapt, depressed mood. Various severe, possibly life-endangering complications can occur, such as pneumonia, bedsores, deep vein thrombosis, urinary tract infection. The following measures can be used to control the early replantation for upper limb injury: postoperatively, the patient must stay in bed for a week, up to no special circumstances after a week; bed exercises, including the active movement of the bed, deep breathing, uninjured limbs, the chest, the waist, can be combined and incorporated into the routine nursing care; the aerobic exercise, including walking, jogging, going downstairs, with the help of sports equipment.
4. *Sensory training*: Sensory reeducation means educating patients to keep their fingers off hot or sharp objects. In order to restore the touch, the eye looks at and uses proper pressure to press the surrounding skin with a rubber cylinder, then stops and the eyes are closed to realize the difference between the front and back. Then the patient focuses on exercising, moving the eyes, looking at the fingers at the right point, then stopping and feeling the difference. These two tactile movements were restored twice a day, each time for 10 min. This is called tactile training. The third method is the temperature sense training: the patient uses the fingers to touch two bottles of cold water and warm water respectively, and to touch two small bottles with the fingers respectively, with open eyes and closed eyes, and feel the difference between the two (10 min per time, twice a day). Complex sensory training consists of glass marbles, small pieces of wood, red dates, six angle nuts, rubber, a peanut, a screw, sandpaper, and a coin, a total of nine different objects, being embedded in rice, and the patients test whether they can correctly judge the objects they touch.

9.2.3 Occupational Therapy

Occupational therapy for the restoration of severed finger function has the purpose of training for the selection of some of the activities of daily life, e.g., labor, cognitive activity, as an effective method of treatment to relieve symptoms and improve the function of the finger. It is an important component of rehabilitation therapy and a link between the patient's family and society. Occupational therapy is a bridge for patients to move from hospital to society. These activities include self-care skills, career values, and recreational activities that can create value. The method of occupational therapy should meet the following requirements: (1) Purposeful and meaningful activities; the right difficulty can play the role in training; by the patient's subjective efforts can be reached; the amount of activity can be interesting; the appropriate adjustment. The content of occupational therapy in general includes the following: training in the activities of daily living, such as wearing clothing and footwear, washing, combing, and eating; occupation skills training, such as carpentry, sewing, typing, computer operation; housework: cleaning, cooking, and using electrical appliances; (2) production process: carving, embroidery, knitting process; (3) playing cards, entertainment, games, chess, calligraphy, and painting. The more perfect process of occupational therapy should begin with functional evaluation, defining the nature and range of the functional damage of the hand, selecting proper training content and methods, and then guiding the patients to practice these.

9.2.4 Application of a Brace

The brace is also an orthotic device that aids the motor organs with the aid of external mechanical structures. It can be relatively or strictly braked to ensure tissue healing, anti-inflammatory and pain relief, and to facilitate the activities of the other joints, creating conditions for early movement of the entire limb. Continuous correction of certain deformed joints, or prevention of deformity should be carried out. With development over time, the brace has been made more beautiful and convenient, comfortable, detachable for washing, and is acceptable to the public.

9.2.5 Occupational Rehabilitation

The occupation of the patient should be found out and the job demands analyzed, the patient's function and work requirements should be carried out in the corresponding pre-job training, such as vocational rehabilitation training with the BTE Primus system. This is to maximize the recovery and improve the disabled worker's body function and ability for self-care, to restore and improve their occupational ability, and to promote their return to society and return to work as far as possible.

9.2.6 Traditional Rehabilitation Therapy

Traditional rehabilitation therapy guided by the basic theory of TCM, TCM psychology, Chinese medicine, acupuncture and massage, traditional sports, qigong, diet, natural, physical, entertainment and other traditional methods, according to the characteristics of pathological syndromes such as disability, diagnosis, and rehabilitation.

9.2.7 Psychological Counseling

This can be implemented using psychological methods for sleep management, pain management, emotional management, promoting communication, enhancing patient compliance, and self-confidence.

9.3 The Characteristics of Rehabilitation Treatment for Finger Replantation

Compared with exercise after finger replantation, the postoperative rehabilitation is stricter, because the blood supply in early stages of the operation may be unstable, and other complications may occur. Therefore, clinicians should pay close attention to the patient's postoperative condition, and carry out active and optimal treatment and rehabilitation exercises. Focus should be placed on the normal functioning of the affected finger, including finger flexibility, grip strength, pinch strength, endurance, and functional tactile recovery (Figs. 9.4 and 9.5).

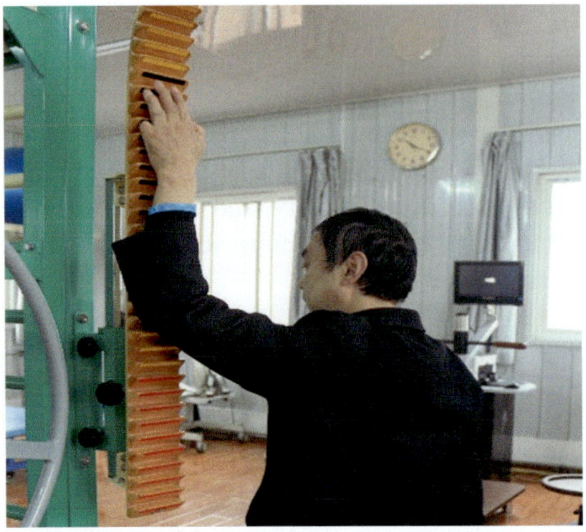

Fig. 9.4 Pay close attention to both active and passive activity of the close joint

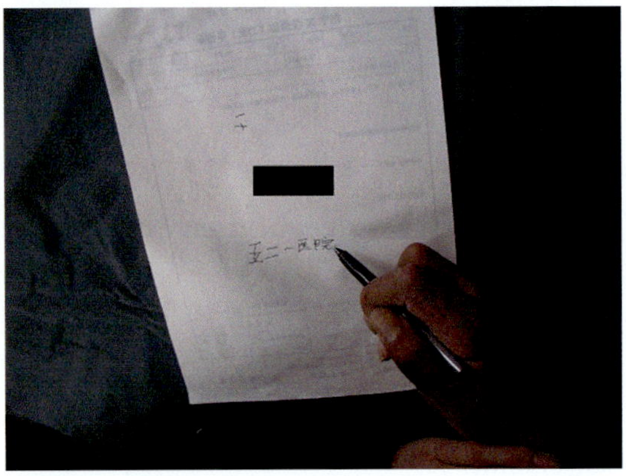

Fig. 9.5 ADL training

9.4 The Meaning of Functional Rehabilitation

The hand is an important organ of labor; it is also an important organ of expression after replantation. To obtain successful results and avoid joint stiffness, deformity, pain, the patient must pass through the physical rehabilitation system. In summary, the individuality of the patient and the individuality of the hand among human organs, once it has lost its function, is likely to cause a family predicament and increase the social burden. As a clinician, technically not confined to the immediate surgery, physicians should pay more attention to the future, to achieving hand injury recovery and reconstruction to the maximum extent possible, enabling the patient to make a physical, mental, social, and financial recovery, bringing them back to life, back to work (WHO).

Part II

The Special Types of Finger Replantation

The so-called special types of finger replantation are also known as complex finger replantation. They are different from the traditional simple cases, of which the injured fingers are much more complex. If the patient is in a good condition with one injury, replantation is easily performed. Based on the traditional concepts, the number of techniques for the special types of finger replantation is growing, together with further improvement and innovation, and top technology in finger replantation. With the progress in microsurgical technology, finger replanting technology is also improving. With the accumulation of doctor's clinical experiences day by day, the special types of finger replantation have made the following breakthroughs:

1. Boundaries of the replanting plane; in theory in any part of the finger, from the root to tips, is replantable.
2. Age limit; patients aged from 5 months to more than 70 years have achieved successful replantation and functional recovery.
3. Successful multiple finger replantation, i.e., cases in which up to ten fingers have been completely severed.
4. Limit of the broken structure of the fingers, making a multiple-planed, ring-shaped, or vertical replantation.
5. Achieving a successful replantation with a combination of multiple tissue defects and composite broken tissues via means of tissue transplantation.
6. Time limit of finger replantation, how long the severed fingers can be kept at room temperature (without special cryopreservation); with an ischemic period more than 15 h, or even more than 24 h, successful replantation can still be achieved.

With the traditional theory, it was believed that it was impossible to replant those overdue fingers. Now this is possible and the success rate is also rising, up to 90–95% or more. The functioning of the replanted finger has also gradually improved, which is the inevitable result of the development of microsurgical technology and increased living standards.

We investigate the re-classification method of the special types of finger replantation according to the domestic and foreign scholars, and combine this with our own 20-year experience of clinical microsurgery. We summarize the current complex finger replantation as 13 special types of replantation, and discuss and classify as technical clinical cases. They are:

1. Replantation of the distal part of the fingers, when the severed plane is over the final finger joints, including fingertip replantation (some scholars classify the replantation of the tissues distal to the nail root as fingertip replantation). Although the blood vessels of the distal part of the fingers are thin, and difficult to replant, the success rate of surgery could reach 90% or more.
2. Rotated avulsion finger replantation, due to high-speed operation and pulling of a machine. Various tissues vary greatly in the extent to which the resist violence in finger replantation; different severed planes are in different situations, but the degree of damage can be very complex. This type of finger replantation often requires transplantation of tendons, blood vessels, nerve transposition, or transplantation reconstruction to achieve successful functioning.
3. Replantation of multiple fingers: In this type, more than one finger is severed from the hand. Surgery is time consuming and it is technically difficult to achieve success. Reliable techniques and good teamwork are necessary.
4. Replantation of multiple fingers and multiple segments: When there are more than two replantations on the same severed plane. It is divided into multiple segments in one finger and multiple segments in multiple fingers. The surgery is also difficult, and requires elaborate surgical techniques.
5. Replantation of fingers in children: When the patients are children under 12 years old. In this section, we choose only <3-year-old, who are characterized by thinner blood vessels, less anti-tension, they more easily spasm, more difficult to break, and replantation surgery will probably fail.
6. Transplantation and replantation of fingers: When the part between the fingers and the palm, and the part between the palm and wrist are damaged, it is impossible to replant the broken fingers directly. We need to make good use of the broken fingers to revise and shift to replant. We can replant onto the stump of the forearm, wrist or palm, rebuilding the extension, flexion, pinch, fold, and other important functions of the hands.
7. Replantation of the fingers with skin and soft-tissue defects: Cases in which there are severed fingers combined with defects of the skin and soft tissue, and even blood vessels, nerves, and tendon. We can use a flap to repair the wound. In some cases, we can also use the blood vessel of the axis flap to connect the injured vasculature, reconstructing the blood supply of the damaged fingers. At the same time, we can reconstruct the flexion and extension powers of the fingers via tendon transposition, and repair sensation by nerve transplantation.

8. Replantation of the hand tissues: Hand injury often leads to an intermittent skin interruption of certain parts of the body, the broken-off parts often include the bones, joints, tendons, and other complex tissues, and the skin tissues cannot survive without anastomosis of the blood vessels. Although it is difficult to perform replantation surgery, both the function and the shape are satisfactory after surgery.
9. Replantation in the self-mutilating patients, for various reasons such as out-of-control emotions, depression, or being inebriated. The patients often use sharp knives or other sharp items to cut his or her fingers. These cases are characterized by neat and regular incisions, and the nerves and blood vessels are often in the same severed plane. The severed fingers are often complete, with no more bruises. The replantation surgery itself is not difficult; however, the postoperative vascular crisis rate is high, affecting replantation success.
10. Finger replantation in the elderly. Generally, this section often refers to patients over 60 years old. As China has a progressively aging society, the number of patients with severed fingers is increasing. The poor vascular condition of the elderly, plus the drug safety problems combined with many complications, and the unideal rehabilitation, all these factors result in replantation difficulties.
11. Replantation of crushed fingers. Compared with the avulsed severed fingers, crushed fingers indicate when the patient attempts to withdraw his or her hands when the fingers are caught in a fast-moving machine. In this case, the soft tissues of the whole finger, including the skin, subcutaneous tissues, and vascular nerves, are torn off completely like gloves. The remaining fingers are only the phalanges, joints, and flexor tendons, and sometimes even include avulsion of the distal segment and the flexor tendon in the most serious cases. The patients in this section are characterized by contraction, serious damage to the vascular beds, and the blood vessels, nerves, tendons, bone and joints after the avulsion are not in a plane. The success rate of surgery is low.
12. Ectopic replantation. After the injury, the damage of the proximal limb is very serious, and it is not suitable for replantation under emergency conditions. We can temporarily implant the broken fingers in other normal parts of the body, reconstructing its blood supply to ensure survival. When the conditions of the wound are suitable for replantation, we perform the operations.
13. Late finger replantation. For various reasons, the finger replantation surgery was not performed during the 6–8 h after the injury at room temperature. In this section, patients receive replantation surgery more than 10 h after the injury. Although there is no absolute time limit, according to the classical theory, it is believed that late replantation consists of cases when replantation is performed after more than 12 h at room temperature and 24 h under refrigerated conditions.

Replantation of Severed Fingers in Children

10

10.1 Overview of Replantation of Severed Fingers in Children

The technology of the replantation of severed fingers makes it possible to achieve normal limb morphology and functional recovery through precise microvascular anastomosis, and sufficient repair of bone, tendons, the skin, and nerves. In 1964, Malt and McKhann reported that they preserved a 12-year-old boy's upper arm in May 1962. In 1963, Kleinert et al. (1963) first reconstructed the blood supply of the thumb by means of arterial anastomosis. In 1965, Komatsu and Tamai (1968) successfully completed the replantation of the first complete amputation of a finger. In 1974, Tamai performed a successful replantation of the left proximal interphalangeal joint of a little finger that had been completely cut off in a 20-month-old child. At that time, Tamai anastomosed the finger artery and finger nerve with the help of a microscope and obtained good clinical results. In 1980, reported a case of a 45-month-old child in whom 2–5 fingers on the left hand had been completely cut off. All the fingers survived after replantation. In 1980, Wang Chengqi et al. (1983) reported a successful case of a 25-month-old child with 2–5 fingers completely severed from the left hand, in which the index and middle fingers were shifted with the amputated middle and ring fingers. In 1982, Cheng Guoliang et al. (1982) reported a 9- to 15-year follow-up study of 26 cases with 45 replanted fingers and found that the postoperative excellent and good rate was 100%. This study truthfully reflected the level of severed finger replantation in children in our country, which has leapt up to the world's advanced level in a short period of time. However, compared with adults, replantation of severed fingers in children still has its peculiarities:

1. The finger blood vessel is small and anastomosis is very difficult.
2. Children's mental development is not complete; thus, they cannot fully cooperate with the treatment after the operation.
3. Limitations of drug use

   The development of the surgical microscope, fine microsurgical instruments, and microsuture hardware laid the foundations for the replantation of severed fingers in children up to the 1970s.

10.2 Case Presentation

Case 1: Replantation of the Avulsion of the Right Ring Finger's Distal Section

An 18-month-old boy, distal section in vitro of the right ring finger, pain, bleeding because of a powder grinder injury, admitted in 1.5 h. Physical examination: The general situation was good; the vital signs were stable. The skin near the palm side of the fourth finger on the right hand was avulsed

J. Lin et al., *Special Type of Finger Replantation*, https://doi.org/10.1007/978-981-10-6229-2_10

about 0.8 cm*0.5 cm, with tendon exposure, an irregular edge, lack of the distal finger section, bone exposure, and defect wound bleeding. In the neurovascular bundle tip an approximately 2-cm-long connecting the palm to the fingers. This looked like a "horsetail," and there was congestion under the nail. The other fingers' blood supply was normal. The operation was successfully performed under general anesthesia. The finger should be ruddy, in moderate tension, after a relaxing tourniquet. The child was brought safely to the ward after the replanted finger had been fixed with a sterile cotton bandage and padded with broken cotton yarn. After the operation, the patient was given conventional treatment, and 10 days later, the replanted severed finger had successfully survived. The growth and function are good after regular follow-up and functional exercise guidance (Figs. 10.1, 10.2, 10.3, 10.4, 10.5, and 10.6).

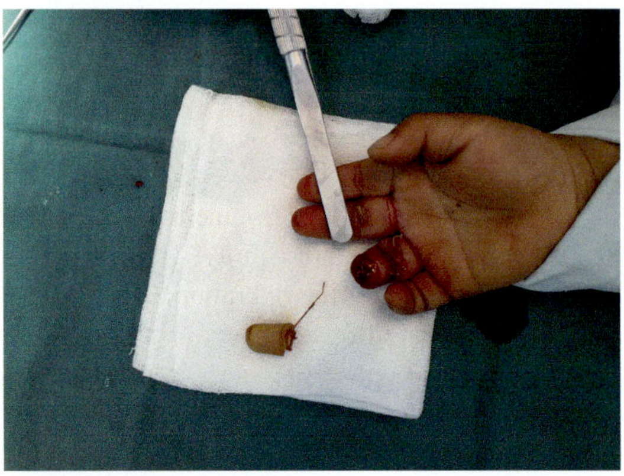

Fig. 10.1 The severed finger

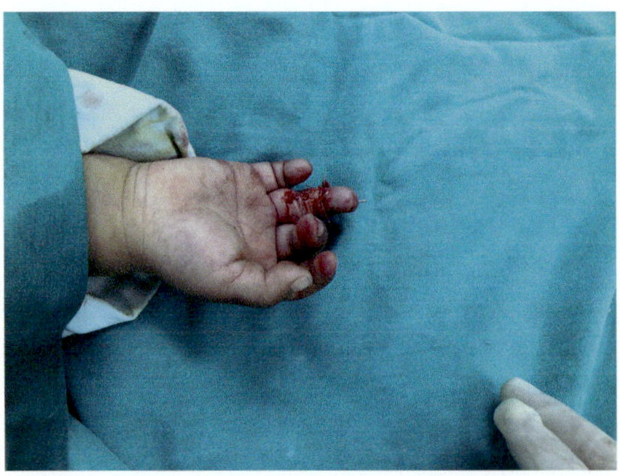

Fig. 10.2 Blood supply situation in the palm side after a successful replantation

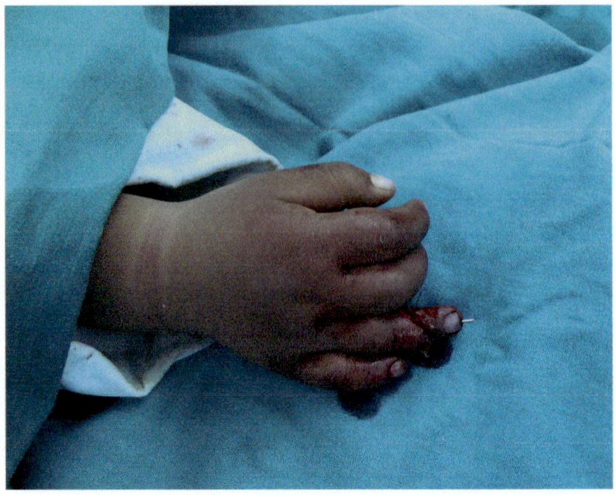

Fig. 10.3 Blood supply situation in the dorsal side after a successful replantation

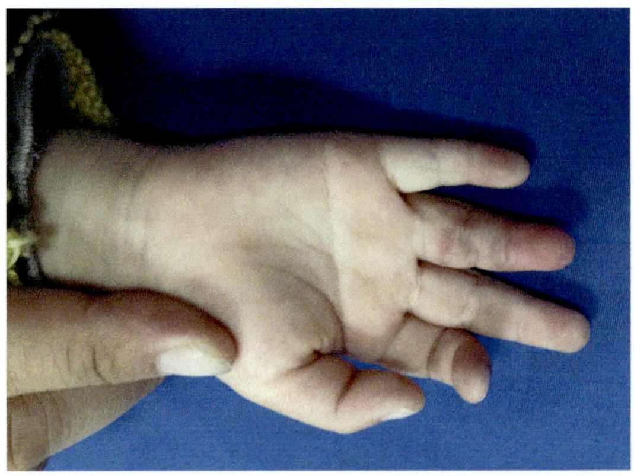

Fig. 10.4 The situation on the palm side 3 months later

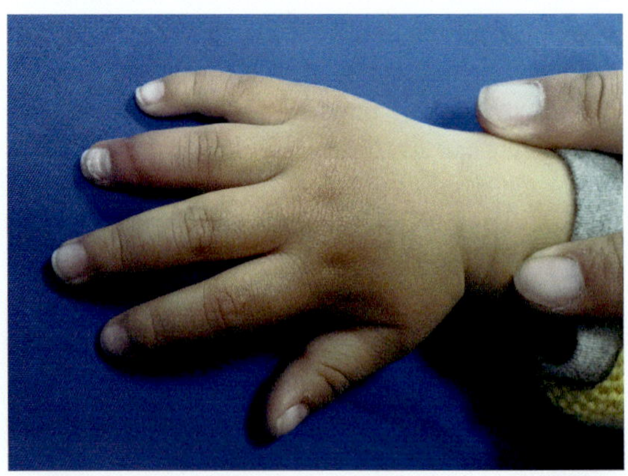

Fig. 10.5 The situation on the dorsal side 3 months later

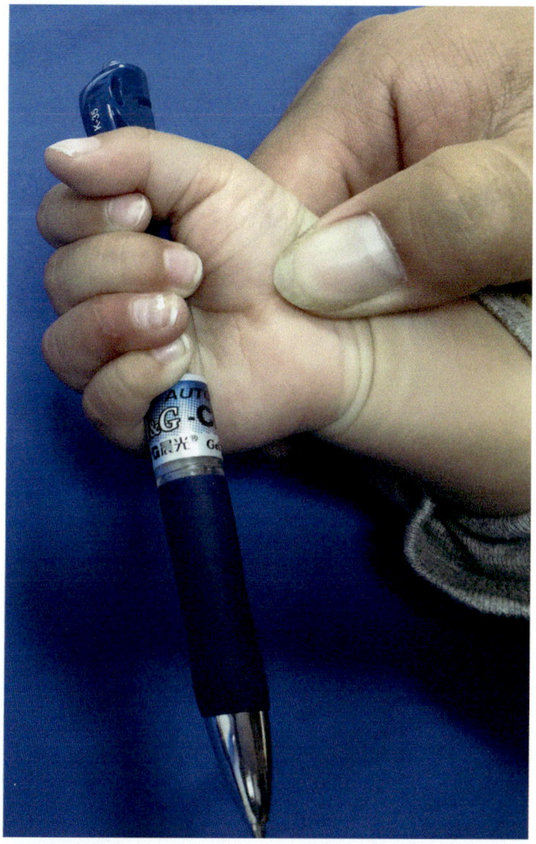

Fig. 10.6 Finger flexor function 3 months later

Case 2: Replantation of Avulsion of the Left Ring Finger's Distal Section

A 23-month-old boy, distal section in vitro of the left ring finger, pain, bleeding because of a lathe cutter chain injury, admitted in 2 h. PE: The general situation was good; the vital signs were stable. Only about 0.1 cm of the skin was in connection with the distal volar of the left ring finger, with tendon retraction, articular surface exposure, and defect wound bleeding. There was congestion under the nail and the other fingers' blood supply was normal. The operation was successfully performed under general anesthesia. The finger should be ruddy, in moderate tension after a relaxing tourniquet. The child was brought safely to the ward after the replanted finger had been fixed with sterile cotton bandage and padded with broken cotton yarn. After the operation, the patient was given conventional treatment, and 10 days later, the replanted severed finger had successfully survived. The growth and function were good after regular follow-up and functional exercise guidance (Figs. 10.7, 10.8, 10.9, 10.10, 10.11, 10.12, 10.13, 10.14, and 10.15).

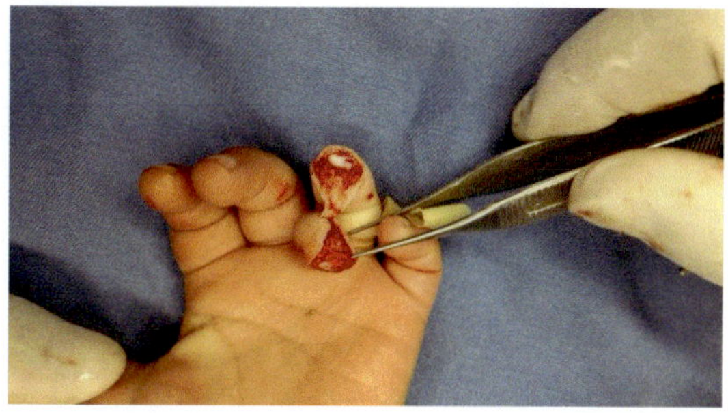

Fig. 10.7 The severed finger

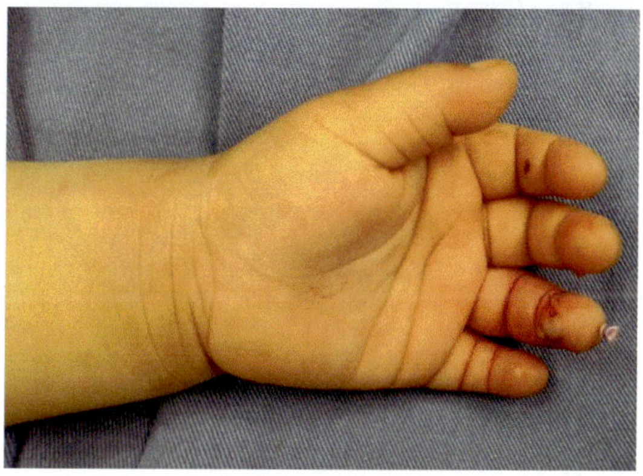

Fig. 10.8 The palm side after replantation

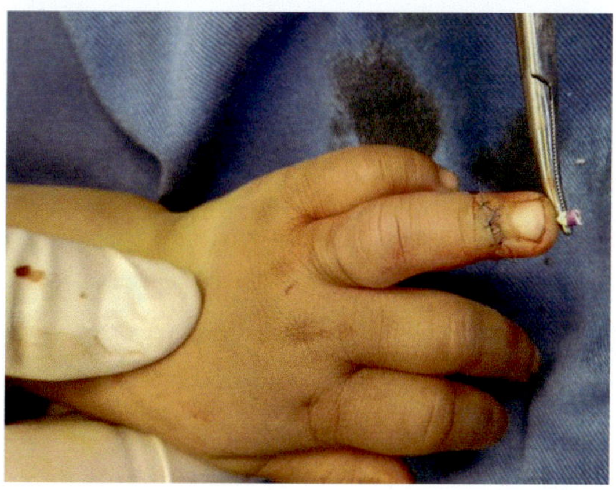

Fig. 10.9 The dorsal side after replantation

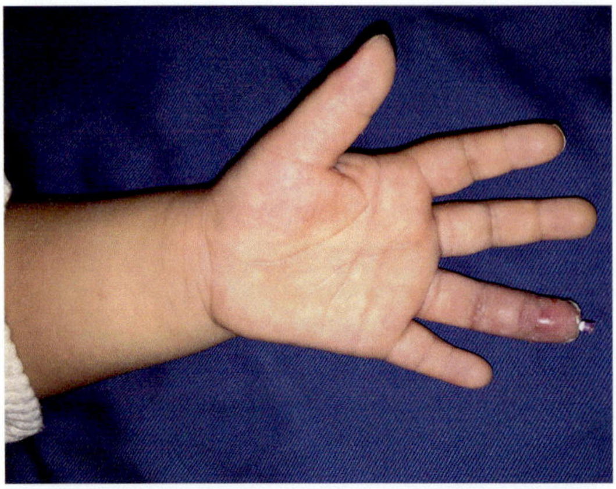

Fig. 10.10 The palm side 3 weeks later

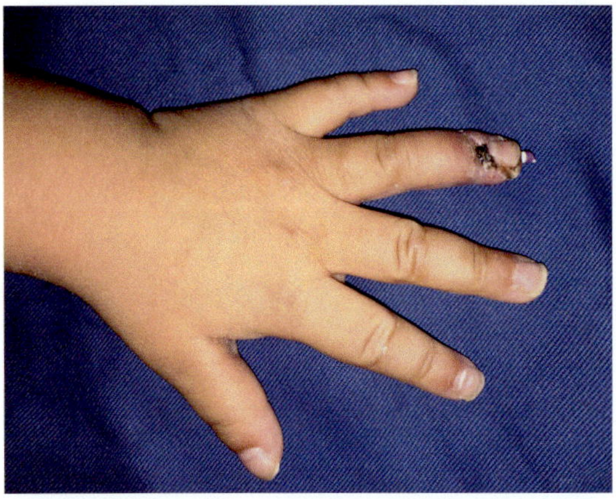

Fig. 10.11 The dorsal side 3 weeks later

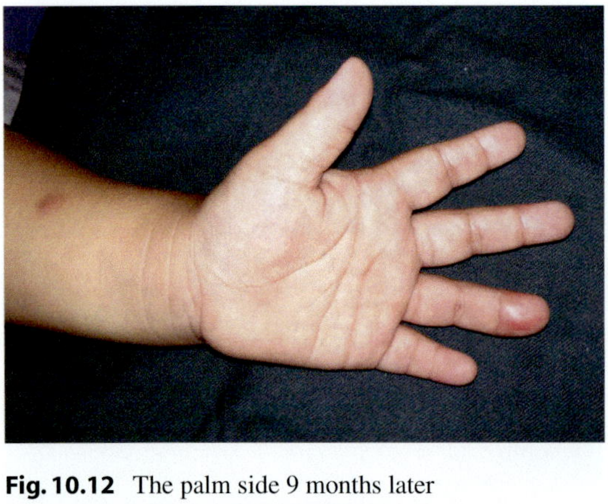

Fig. 10.12 The palm side 9 months later

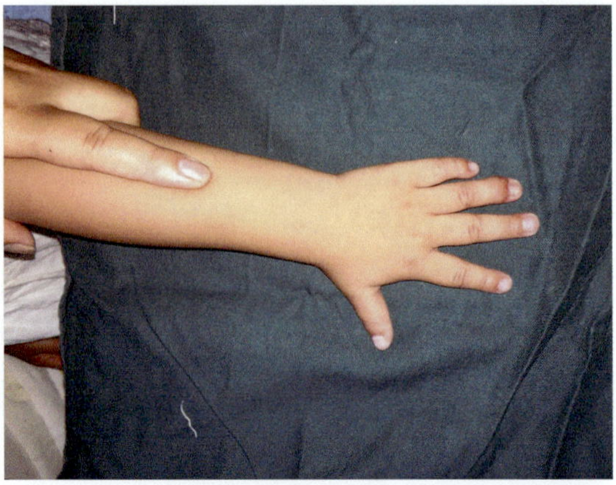

Fig. 10.13 The dorsal side 9 months later

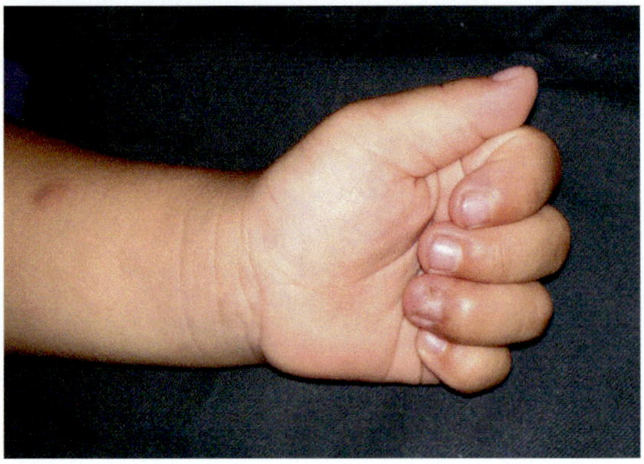

Fig. 10.14 The function 9 months later

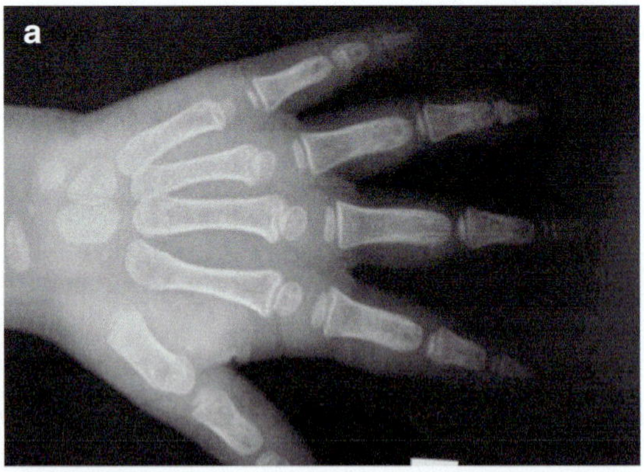

Fig. 10.15 Preoperative and postoperative X-rays

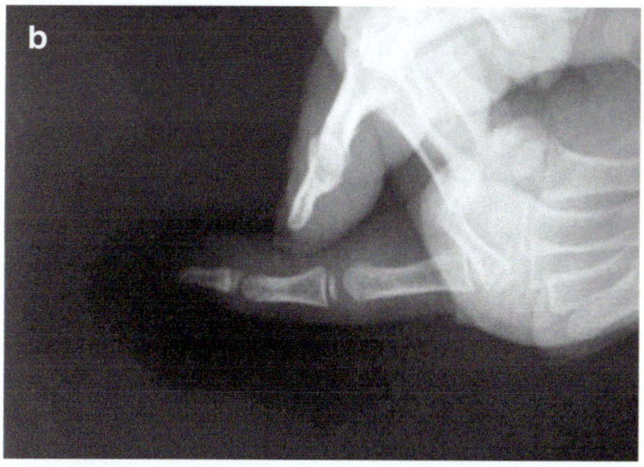

Fig. 10.15 (continued)

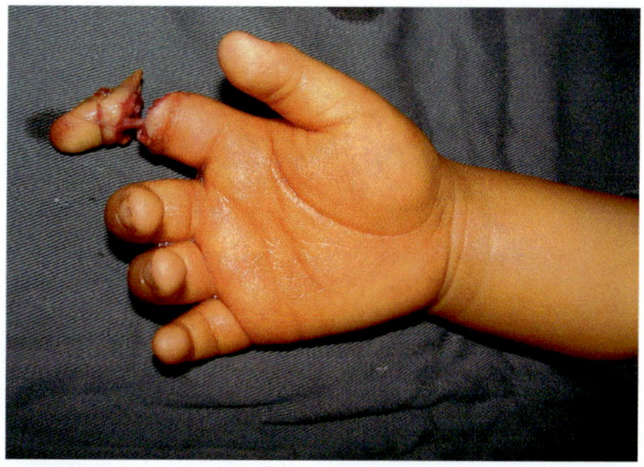

Fig. 10.16 The severed finger

Case 3: Replantation of the Distal and Phalanx Sections of the Right Index Finger

A 35-month-old boy, the distal and phalanx sections of the right index finger were in vitro, pain, bleeding because of a machine tool injury, admitted in 1 h. PE: the general situation was good; the vital signs were stable. There was an oblique wound in the distal and phalanx sections of the right index finger, with an approximately 0.8-cm the palmar flexor tendon tear and exposure, and defect wound bleeding. The neurovascular bundle defect was isolated about 2.5 cm in the palmar ulnar side, like a "horsetail." There was congestion under the nail and the other fingers' blood supply was normal.

The operation was successfully performed under general anesthesia (we found nerve avulsion defects on both sides, which could not be matched). The finger should be ruddy, and in moderate tension after a relaxing tourniquet. The child was brought safely to the ward after the replanted finger had been fixed with a sterile cotton bandage and padded with broken cotton yarn. After the operation, the patient was given conventional treatment, and 10 days later, the replanted severed finger had successfully survived. We transplanted the left sural nerve to reconstruct the finger nerve function 3 months after the first operation. The growth and function were good after regular follow-up and functional exercise guidance (Figs. 10.16, 10.17, 10.18, 10.19, 10.20, 10.21, 10.22, 10.23, and 10.24).

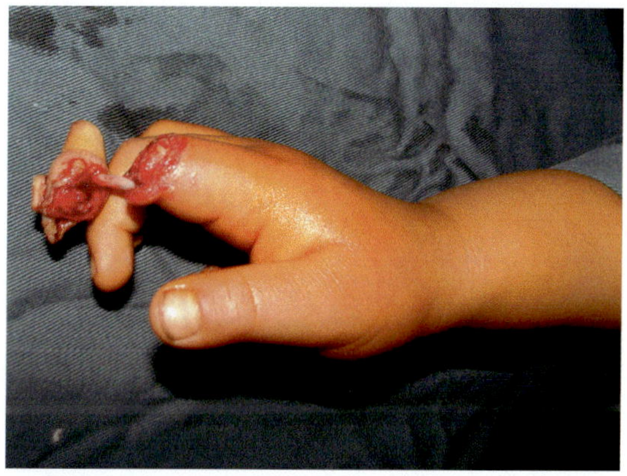

Fig. 10.17 The dorsal side of the severed finger

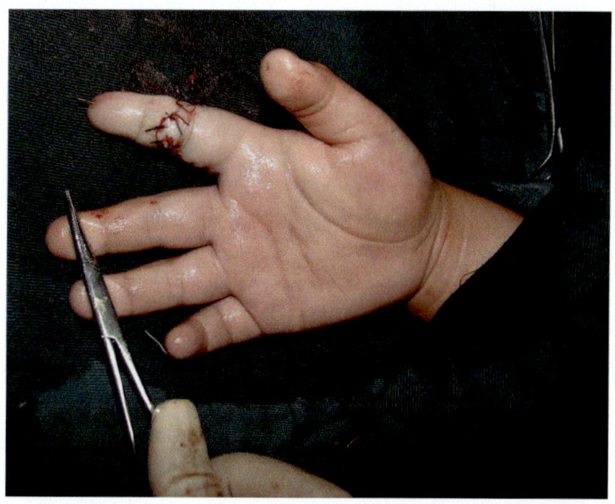

Fig. 10.18 Blood supply situation on the palm side after a successful replantation

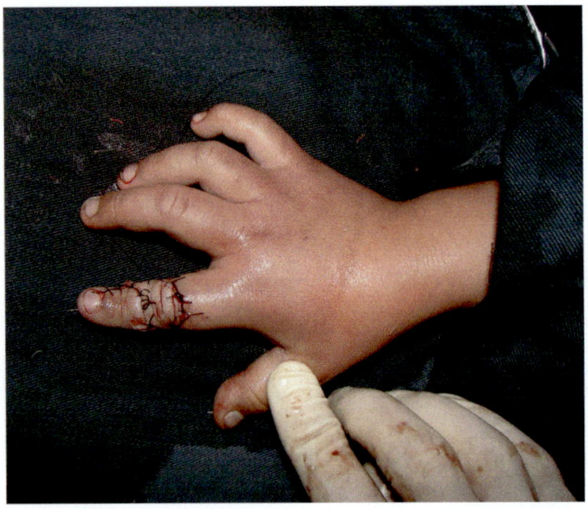

Fig. 10.19 Blood supply situation on the dorsal side after a successful replantation

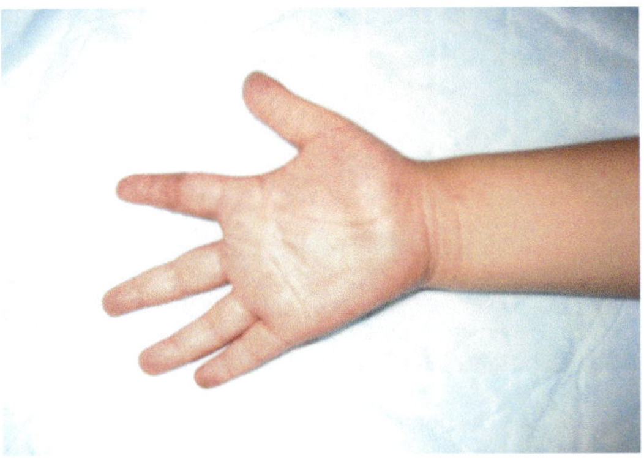

Fig. 10.20 The situation on the palm side 3 months later

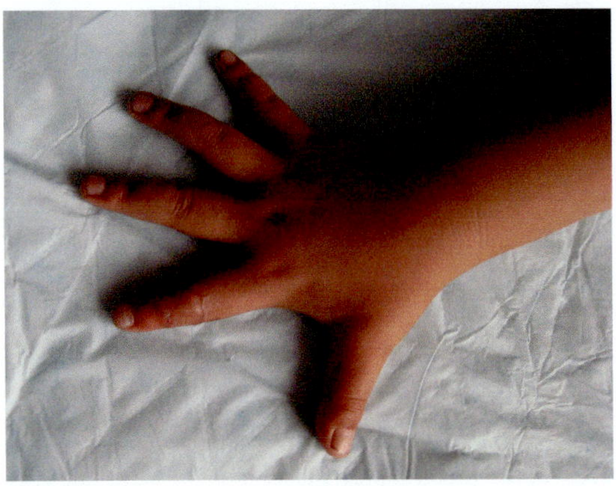

Fig. 10.21 The situation on the dorsal side 3 months later

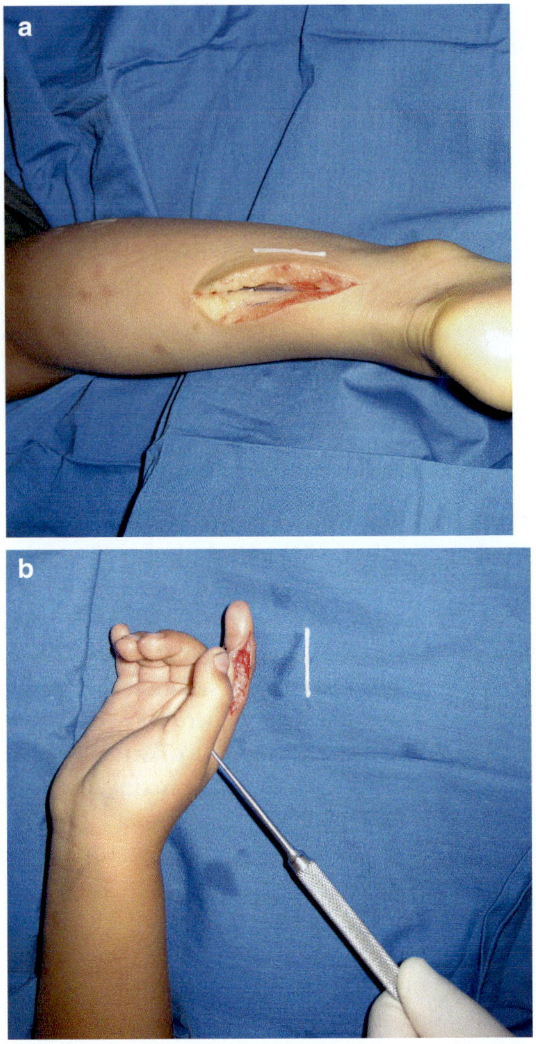

Fig. 10.22 Reconstructed finger nerve function 3 months later

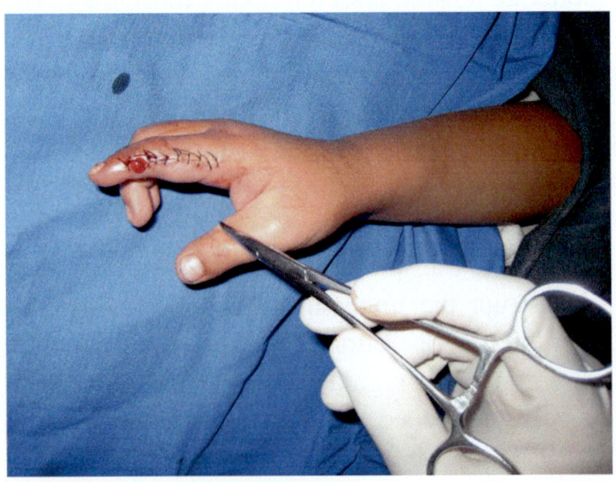

Fig. 10.23 The surgery was over

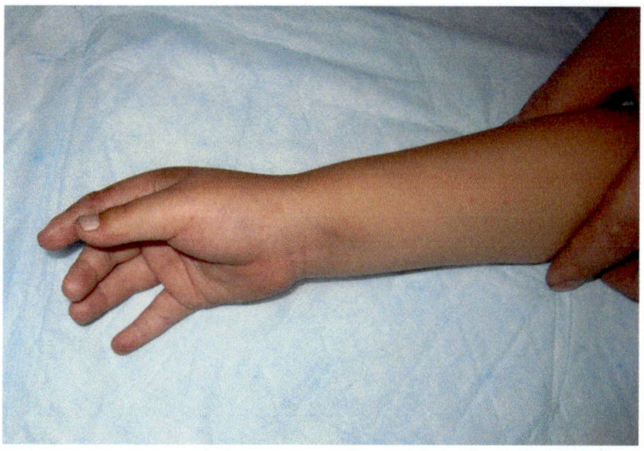

Fig. 10.24 The growth and function were good 9 months later

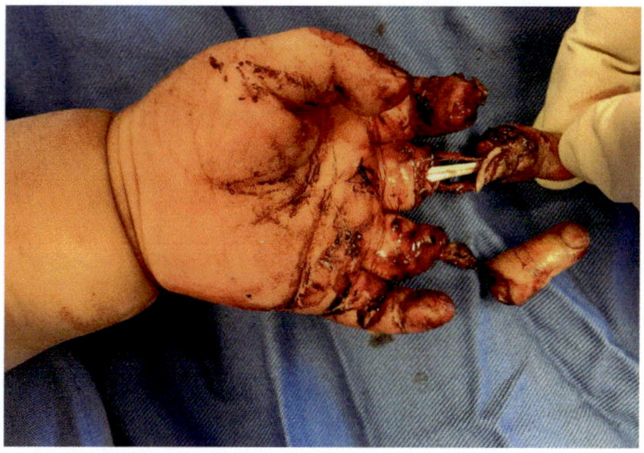

Fig. 10.25 The palm side of the severed fingers

Case 4: Replantation of the Right Index, Middle, and Ring Fingers

A 9-month-old boy, right index, middle, and ring fingers were in vitro, pain, bleeding because of a machine tool injury, admitted in 1.5 h. PE: the general situation was good; the vital signs were stable. The distal and phalanx sections of the left index finger were defect, with wound bleeding and exposed bone; the proximal and middle segments of the middle and ring fingers were avulsed. Only a flexor tendon and the radial nerve were attached to the middle finger, and the distal end did not have any blood supply. The operation of the index finger stump repair, replantation of the middle and ring fingers, and interphalangeal joint fusion were carried out under general anesthesia. The finger should be ruddy, and in moderate tension after a relaxing tourniquet. The child was brought safely to the ward after the replanted finger had been fixed with a sterile cotton bandage and padded with broken cotton yarn. After the operation, the patient was given conventional treatment, and 10 days later, the replantation of the severed finger had successfully survived. We transplanted the left sural nerve to reconstruct the finger nerve function 3 months after the first operation. The growth and function were good after regular follow-up and functional exercise guidance (Figs. 10.25, 10.26, 10.27, 10.28, 10.29, 10.30, 10.31, 10.32, and 10.33).

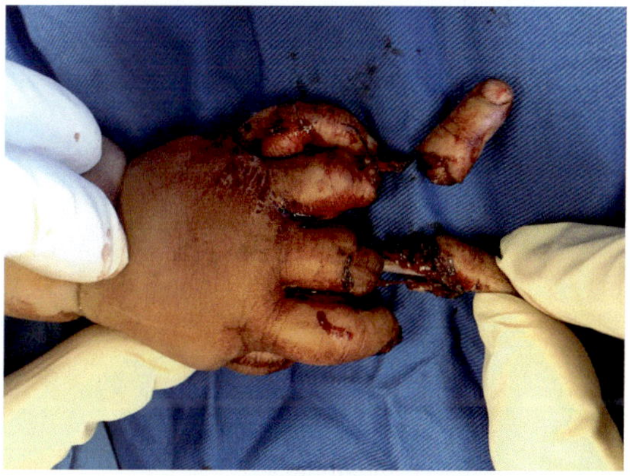

Fig. 10.26 The dorsal side of the severed fingers

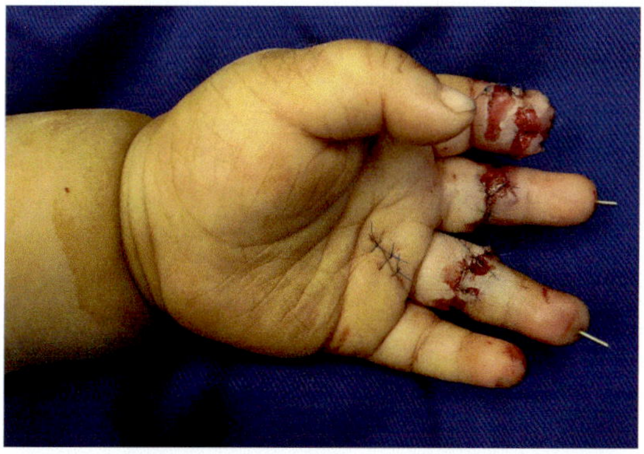

Fig. 10.27 Blood supply situation on the palm side after a successful replantation

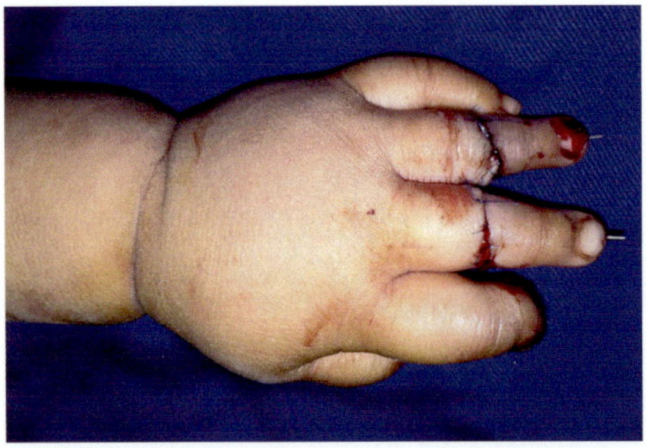

Fig. 10.28 Blood supply situation on the dorsal side after a successful replantation

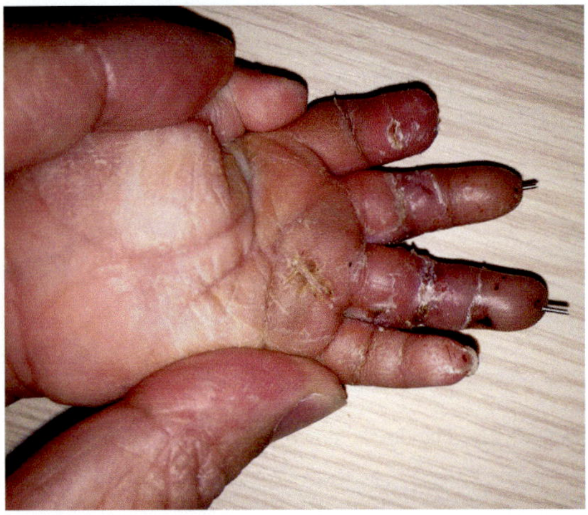

Fig. 10.29 The situation on the palm side 2 weeks later

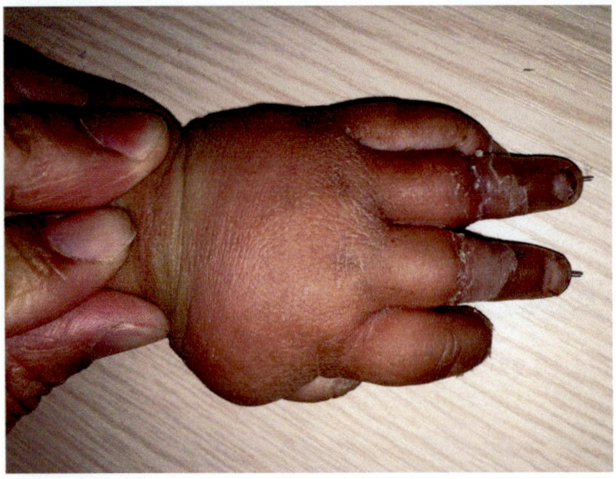

Fig. 10.30 The situation on the dorsal side 2 weeks later

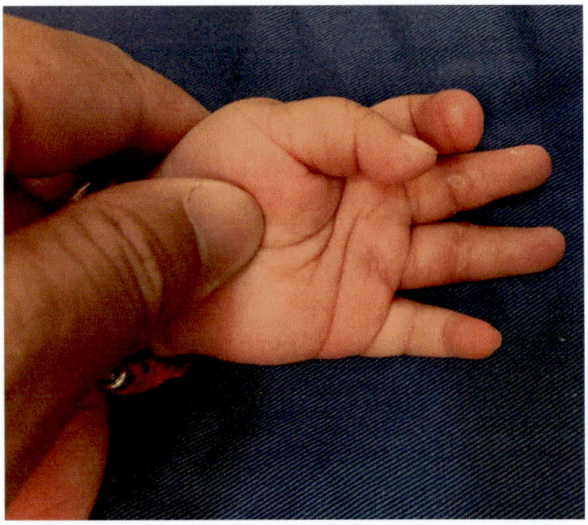

Fig. 10.31 The situation on the palm side 3 months later

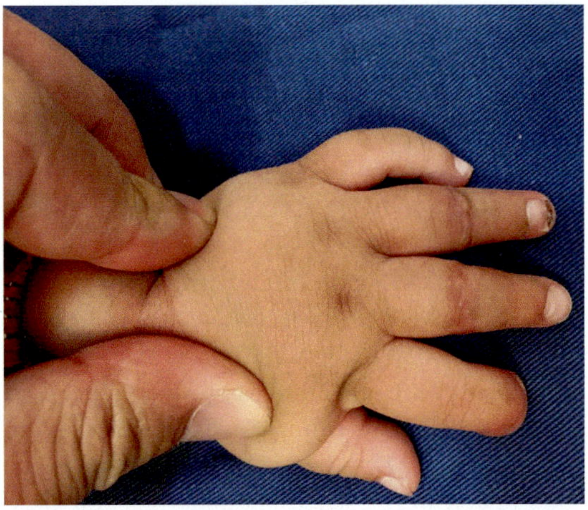

Fig. 10.32 The situation on the dorsal side 3 months later

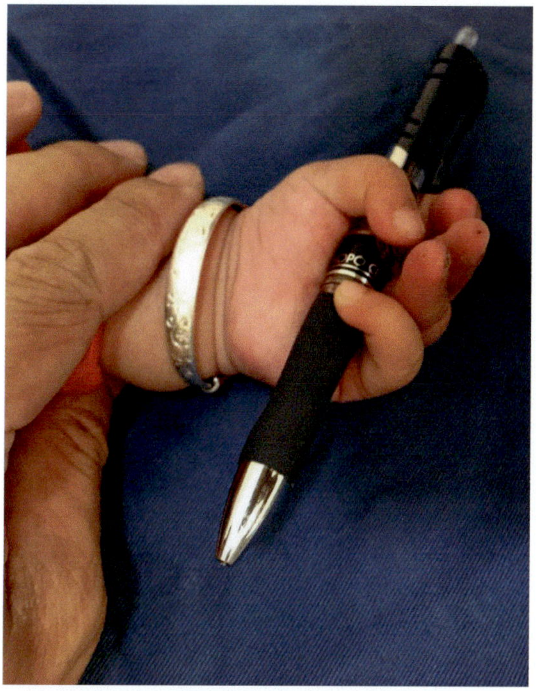

Fig. 10.33 The functional situation 3 months later

Case 5: Replantation of the Left Middle and Ring Fingers

A 27-month-old boy, proximal section of the left middle and ring fingers, pain, bleeding because of a triangle, admitted in 1 h. PE: The general situation was good; the vital signs were stable. The proximal section of the left middle and ring fingers was completely severed with tendon exposure, an irregular edge, lack of bone exposure of the distal finger section; the other fingers' blood supply was normal. The operation was successfully carried out under general anesthesia. The finger should be ruddy, and in moderate tension after a relaxing tourniquet. The child was brought safely to the ward after the replanted finger had fixed by a sterile cotton bandage and padded with broken cotton yarn. After the operation, the patient was given conventional treatment, and 10 days later, the replanted severed fingers had successfully survived. The growth and function were good after regular follow-up and functional exercise guidance and the family are satisfied. (Figs 10.34, 10.35, 10.36, 10.37, 10.38, 10.39, and 10.40).

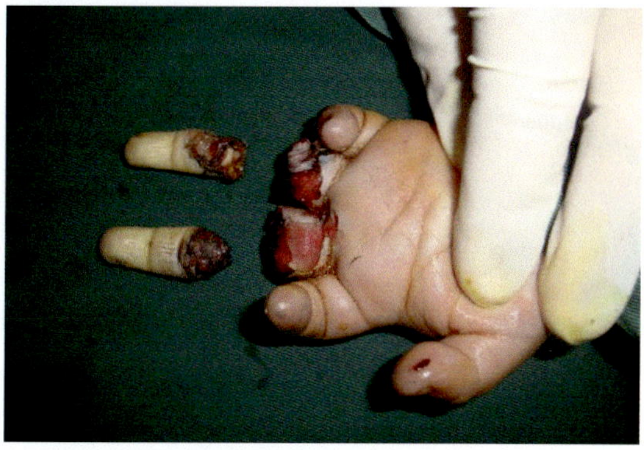

Fig. 10.34 The palm side of the severed fingers

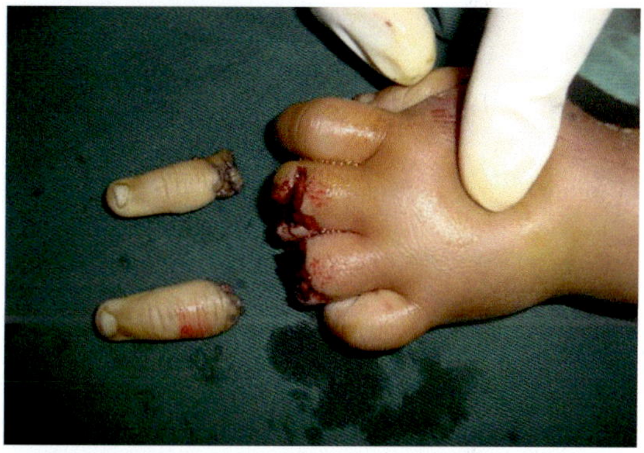

Fig. 10.35 The dorsal side of the severed fingers

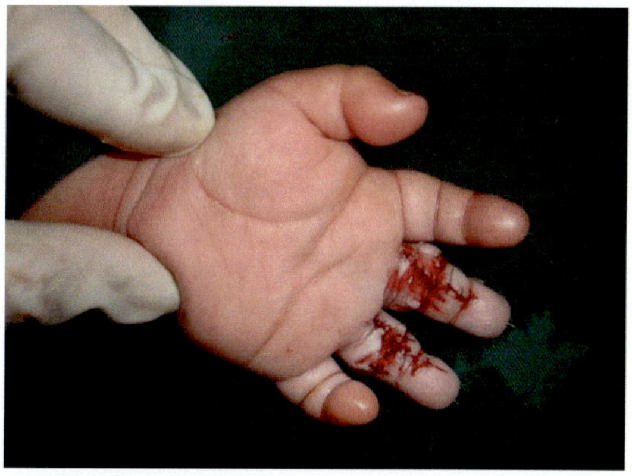

Fig. 10.36 The palm side after replantation

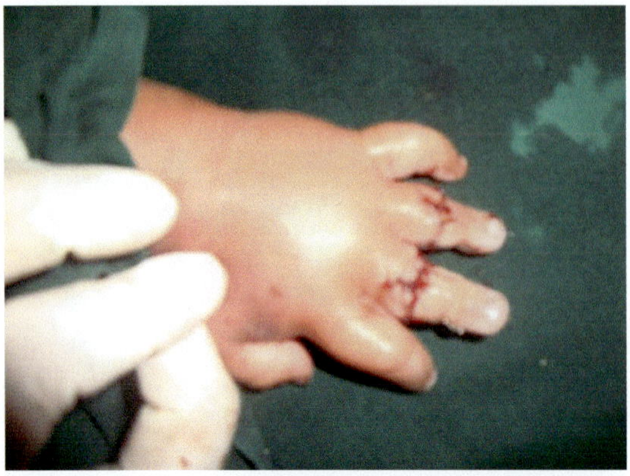

Fig. 10.37 The dorsal side after replantation

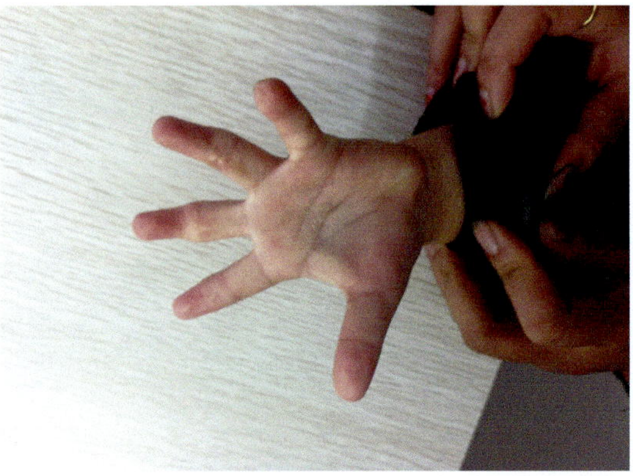

Fig. 10.38 The palm side 2 weeks later

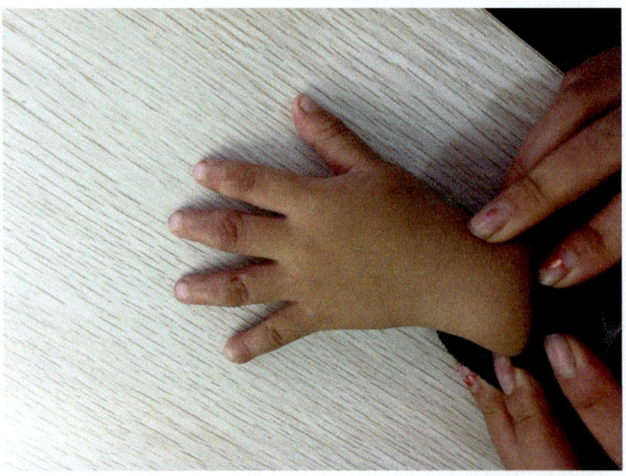

Fig. 10.39 The dorsal side 2 weeks later

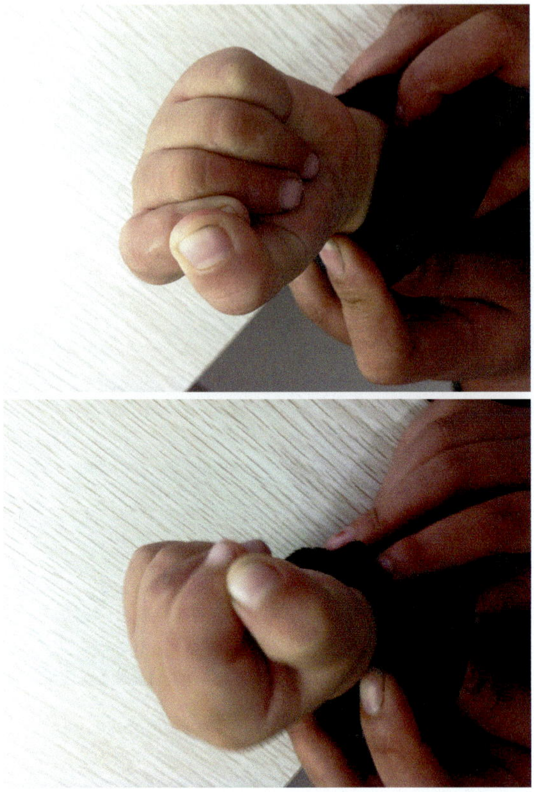

Fig. 10.40 Function 3 months later

10.3 Key Points of the Operation

1. To thoroughly clean and prevent infection. Remove the necrotic tissue under general anesthesia under a ×12 microscope. To find the arterial and venous blood vessels and nerve carefully, clear and cut off the excess adventitia, marking, and for standby application.
2. Shorten the end of the fracture appropriately. Retain the distal phalanx base joint and flex tendon as far as possible to maintain the integrity of the distal interphalangeal joint. Fix the fracture with a single Gram's needle (0.8–1 mm) longitudinally.
3. The smaller the child is, the smaller the diameter of the blood vessel, and the thinner the blood vessel wall will be. It is difficult to perform anastomosis as the base of the finger the distal vascular diameter is approximately 0.15–0.3 mm, and vascular strength is poor

under the age of 3. We use 11-0 or 12-0 non-invasive thread, under tourniquet control for anastomosis, operate using not only strictly non-invasive technology, grasp the good blood vessel and nerve anastomosis spacing, margins, but we also use a "stable, accurate and precise, skillful" small vascular anastomosis technique.

4. The tightness of the skin should be appropriate to avoid the oppression of vascular anastomosis after the success of reconnecting the blood supply.
5. Suture the incisions appropriately, not pressing the vessels.
6. Postoperative low-dose heparin sodium intravenous anticoagulant, anticonvulsant, sedative (heparin sodium by 100–150 U/kg with physiological saline 500 mL, disposable intravenous infusion with a micro-pump 24 h uninterrupted sustained input, drop speed is stable and uniform, decreasing after 3 days. The drugs should be continued for 5–7 days and to combat infection, cefuroxime should be administered for 3–5 days.

10.4 Notes

1. Parents' demands and expectations are generally high, and detailed preoperative talk and education must be emphasized.
2. The mechanism of injury and wound conditions must be understood and should be judged by the experience of the physician who makes a prognosis and decides whether to carry out the surgery.
3. Nursing is most important. Let the parents actively cooperate with the treatment, so that children can try to achieve good medical progress, to obtain the best curative effect.
4. Children face injury, fear, pre-operative and post-operative pain, postoperative brake position brings psychological tension, fear, crying, touch, and other complex treatments. They are prone to vascular spasm, which affects the replantation with regard to the blood supply. Give children a warm therapeutic environment and personalized care.
5. Ensure that the blood vessels are not distorted, that they are not under pressure, and that there is no leakage of blood. In addition, if the right side cannot find if the right side of the artery can not be found, the proximal arteriovenous defect can be transplanted to the finger or the dorsal hand vein can be used.
6. The margin should be accurate and uniform, the knot should be gently lifted, preventing anastomotic varus. The operation requires stability, and should be light and fast.
7. Protect the epiphysis and avoid injury that will affect the later development of the finger.
8. Regarding liver and kidney function in children, some enzymes and blood–brain barrier development are not perfect. As for drug metabolism and detoxification function, drugs easily pass through the blood–brain barrier arriving in the central nervous system and produce toxic side effects. Small, individualized doses, avoiding multidrug combinations, should be the principle.
9. As sensation has not yet been fully restored to the replanted finger, attention should be paid during the rehabilitation period to avoid secondary injury, such as scalds, frostbite, and wounds.
10. Survival should not be the only sign of success. The definition of "success" should be associated with a good appearance and functional recovery. Children should be encouraged to use the hand to recover functioning.

References

Cheng GL, Pan ZD, Xu PC. Severed finger replantation in children. Natl Med J China. 1982;62(5):303–4.

Kleinert HE, Kadsan ML, Romero JL. Small blood vessel anastomosis for salvage of severely injured upper extremity. J Bone Joint Surg [Am]. 1963;45:788.

Komatsu S, Tamai S. Successful replantation of a completely cutoff thumb: case report. Plast Reconstr Surg. 1968;42:374–7.

Wang CQ, Fan QS, Cai JF. Severed finger replantation in children. Chin J Orthopaed. 1983;3(6):349–51.

11 Transpositional Replantation of Severed Fingers

11.1 Summary

Transpositional replantation is also known as ectopic replantation, when the hand suffers severe trauma, the digital body, such as the palm and fingers, is partially preserved relatively intact, but without being able to undergo in situ replantation. To restore the function of the hand as far as possible, make use of the severed fingers, and, according to the function, of the need to shift the area. The relatively minor finger is shifted to a relatively important position or to reconstruct a hand shape in a proximal limb. Reconstructing the hand function and utility avoids a second-stage operation and reduces the patient's pain and burden.

With the development of microsurgery techniques in recent years, transpositional replantation is not only a special type of reconstruction technique, but also a form of cosmetic plastic surgery. Doctors must have good clinical thinking and a precise microvascular anastomosis technique to accurately assess that the digital part could not be replanted in situ or good recovery of finger pinching and grasping would not be obtained, that the gripping and the main functions could even be replanted in situ, and full use should be made of the digital part to undertake transposition replantation to achieve relatively satisfactory limb morphology and functional reconstruction.

11.2 Case Presentation

Case 1: Transpositional Replantation of the Residual Thumb, Ring Finger, and Little Finger
Female patient, 38 years old, whose left hand was in pain and bleeding because of extrusion by an injection molding machine, was admitted within an hour. Physical examination: The general situation was good; the vital signs were stable. The left wrist had a serious defect, only the thumb and the proximal distal parts of the ring and little fingers were completely residual. We could see a bleeding, irregular wound with multiple fractures, tendon, blood vessel, and broken nerve ends. The residual fingers were without blood supply. The residual thumb, ring finger, and little finger were shifted and reset with metacarpal and radial alignment after satisfactory debridement under anesthesia, and fixed with 1.0-mm Kirschner wire. Then, the tendons, blood vessels, and nerves were anastomosed. The operation was successful and the tourniquet was relaxed. The fingers should be ruddy, with moderate tension. The patient was brought safely to the ward after the replanted fingers had been fixed with a sterile cotton bandage and padded with broken cotton yarn. After the operation, the patient was given conventional treatment, and by 2 weeks later, the replanted severed fingers had successfully survived. The growth and function were good after regular follow-up and functional exercise guidance (Figs. 11.1, 11.2, 11.3, 11.4, 11.5, 11.6, 11.7, 11.8, and 11.9).

J. Lin et al., *Special Type of Finger Replantation*, https://doi.org/10.1007/978-981-10-6229-2_11

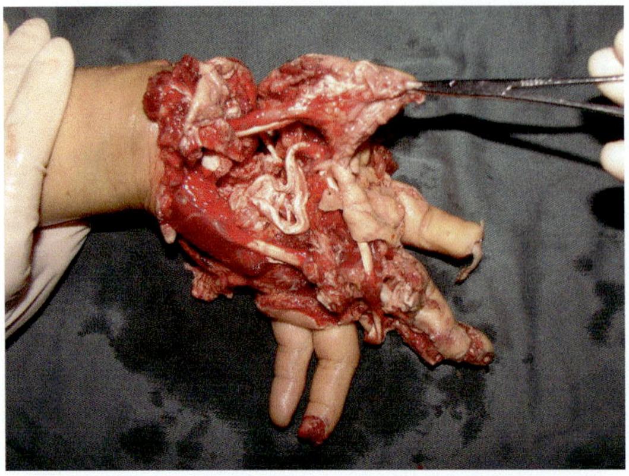

Fig. 11.1 The lateral view of the hand

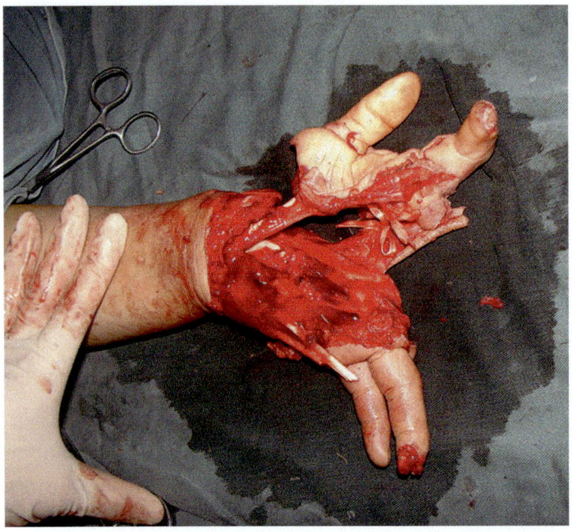

Fig. 11.2 The palm view of the hand

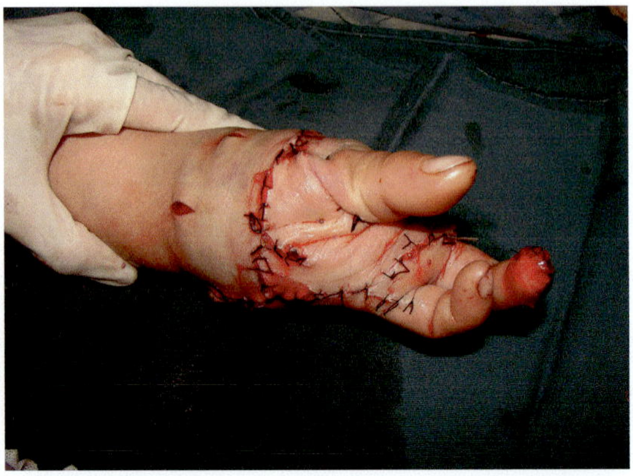

Fig. 11.3 The situation of the palm side after transpositional replantation

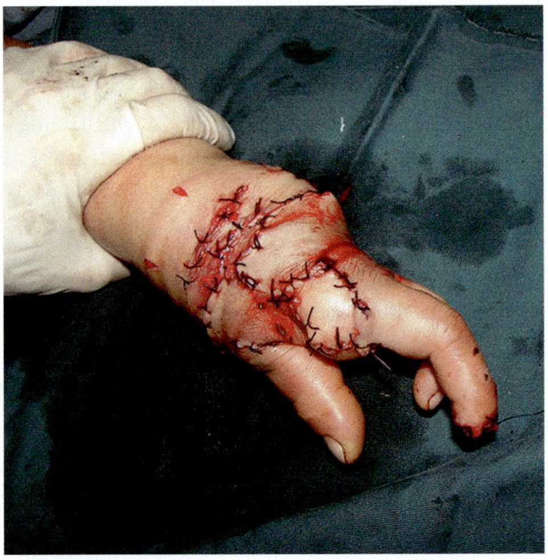

Fig. 11.4 The situation of the radial side after transpositional replantation

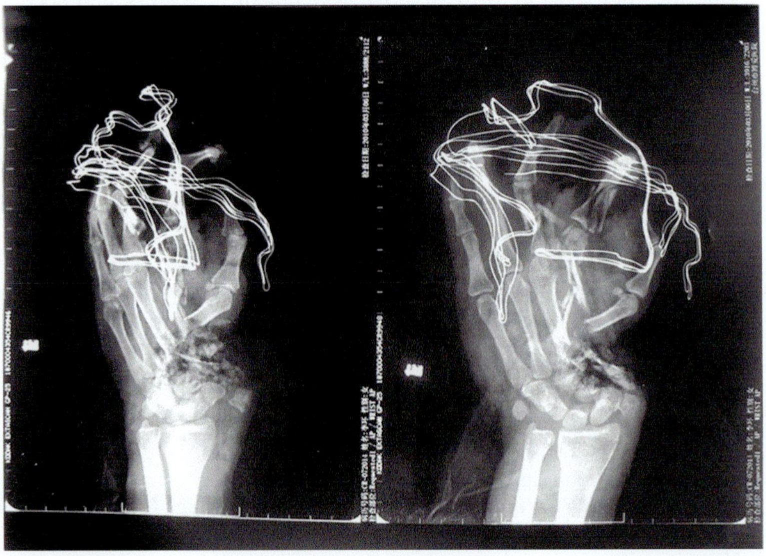

Fig. 11.5 The X-ray before surgery

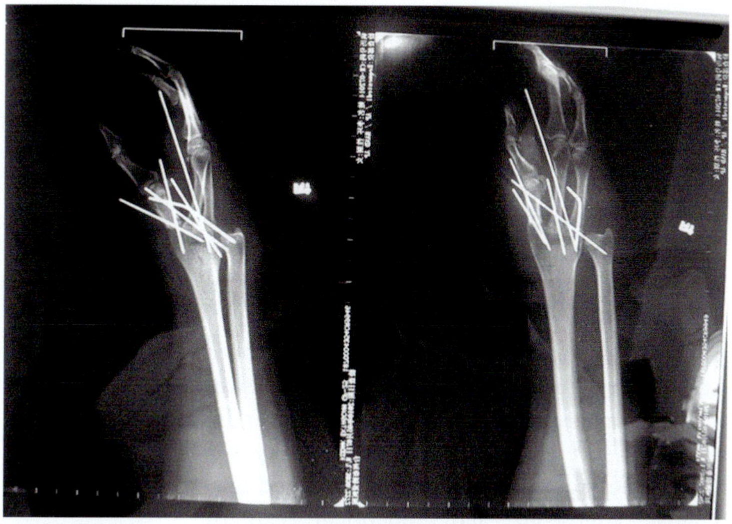

Fig. 11.6 The X-ray after surgery

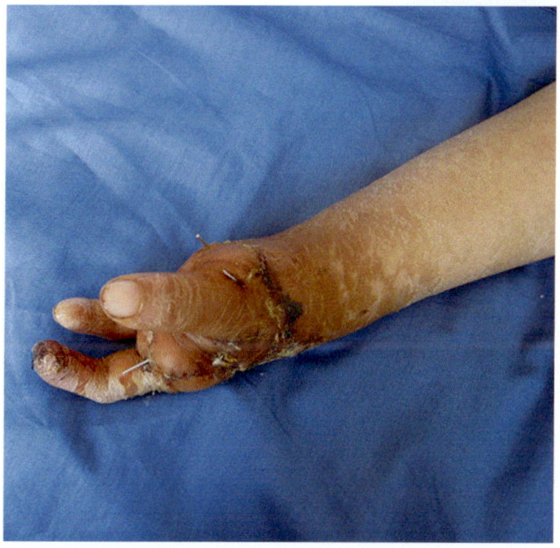

Fig. 11.7 Completely survived 2 weeks after surgery

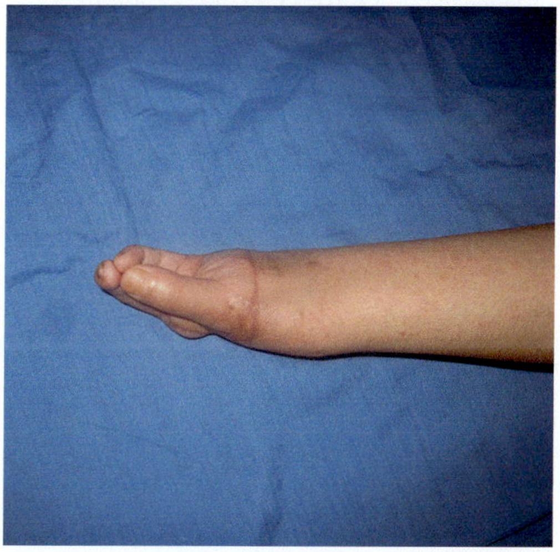

Fig. 11.9 The holding function of the fingers 15 months later

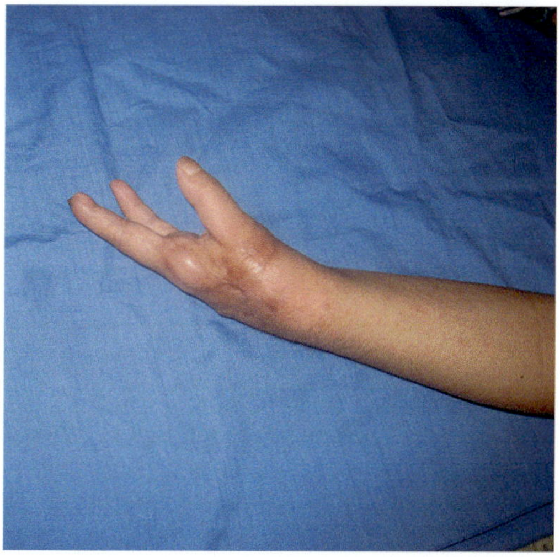

Fig. 11.8 The open function of the fingers 15 months later

Case 2: Transpositional Replantation of the Residual Part of the Ring and Little Finger to Reconstruct the Index Finger

Male patient, 35 years old, whose right hand was in pain and bleeding because of a punch, was admitted within 2 h. PE: The general situation was good; the vital signs were stable. The right palm stripes had a serious defect; only the thumb and the proximal distal parts of the middle and ring fingers were completely residual. Right palm, index finger, little finger, the proximal part of the middle and ring fingers were defective. We could see a bleeding, irregular wound with multiple fractures, tendon, blood vessels, and broken nerve ends. The residual fingers were without blood supply and seriously polluted. The residual proximal part of the ring and little fingers were shifted and reset with the second and third metacarpal after satisfactory debridement under anesthesia, and fixed with 1.0-mm Kirschner wire. Then, the tendons, blood vessels, and nerves were anastomosed. The operation was successful and the tourniquet was relaxed. The fingers should be ruddy, with moderate tension. The patient was brought safely to the ward after the replanted fingers had been fixed with a sterile cotton bandage and padded with broken cotton yarn. After the operation, the patient was given conventional treatment, and by 2 weeks later, the replanted severed fingers had successfully survived. The growth and function were good after regular follow-up and functional exercise guidance (Figs. 11.10, 11.11, 11.12, 11.13, 11.14, 11.15, 11.16, 11.17, and 11.18).

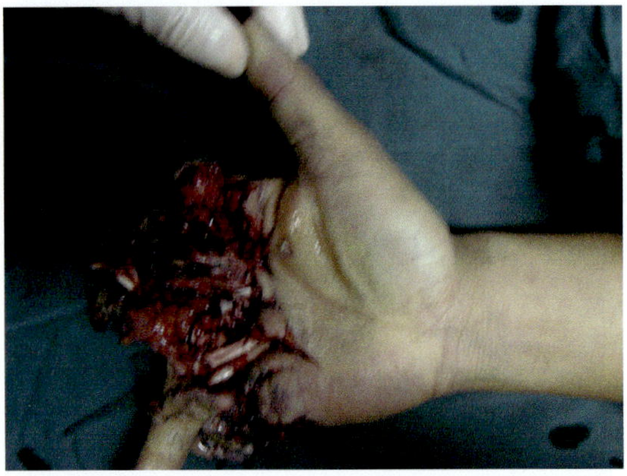

Fig. 11.10 The situation of the palm side

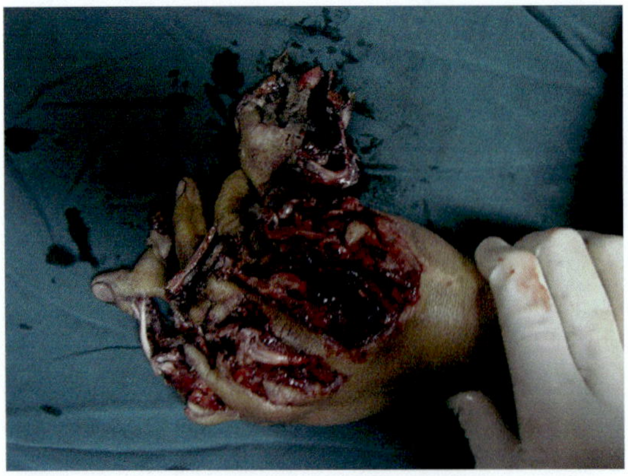

Fig. 11.11 The situation of the dorsal side

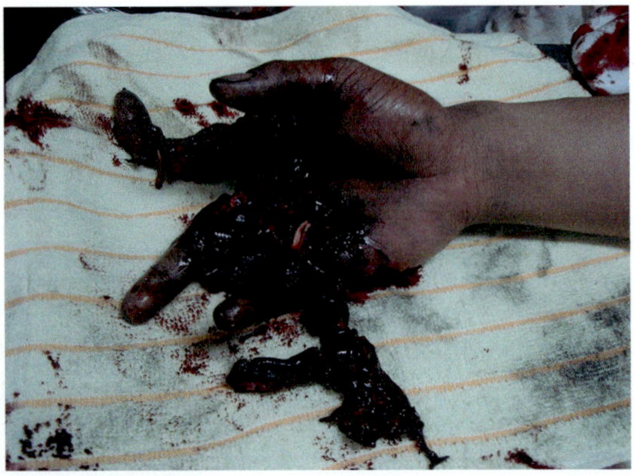

Fig. 11.12 The hand was seriously polluted

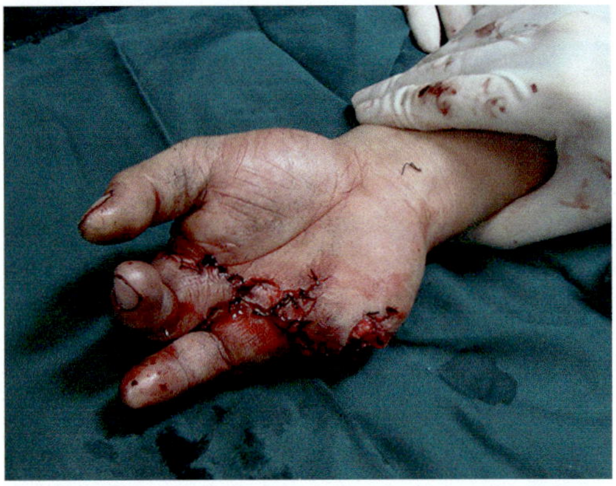

Fig. 11.13 The situation of the palm side after transpositional replantation

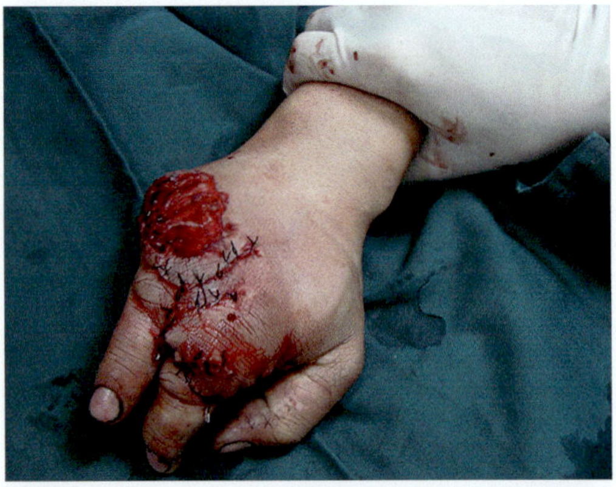

Fig. 11.14 The situation of the dorsal side after transpositional replantation

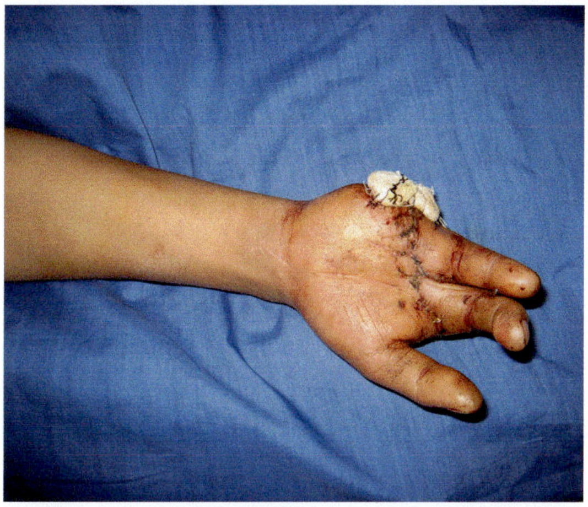

Fig. 11.15 The situation of the palm side after free skin graft

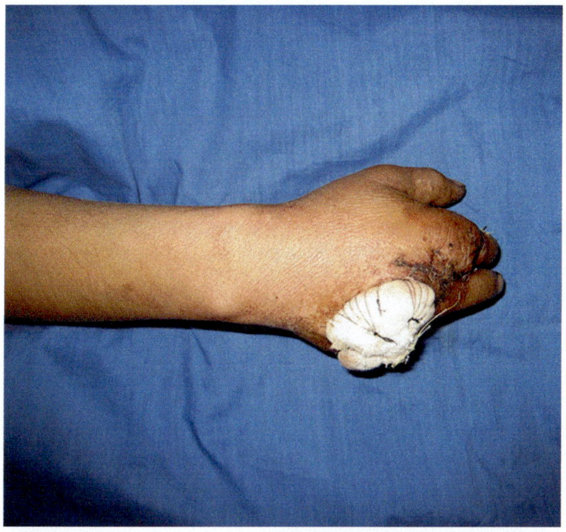

Fig. 11.16 The situation of the dorsal side after free skin graft

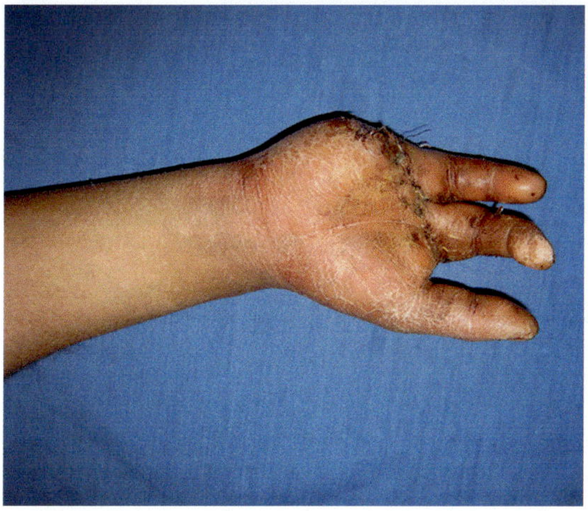

Fig. 11.17 The shape and functional guidance 2 months later

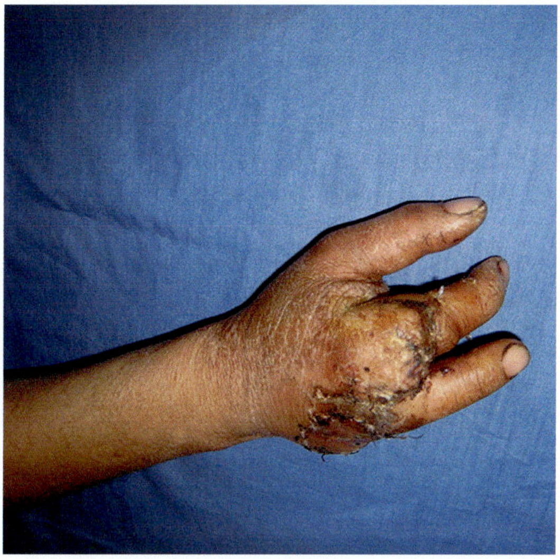

Fig. 11.18 The shape and functional guidance 2 months later

Case 3: Transpositional Replantation of the Residual Part of the Ring and Little Fingers to Reconstruct the Middle and Ring Fingers
Male patient, 20 years old, whose right hand was in pain and bleeding because of an electric saw, was admitted within 1.5 h. PE: The general situation was good; the vital signs were stable. There was a longitudinal oblique wound in the right hand. Fingertips of the index finger, proximal distal part of the middle finger were defective. The ring and little fingers were broken off. Only the skin of the ulnar side of the palm was connected. The proximal distal parts of the ring and little fingers were completely residual but without blood supply. We could see a bleeding, irregular wound with multiple fractures, tendon, blood vessels, and broken nerve ends. The residual proximal part of the middle, ring, and little fingers and the middle section of the ring finger were shifted and reset to reconstruct the middle and ring fingers after satisfactory debridement under anesthesia, and fixed with 1.0-mm Kirschner wire. Then, the tendons, blood vessels, and nerves were anastomosed. The operation was successful and the tourniquet was relaxed. The fingers should be ruddy, and with moderate tension. The patient was brought safely to the ward after the replanted fingers had been fixed with a sterile cotton bandage and padded with broken cotton yarn. After the operation, the patient was given conventional treatment, and by 2 weeks

later, the replanted severed fingers had successfully survived. The growth and function were good after regular follow-up and functional exercise guidance (Figs. 11.19, 11.20, 11.21, 11.22, 11.23, 11.24, 11.25, 11.26, and 11.27).

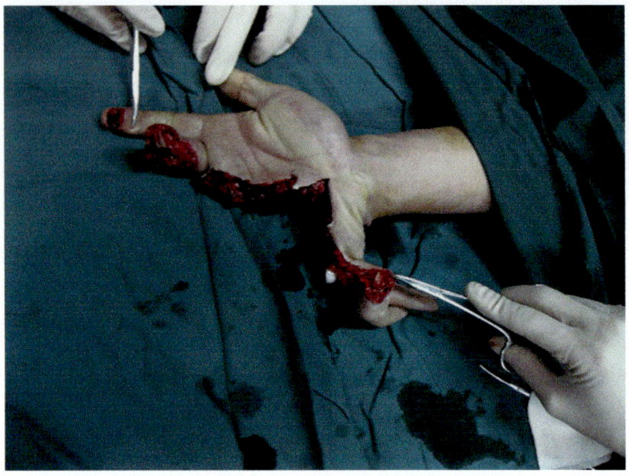

Fig. 11.19 The palm side of the hand

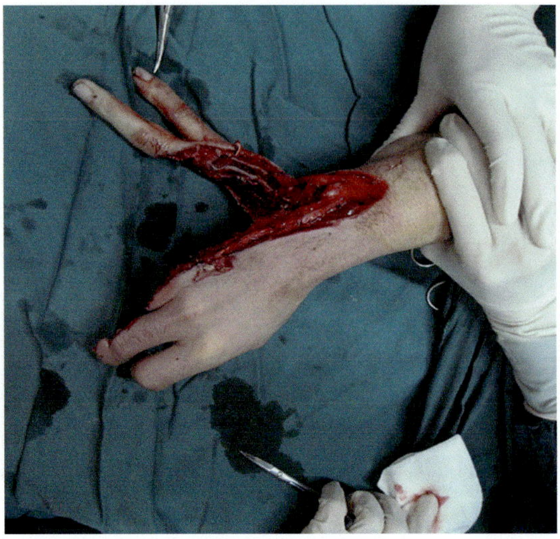

Fig. 11.20 The dorsal side of the hand

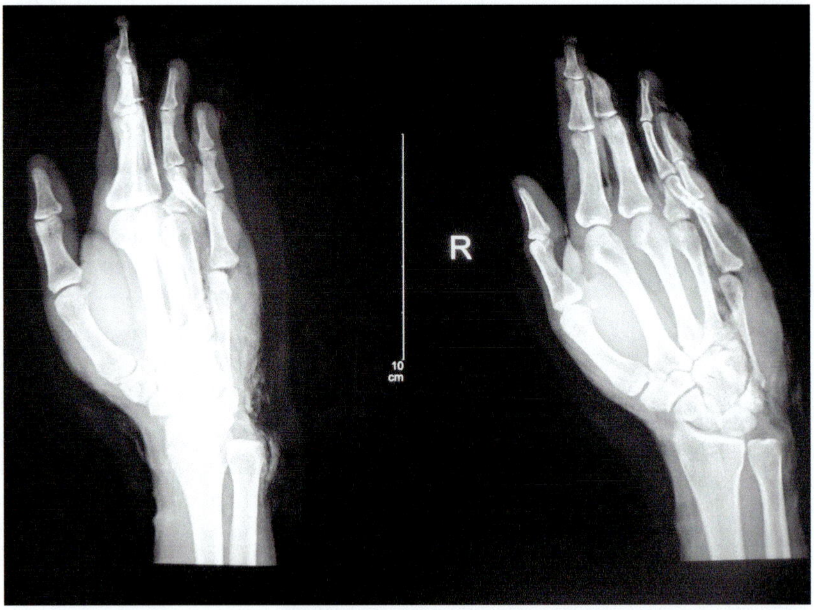

Fig. 11.21 The X-ray before surgery

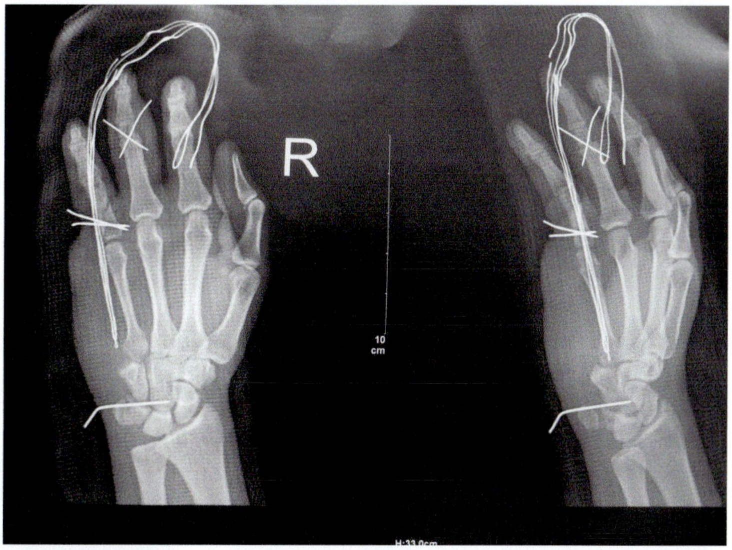

Fig. 11.22 The X-ray after surgery

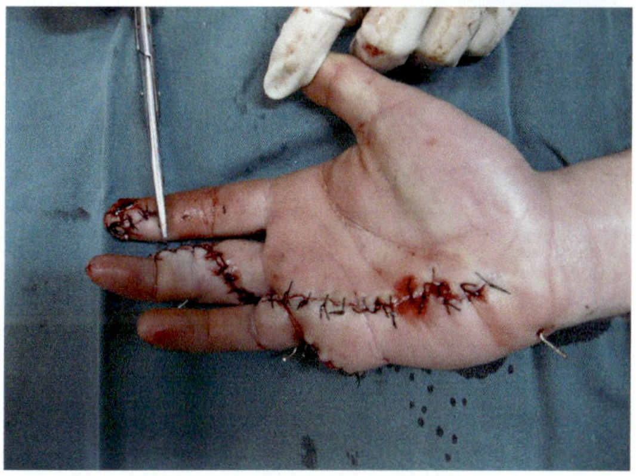

Fig. 11.23 The palm side after the surgery

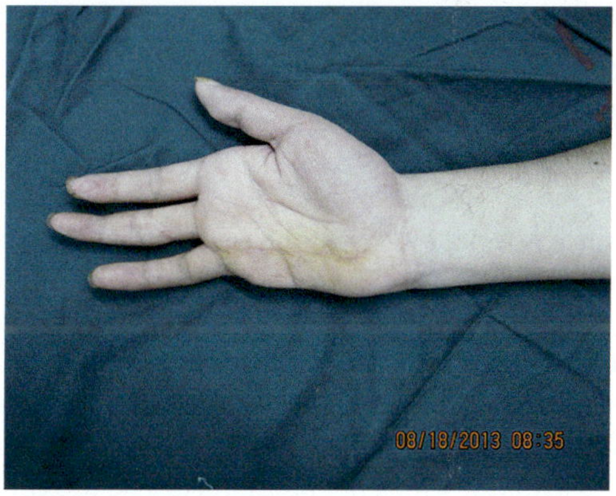

Fig. 11.25 The open function of the fingers 12 months later (palm side)

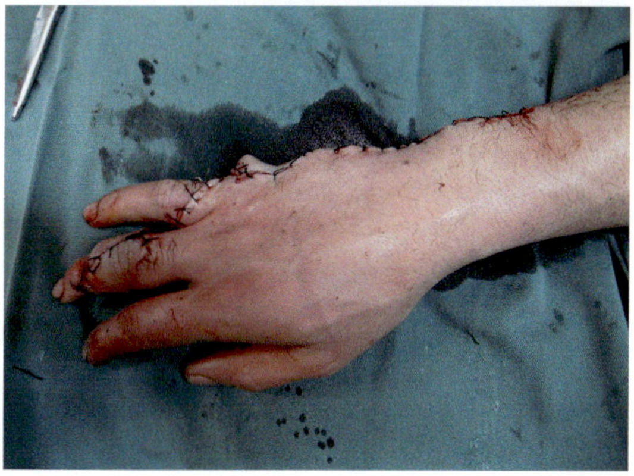

Fig. 11.24 The dorsal side after the surgery

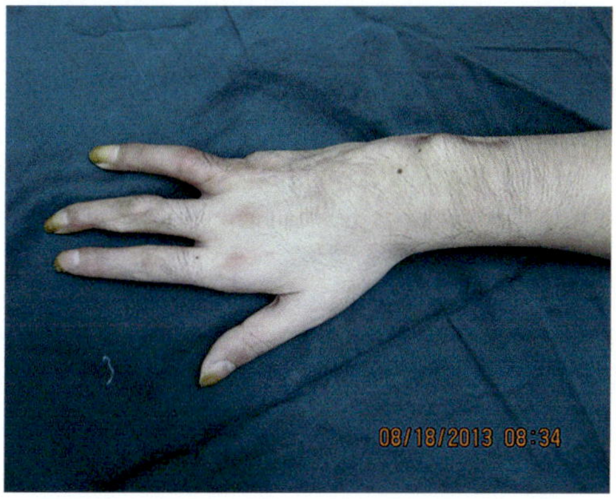

Fig. 11.26 The open function of the fingers 12 months later (dorsal side)

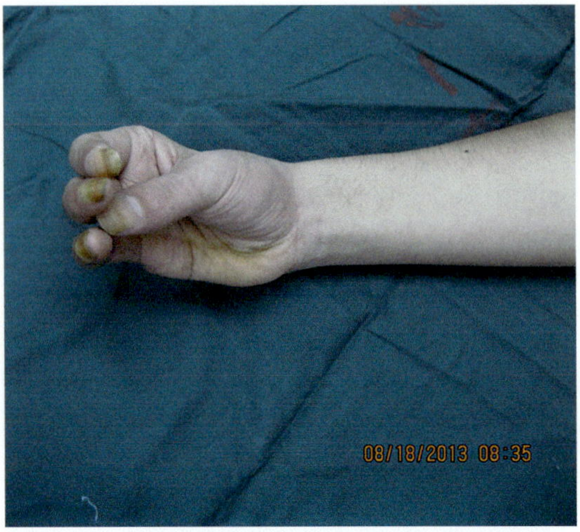

Fig. 11.27 The holding function of the fingers 12 months later

Case 4: Transpositional Replantation of the Residual Part of the Index Finger to Reconstruct the Thumb

Male patient, 46 years old, whose right hand was in pain and bleeding because of a die hot press injury, was admitted within 1 h. PE: The general situation was good; the vital signs were stable. There was a longitudinal oblique wound in the right hand (from the second fingerwebs to the ulnar wrist crease), about 7 cm*2 cm. The soft tissue of the proximal distal part of the thumb was avulsed, with a hot press trace. The proximal part of the index finger was defective (metacarpophalangeal joint was seriously damaged), the proximal distal\part of the index finger was complete, but without blood supply. We could see a bleeding, irregular wound with multiple fractures, tendon, blood vessels, and broken nerve ends. The blood supply of the third to fifth fingers was not good. The residual middle part of the index finger was shifted and reset to the proximal part of the thumb after satisfactory debridement under anesthesia, and was fixed with 1.0-mm Kirschner wire. Then, the tendons, blood vessels, and nerves were anastomosed. The operation was successful and the tourniquet was relaxed. The finger should be ruddy, and with moderate tension. The patient was brought safely to the ward after the replanted finger had been fixed with a sterile cotton bandage and padded with broken cotton yarn. After the operation, the patient was given conventional treatment, and by 2 weeks later, the replanted severed finger had successfully survived. The growth and function are good after regular follow-up and functional exercise guidance (Figs. 11.28, 11.29, 11.30, 11.31, 11.32, 11.33, 11.34, 11.35, and 11.36).

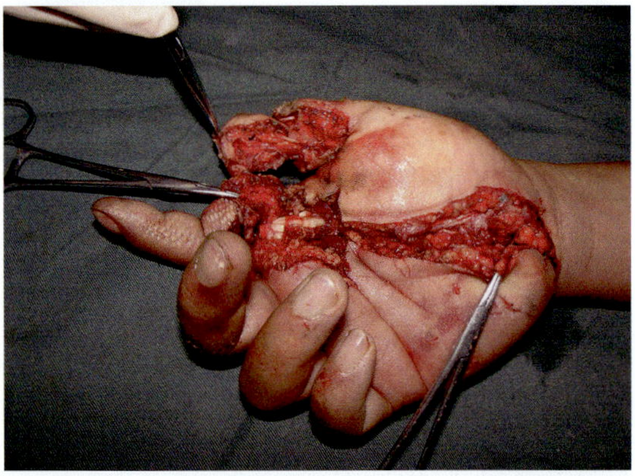

Fig. 11.28 The palm side of the hand

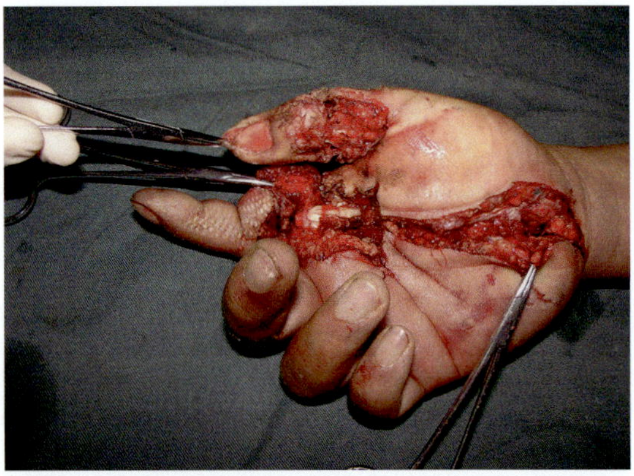

Fig. 11.29 Damage to the dorsal surface of the right thumb

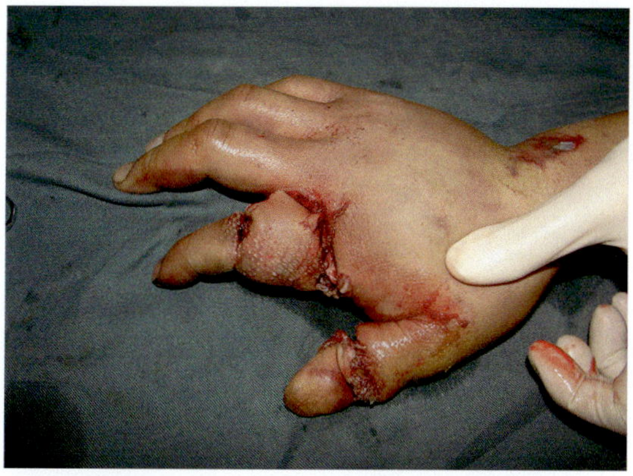

Fig. 11.30 The dorsal side of the hand

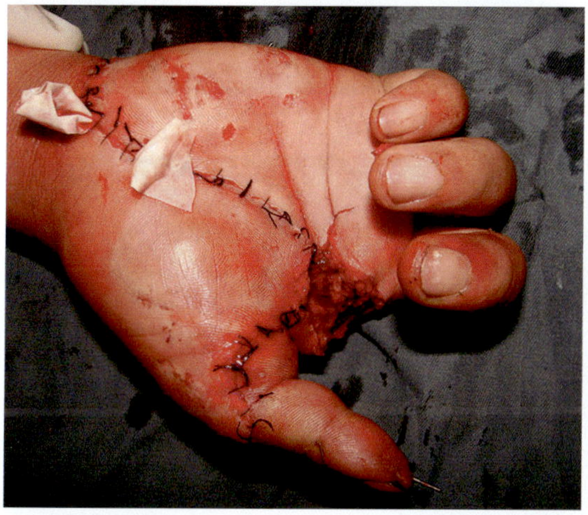

Fig. 11.31 The palm side after surgery

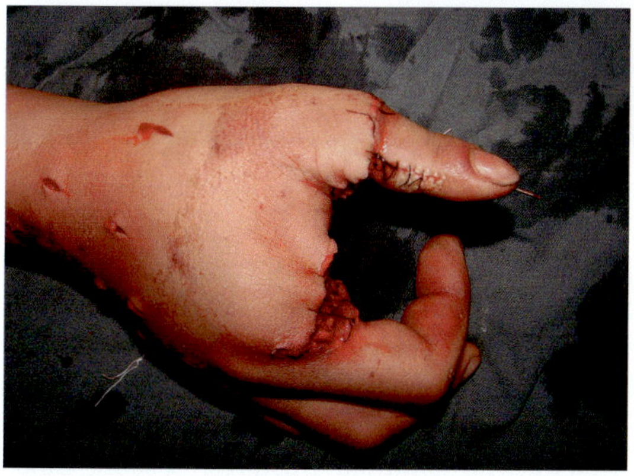

Fig. 11.32 The dorsal side after surgery

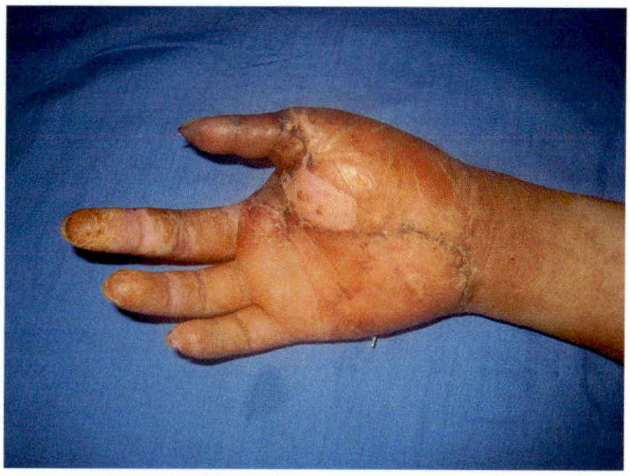

Fig. 11.33 The palm side 3 months later

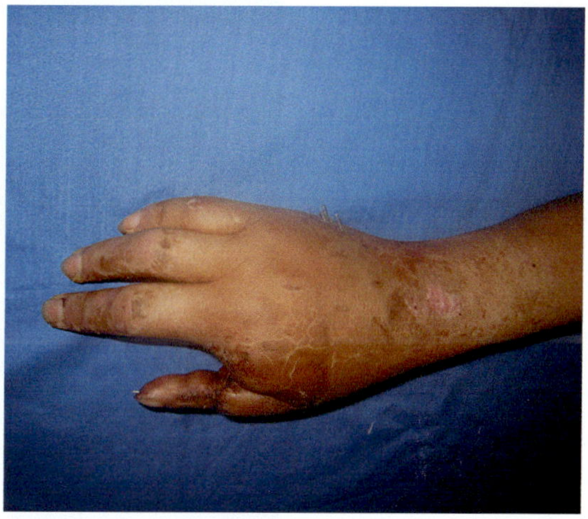

Fig. 11.34 The dorsal side 3 months later

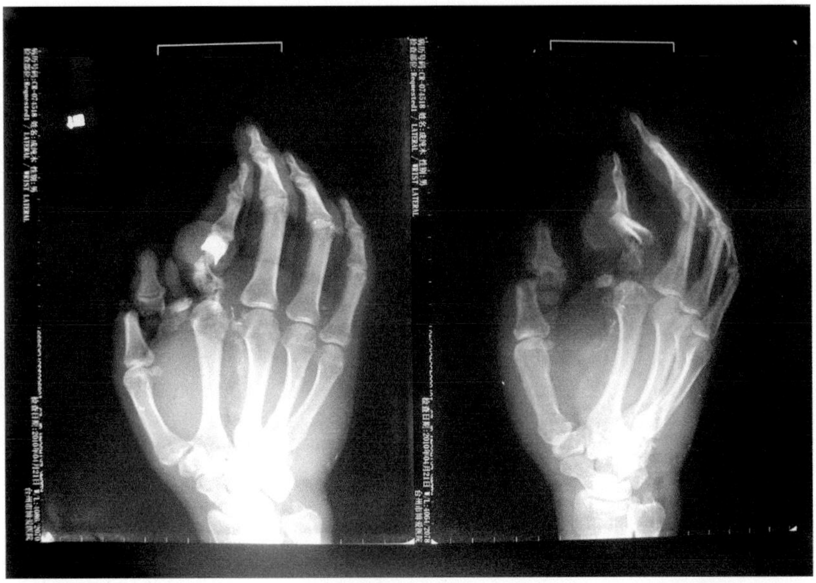

Fig. 11.35 The X-ray before surgery

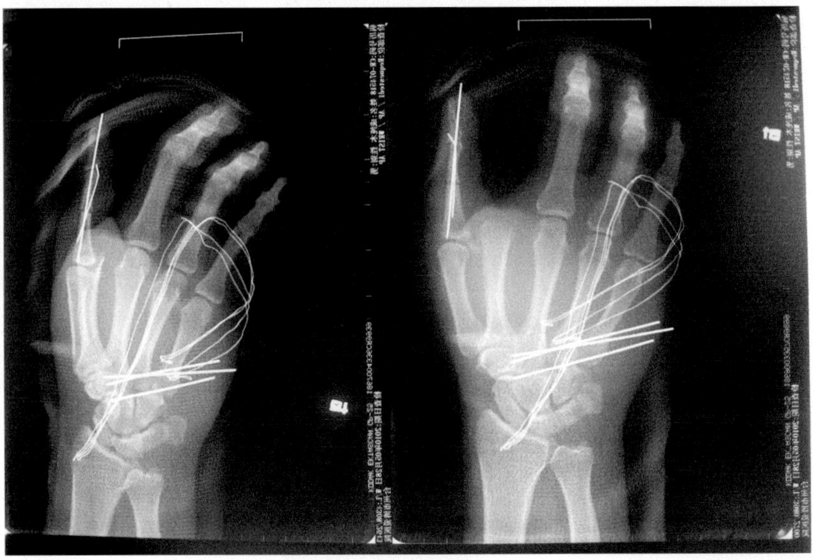

Fig. 11.36 The X-ray after surgery

Case 5: Transpositional Replantation of the Residual Part of the Middle and Little Fingers to Reconstruct the Hand Function

Male patient, 53 years old, whose right hand was in pain and bleeding because of a lathe injury, was admitted within 3 h. PE: The general situation was good; the vital signs were stable. The right proximal palmar crease to the proximal distal part of the index finger was destroyed, whereas the middle and little fingers were relatively complete. They were connected by the proximal end of the tendon, blood vessels, and nerves. The skin of the ring finger was contused and the tendon, blood vessels, and nerves were avulsed. Most of ulnar side of the palm was defective; the thumb was intact. We could see a bleeding, irregular wound with multiple fractures, tendon, blood vessels, and broken nerve ends. The residual proximal parts of the middle and little fingers were shifted and reset to the third and fourth metacarpals after satisfactory debridement under anesthesia, and fixed with 1.0-mm Kirschner wire. Then, the tendons, blood vessels, and nerves were anastomosed. The operation was successful and the tourniquet was relaxed. The fingers should be ruddy, with moderate tension. The patient was brought safely to the ward after the replanted fingers had been fixed with a sterile cotton bandage and padded with broken cotton yarn. After the operation, the patient was given conventional treatment, and by 2 weeks later, the replanted severed fingers had successfully survived. The growth and function were good after regular follow-up and functional exercise guidance (Figs. 11.37, 11.38, 11.39, 11.40, 11.41, 11.42, 11.43, 11.44, and 11.45).

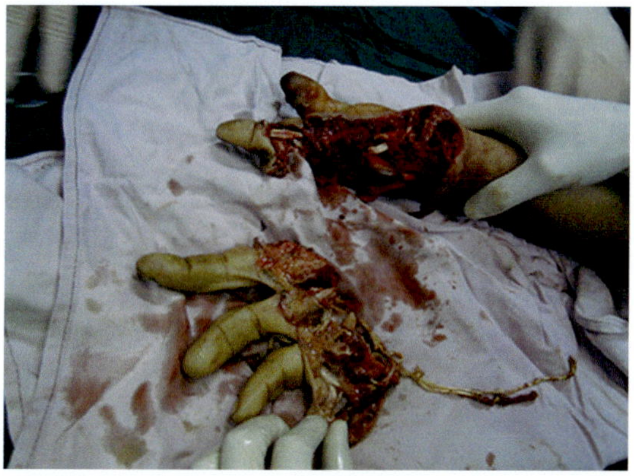

Fig. 11.37 The palm side of the hand

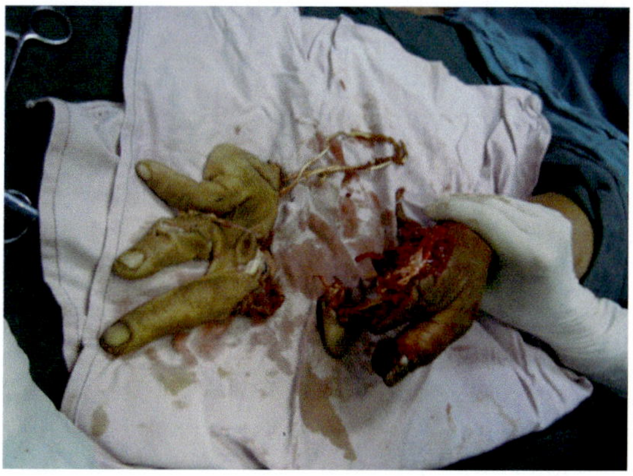

Fig. 11.38 The dorsal side of the hand

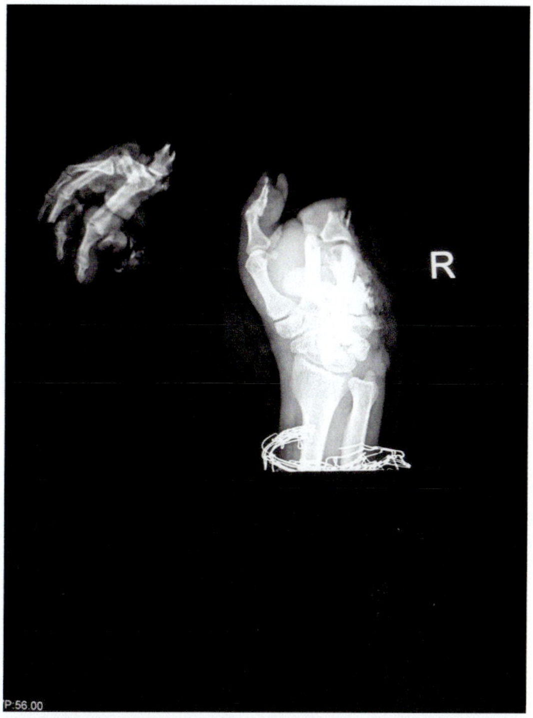

Fig. 11.39 The X-ray before surgery

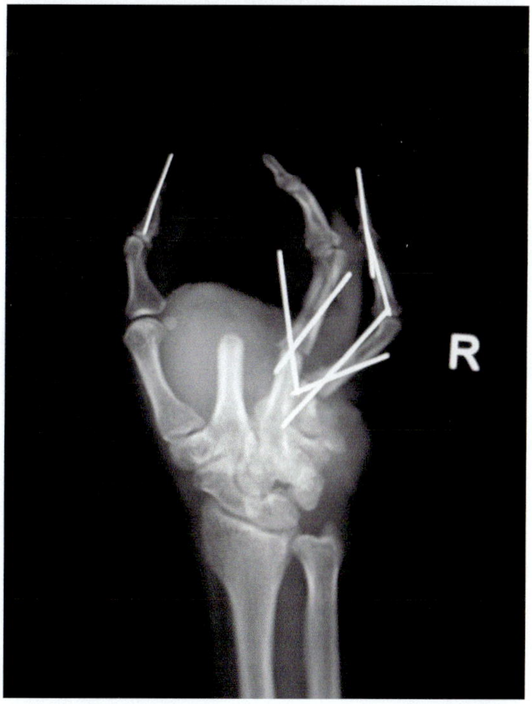

Fig. 11.40 The X-ray after surgery

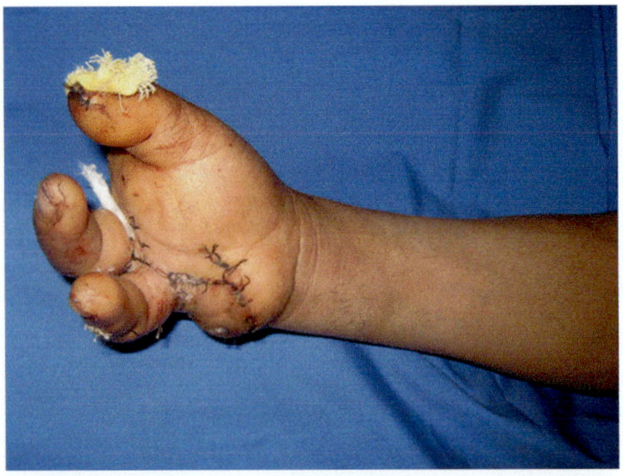

Fig. 11.41 The palm side 2 weeks later

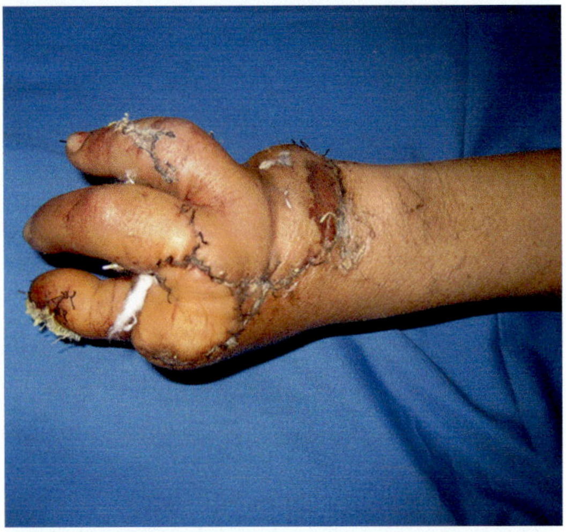

Fig. 11.42 The dorsal side 2 weeks later

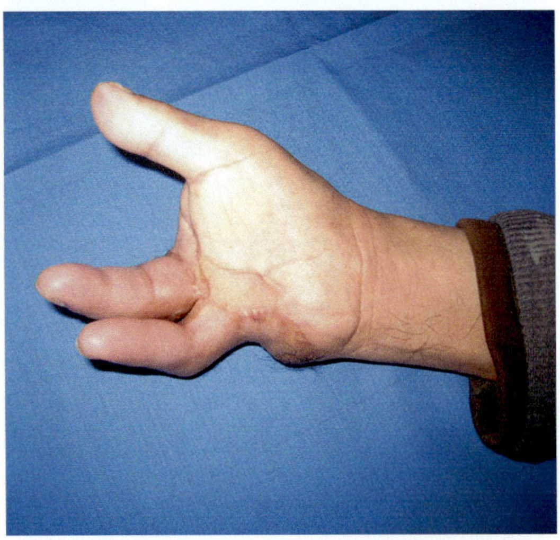

Fig. 11.43 The open function of the fingers 18 months later (palm side)

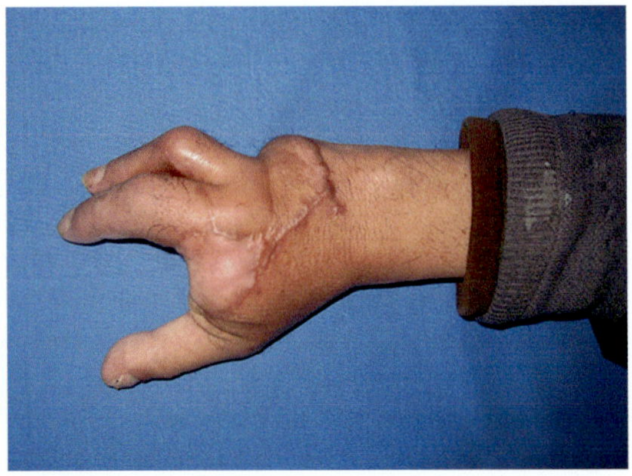

Fig. 11.44 The open function of the fingers 18 months later (dorsal side)

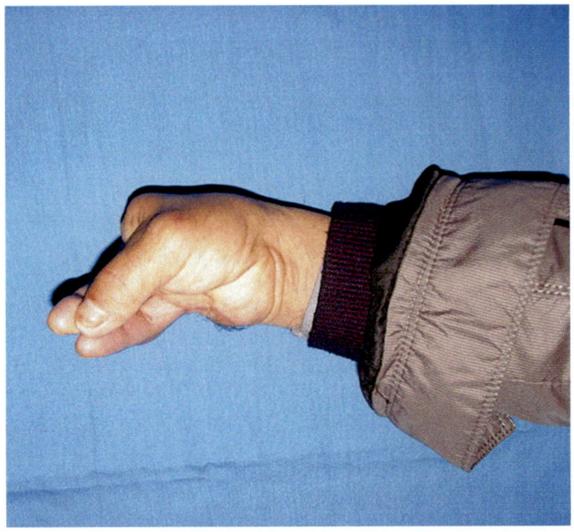

Fig. 11.45 The holding function of the fingers 18 months later

11.3 Key Points

(a) The transpositional replantation of the thumb should be first considered, then the index finger, middle finger, ring finger, and little finger in sequence.

(b) When we select the severed body, we should focus on the site near the joint, and the whole joint will be even better. Phalanxes have different diameters, in which the thumb is bigger than that fixed with Kirschner wire. We should pay attention to the phalanges of the flush, so that the back flat and dorsal digital vein anastomosis have a good vascular bed.

(c) Retain the organization as far as possible to avoid the excision being too short. Nerves and blood vessels cannot be free too long to be cut out. The length of a phalanx should be more than 0.5 cm shorter than the retained tendon, blood vessels, nerves, skin, and soft tissue.

(d) The bone can be fixed not only with Kirschner wire, but also with wire wrapped in and "figure of 8" shape and screws. In the practical operation, the longitudinal fixation of the needle is simple and reliable, and can save the operating time, although it has a certain effect on postoperative joint activity.

(e) Choose the less injured tendon to be sutured to the tendon of the severed finger. The tension should be appropriate, without corner and wrinkles, using a 3-0 non-invasive suturing needle. To avoid bone–tendon adhesion, the tendon bed is repaired with a deep fascia, so that the tendon can be isolated from the bone.

(f) Vascular anastomosis: The proximal vein is easy to find, mostly in the dorsal part; also, the finger vein in the back of the hand. Choose a suitable diameter and make an end-to-end anastomosis in 10–12 stitches. Choose the radial or ulnar artery to anastomose with the total artery or the finger artery of the replantated finger. There are always difficulties with the wide gap, which can be solved by the end-to-side method and the blood vessel. In addition, if the arteriovenous blood vessel is not directly anastomosed, it is necessary to transfer the remaining vein or forearm vein to reconstruct the arteriovenous vessel.

(g) Nerve repair: Special attention should be paid to nerve repair. The nerves on both sides should be anastomosed as far as possible and early functional exercise should be undertaken as soon as possible. If the nerve defect cannot be directly identified, the finger function can be reconstructed by using a healthy residual nerve or the transplanted gastrocnemius nerve.

(h) Skin sutures should not be too tight: A rubber piece should be left for drainage to prevent local bleeding or hematoma formation and oppress the venous drainage. This can be removed after 48 h. We should pay attention to the maintenance of the finger when dressing, and immobilize the hand with the front and rear plaster.

11.4 Notes

(a) The physician should understand the mechanism of injury and wound conditions and should make a prognosis and decide whether to perform the surgery.

(b) This type of finger may be seriously compressed and polluted. In the emergency department we should not only completely remove the loss of living tissues, but we should also not remove too much of the normal tissue, as this is important in preventing infection and ensuring the success of the operation.

(c) When the fingers are connected, we should pay attention to the vein near the dorsal part to prevent damage.

(d) The margin must be accurate and uniform, and the knot should be gently lifted, preventing varus anastomosis. Operation requires stability, lightness, and speed.

(e) After transposition, the size of the finger and blood vessels will be a problem. We should adjust and match them according to the anatomical characteristics and a variety of vascular anastomosis methods should be undertaken, especially at the site of vascular anastomosis. Anticoagulant use should be strengthened to prevent a blood circulation crisis.

(f) Survival should not be the only sign of success. The definition of "success" should be associated with good appearance and functional recovery. Children should be encouraged to use the hand and recover the function.

(g) The nursing of the patient is most important. Let the parents actively cooperate with the treatment to get the best results.

Suggested Reading

Cai JF, Wang CQ. Transposition replantation of severed finger. Chin J Orthopaed. 1987;7:101.

Cai YM, Lin CZ, Qu XY, et al. To summarize the clinical special type of replantation. Chin J Microsurg. 2004;27(3):219–20.

Chen XM, Feng CC, Liu MW, et al. First phase shift finger blast injury 8 cases of thumb reconstruction. Peoples Mil Surg. 1996;11:62.

Chen JZ, Yin DC, Wu KJ. Palmar wrist severed finger replantation ectopic lesion emergency hand reconstruction. Chin J Hand Surg. 2000a;16(2):104.

Chen JZ, Wu KJ, Zhang YW, et al. Palmar wrist severed finger replantation ectopic lesion emergency hand reconstruction. Chin J Microsurg. 2000b;23(1):54.

Cheng GL. Review and prospect of finger replantation. Chin J Hand Surg. 2000;16(2):65–7.

Cheng GL, Pan ZD, Xu PC. Severed finger replantation in children. Natl Med J China. 1982;62(5):303–4.

Cheng GL, Pan DD, Zhang NP, Fang GR. Digital replantation in children: a long-term follow-up study. J Hand Surg Am. 1998;23(4):635–46.

Gong ZF, Gao WY, Zhi L, et al. 28 reports of transposition replantation of severed fingers. J Wenzhou Med Coll. 1997;27(3):135–6.

Jian F. The application of finger tip bloodletting in replantation of distal section of finger of children. Jilin Med J. 2014;35(21):4705–6.

Kleinert HE, Kadsan ML, Romero JL. Small blood vessel anastomosis for salvage of severely injured upper extremity. J Bone Joint Surg [Am]. 1963;45:788.

Komatsu S, Tamai S. Successful replantation of a completely cutoff thumb: case report. Plast Reconstr Surg. 1968;42:374–7.

Liao JW, Zhang ZW, Zhuang JC, et al. A case of double forearm stump finger ectopic replantation and reconstruct hand function. Chin J Hand Surg. 2009;25(2):88.

Lin YQ, Wu JF, Zhen JZ. Experience of transposition replantation of the residual part of the severed fingers to reconstruct the thumb and index finger. Fujian Med J. 2000;22(5):42.

Shou KS, Lei X, Rui YJ, et al. Follow up of functional reconstruction of thumb subemergency. Chin J Microsurg. 1999;15(4):228.

Wang YH, Fu SH. The cooperation and experience of replantation in a one year and a half child. Chin Med Mod Dist Educ China. 2011;9(6):130.

Wang CQ, Fan QS, Cai JF. Severed finger replantation in children. Chin J Orthopaed. 1983;3(6):349–51.

Zhang GL, et al. The stump of the forearm and finger transposition replantation: report of six cases. Chin J Orthopaed. 1990;10(4):249.

Zhang WW, Hong C, Xin W, et al. Severed finger replantation of special types. Chin J Hand Surg. 2003;19(3):135–8.

Zhang FH, Hu YX, Jiang X. Clinical observation of 10 cases of forearm stump finger ectopic replantation and reconstruct hand function. Zhejiang Clin Med J. 2014;3:377–8.

Zhao ZW, Zhou ZH, Liu XL, et al. The treatment of severed fingers under 3 year-old children. Inner Mongolia Med J. 2006;38(9):815–7.

Zhou JH, Wang FP, Li GQ. 2 cases of ectopic joint replantation using left palm. Chin J Pract Hand Surg. 2011;25(1):71.

12 Replantation of the Final Segment of the Finger (Finger Tip)

12.1 Summary

The final segment of the finger is the furthest structure of the hand, the most frequently used in daily life, and has the highest rate of injury; thus, replantation of the final segment of the finger (fingertip) is common. The functioning of the finger will be seriously affected if the final segment is missing, even though it is small. Compared with the flap method of retaining the length of the finger, replantation is irreplaceable in the recovery of appearance, movement, and feeling. In principle, if the systemic condition of the patients permitted it, if the structure of the severed finger was more or less complete, and if patients and their families required replantation, replantation should be chosen whenever possible.

According to the anatomical features of the fingers, Grayson's ligament of the final segment is relatively weak. Most finger arteries and veins will be severed with the distal tissue and the risk of disengaged injury is low; thus, the microcirculation of the severed part will be complete or partially damaged. Replantation of the final segment of the finger (fingertip) will survive with low blood supply as it is small and the tolerance of ischemia and lack of oxygen is strong. Since then, the survival rate of the replanted final segment (fingertip) will be higher, but microsurgical techniques will be more frequently required, especially in multiple severed fingers and multi-plane severed fingers, a long-term surgical ability will also be required.

12.2 Case Description

Case 1: Replantation of the Final Segment of the Right Ring Finger

Male patient, 38 years old, was admitted to hospital for the severed final segment of the right ring finger caused by die extrusion and bleeding for 1.5 h. Physical examination: The general situation was good; the vital signs were stable. The distal part was completely severed from the base of the nail of the right ring finger, revealing bone, an uneven wound, and bleeding. The blood supply to the rest of the fingers was good. Successful debridement and replantation were undertaken under anesthesia under emergency conditions. The replanted finger was red and there was moderate tension after relaxing the tourniquet. It was packed with sterile gauze and padded with broken cotton yarn and the patient was brought back to the ward safely. The patient was given conventional treatments after the operation, such as antibiotics, hormones, and antispasmodics. By 10 days later, the replanted severed finger had successfully survived. The appearance and function were good after regular follow-up and functional exercise guidance, and the needle was withdrawn after 8–10 weeks (Figs. 12.1, 12.2, 12.3, 12.4, 12.5, and 12.6).

J. Lin et al., *Special Type of Finger Replantation*, https://doi.org/10.1007/978-981-10-6229-2_12

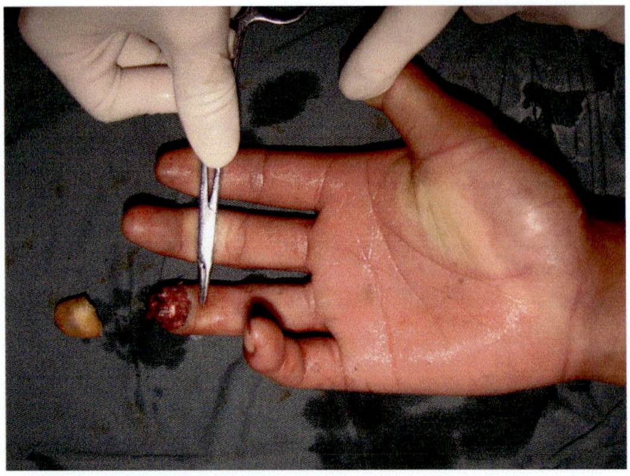

Fig. 12.1 The palm side of the severed finger

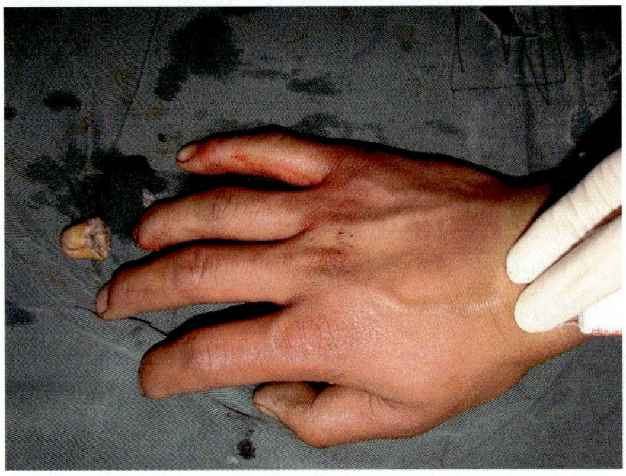

Fig. 12.2 The dorsal side of the severed finger

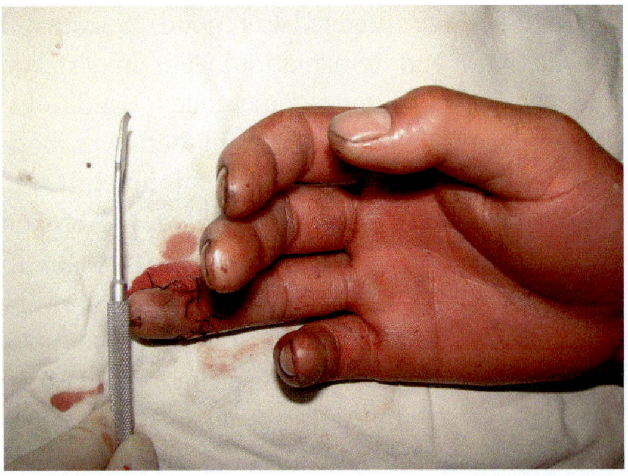

Fig. 12.3 Blood supply situation in the palm side during the operation

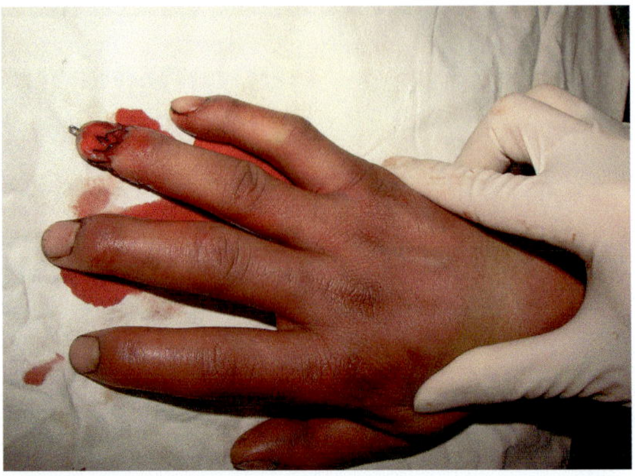

Fig. 12.4 Blood supply situation on the dorsal side during the operation

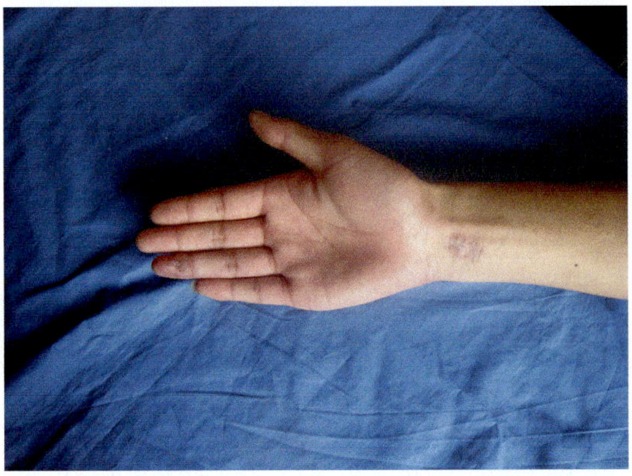

Fig. 12.5 Appearance 8 months later

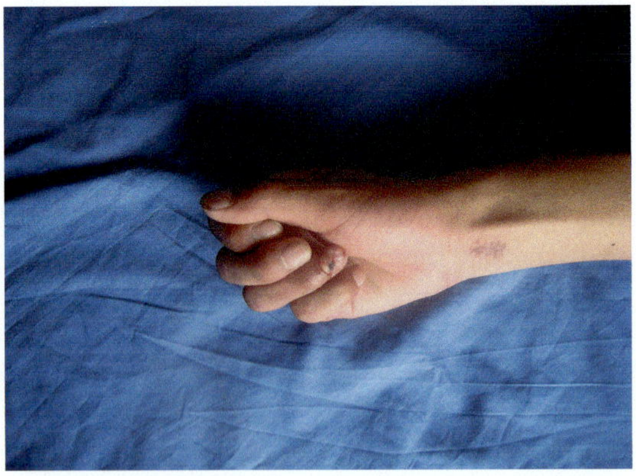

Fig. 12.6 Fist function 8 months later

Case 2: Replantation of Final Segment of the Left Middle and Ring Fingers

Male patient, 33 years old, was admitted to hospital for final-segment severing of the left middle and ring finger caused by a lathe and bleeding for 2 h. PE: The general situation was good; the vital signs were stable. The distal parts were completely severed and the bone was revealed, there were uneven wounds, bleeding, and the blood supply to the rest of the fingers was good. Successful debridement and replantation were performed under anesthesia under emergency conditions. The replanted fingers were red and had moderate tension after relaxing the tourniquet. They were packed with sterile gauze, padded with broken cotton yarn, and the patient was brought back to ward safely. He was given conventional treatments after the operation, such as antibiotics, hormones, and antispasmodic. And By 10 days later, the replanted severed fingers had successfully survived. The appearance and function were good after regular follow-up and functional exercise guidance, and the needles were withdrawn after 8–10 weeks (Figs. 12.7, 12.8, 12.9, 12.10, 12.11, and 12.12).

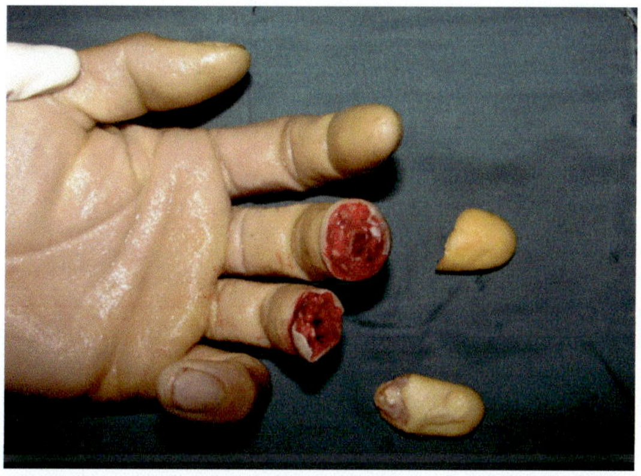

Fig. 12.7 The palm side of the severed fingers

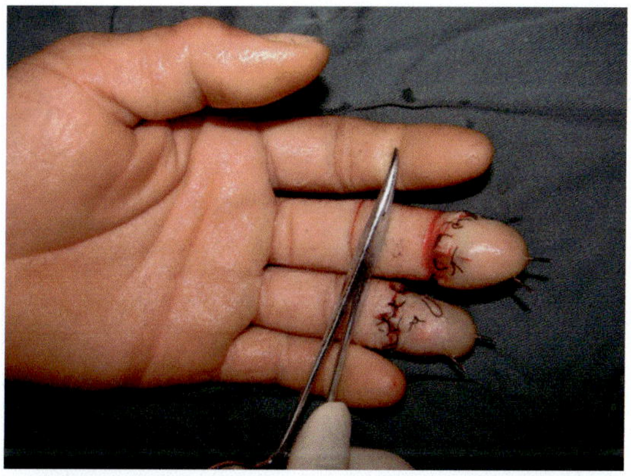

Fig. 12.9 Blood supply situation on the palm side during the operation

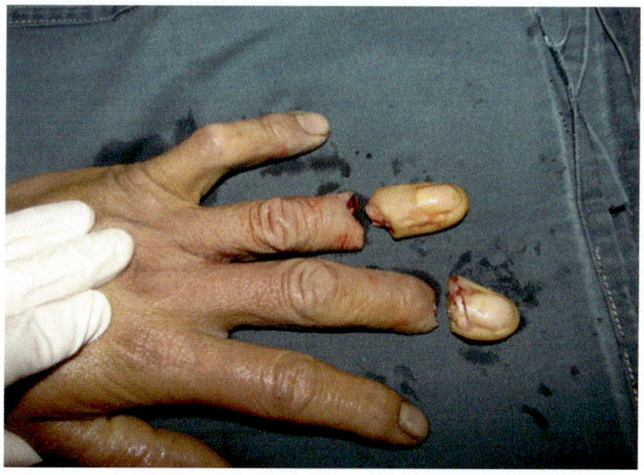

Fig. 12.8 The dorsal side of the severed fingers

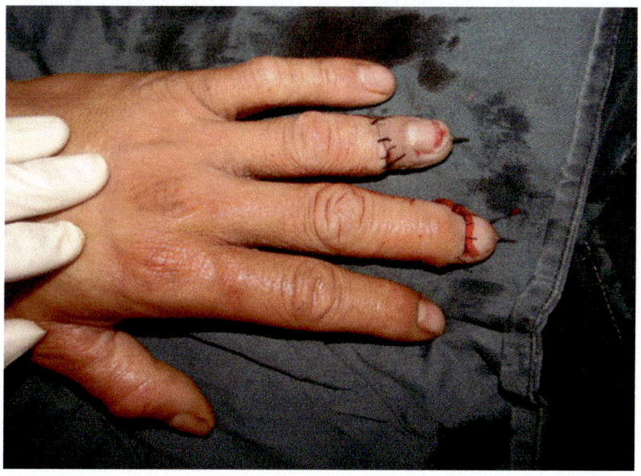

Fig. 12.10 Blood supply situation on the dorsal side during the operation

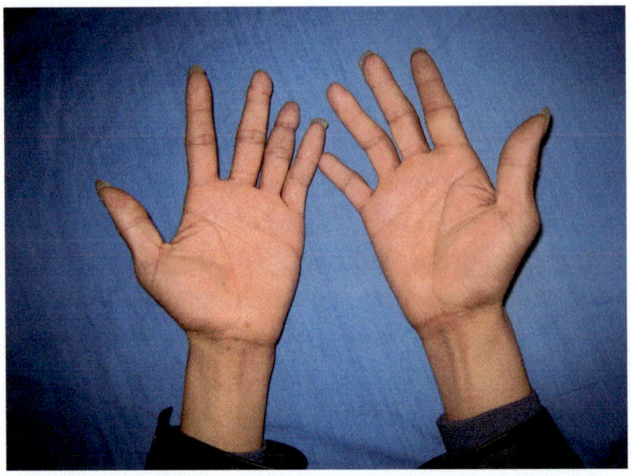

Fig. 12.11 Appearance and function 13 months later

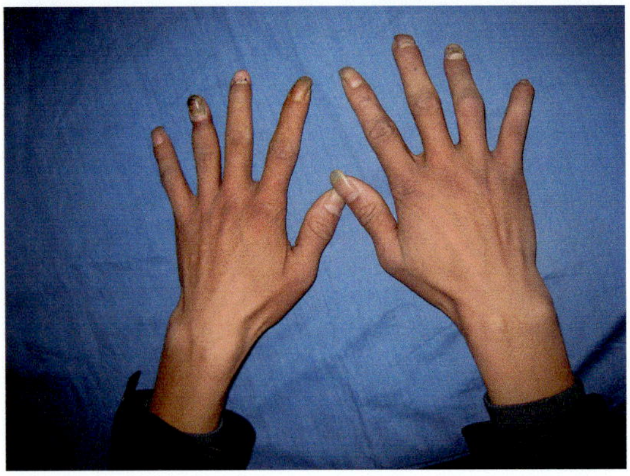

Fig. 12.12 Appearance and function 13 months later

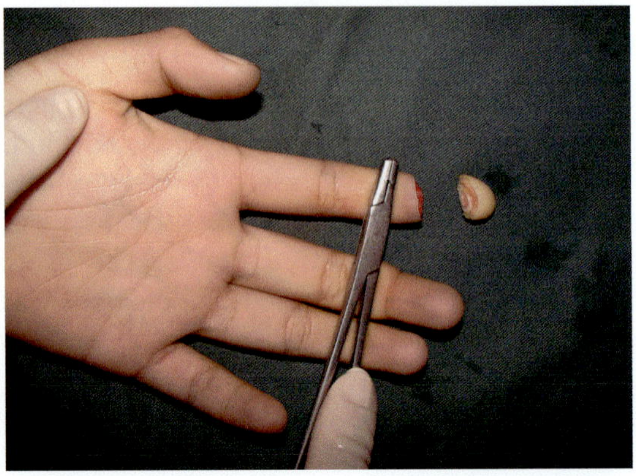

Fig. 12.13 The palm side of the severed finger

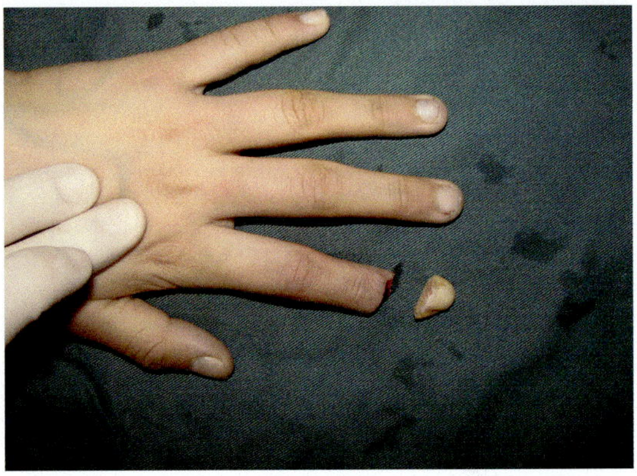

Fig. 12.14 The dorsal side of the severed finger

Case 3: Replantation of the Final Segment of the Left Index Finger

Female patient, 19 years old, was admitted to hospital for a final-segment severing of the left index finger caused by a chainsaw and bleeding for 1 h. PE: The general situation was good; the vital signs were stable. The distal part was completely severed and the bone was revealed, there was a cross-section wound, bleeding, and the blood supply to the rest fingers was good. Successful debridement and replantation were carried out under anesthesia under emergency conditions. The replanted finger was red and had moderate tension after relaxing the tourniquet. It was packed with sterile gauze and padded with broken cotton yarn, and the patient was brought back to the ward safely. She was given conventional treatments after the operation, such as antibiotics, hormones, and antispasmodics. By 2 weeks later, the replanted severed finger had successfully survived. The appearance and function are good after regular follow-up and functional exercise guidance, and the needle was withdrawn after 8–10 weeks (Figs. 12.13, 12.14, 12.15, 12.16, 12.17, and 12.18).

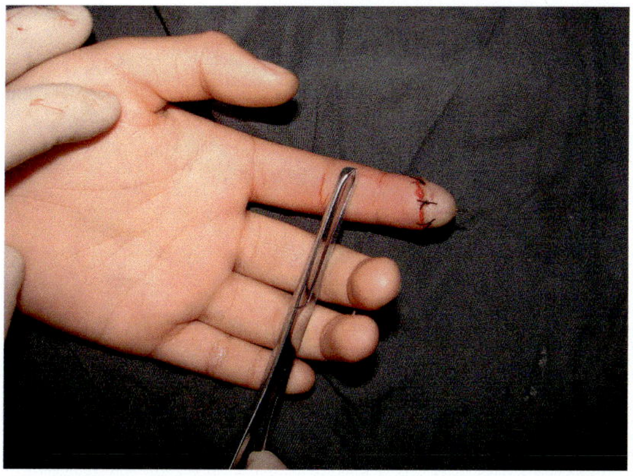

Fig. 12.15 Blood supply situation on the palm side during the operation

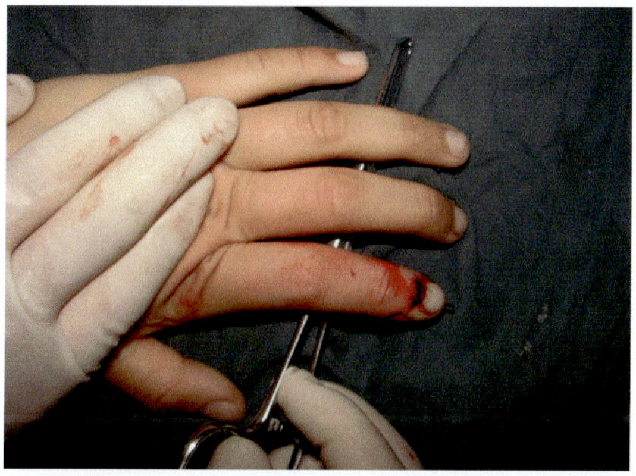

Fig. 12.16 Blood supply situation on the dorsal side during the operation

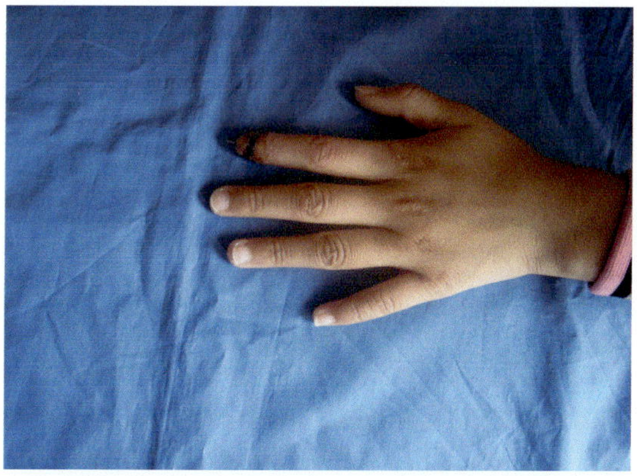

Fig. 12.17 The palm side of the severed finger 15 months later

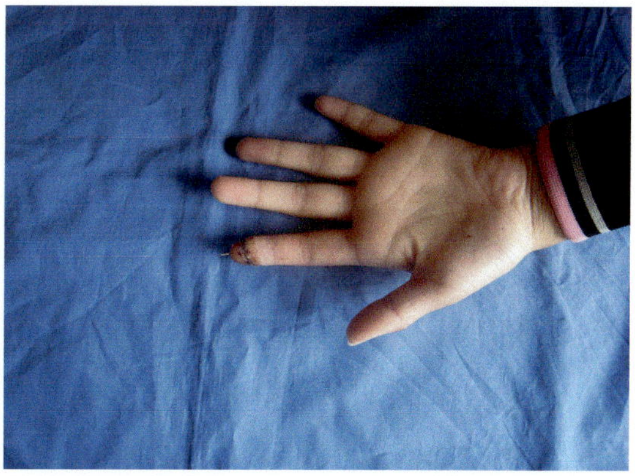

Fig. 12.18 The dorsal side of the severed finger 15 months later

Case 4: Replantation of the Final Segment of the Left Index and Middle Fingers

Female patient, 36 years old, was admitted to hospital for final-segment severing of the left index and middle fingers caused by a lathe and bleeding for 1.5 h. PE: The general situation was good; the vital signs were stable. The distal parts were completely severed and the bone was revealed, with cross-section wounds, bleeding, and the blood supply to the rest of the fingers was good. Successful debridement and replantation were performed under anesthesia under emergency conditions. The replanted fingers were red and had moderate tension after relaxing the tourniquet, and were packed with sterile gauze and padded with broken cotton yarn, and the patient was brought back to the ward safely. The patient was given conventional treatments after the operation, such as antibiotics, hormones, and antispasmodics. By 10 days later, the replanted severed fingers had successfully survived. The appearance and function were good after regular follow-up and functional exercise guidance, and the needles were withdrawn after 8–10 weeks. The patient and family were satisfied with the result (Figs. 12.19, 12.20, 12.21, 12.22, 12.23, and 12.24).

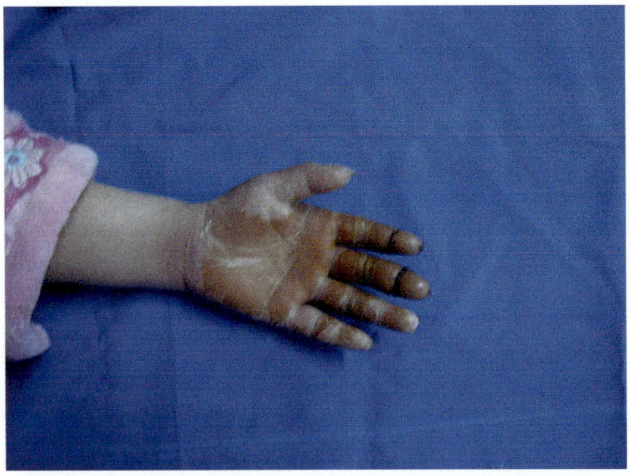

Fig. 12.19 The palm side of the severed fingers

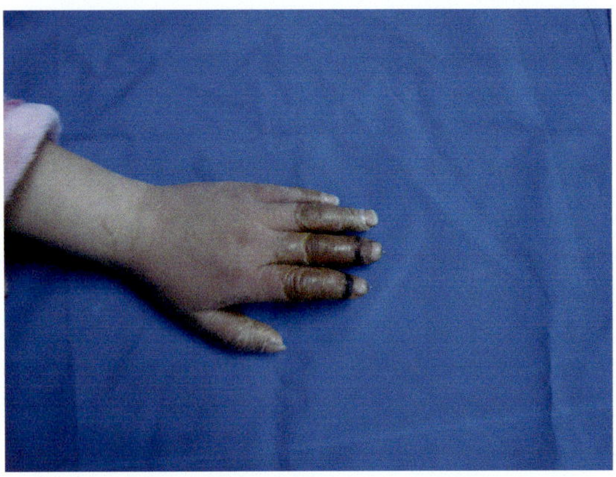

Fig. 12.20 The dorsal side of the severed fingers

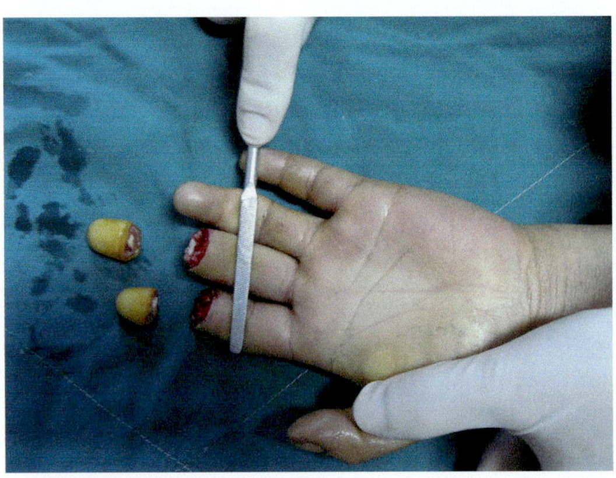

Fig. 12.21 Blood supply situation on the palm side during the operation

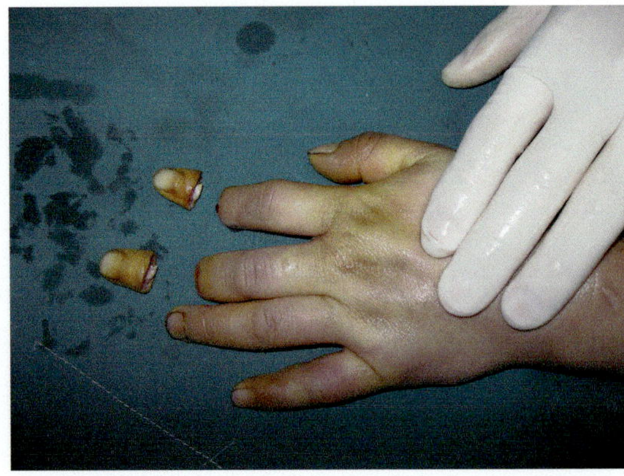

Fig. 12.22 Blood supply situation on the dorsal side during the operation

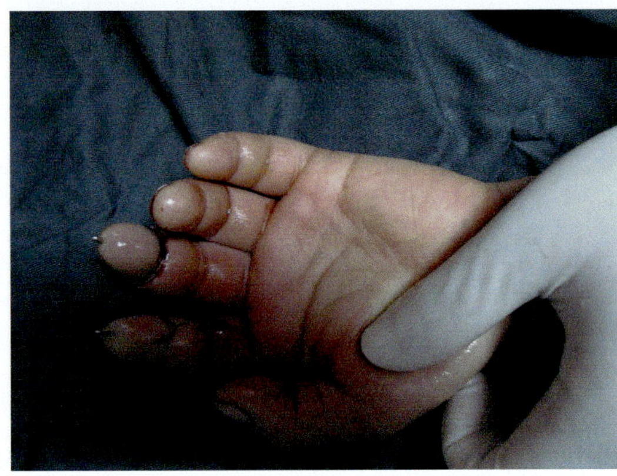

Fig. 12.23 The palm side of the severed fingers 2 months later

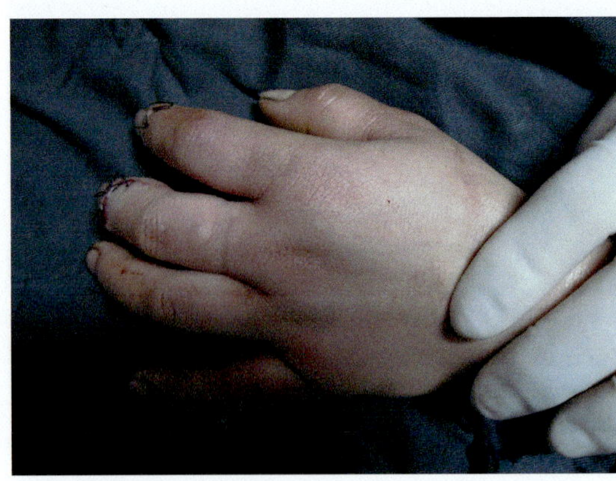

Fig. 12.24 The dorsal side of the severed fingers 2 months later

Case 5: Replantation of the Final Segment of the Right and Left Index and Middle Fingers
Male patient, 23 years old, was admitted to hospital for final segment severing of the right and left index and middle fingers caused by a chainsaw and bleeding for 1.5 h. PE: The general situation was good; the vital signs were stable. The distal parts were completely severed and the bone was revealed, with cross-section wounds, bleeding, and the blood supply to the rest of the fingers was good. Successful debridement and replantation were carried out under anesthesia under emergency conditions. The replanted fingers were red and had moderate tension after relaxing the tourniquet, and were packed with sterile gauze and padded with broken cotton yarn, and the patient was brought back to the ward safely. The patient was given conventional treatments after the operation, such as antibiotics, hormones, and antispasmodics. By 2 weeks later, the replanted severed fingers had successfully survived. The appearance and function were good after regular follow-up and functional exercise guidance, and the needles were withdrawn after 8–10 weeks. The patient and family were satisfied with the result (Figs. 12.25, 12.26, 12.27, 12.28, 12.29, 12.30, 12.31, 12.32, and 12.33).

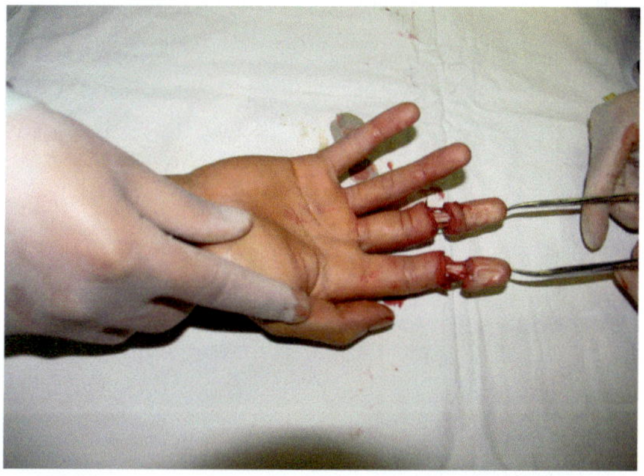

Fig. 12.25 The palm side of the severed fingers of the right hand

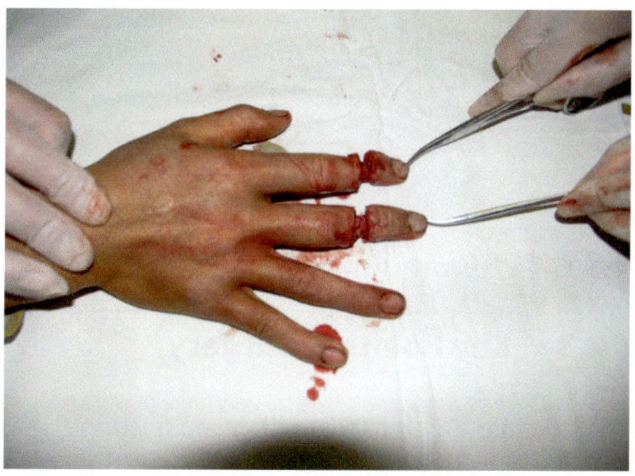

Fig. 12.26 The dorsal side of the severed fingers of the right hand

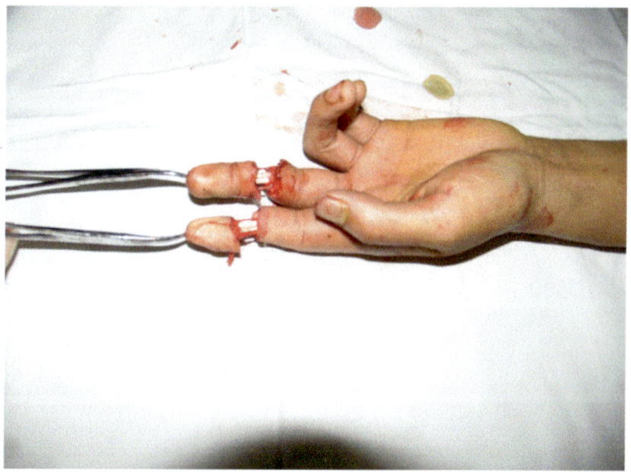

Fig. 12.27 The palm side of the severed fingers of the left hand

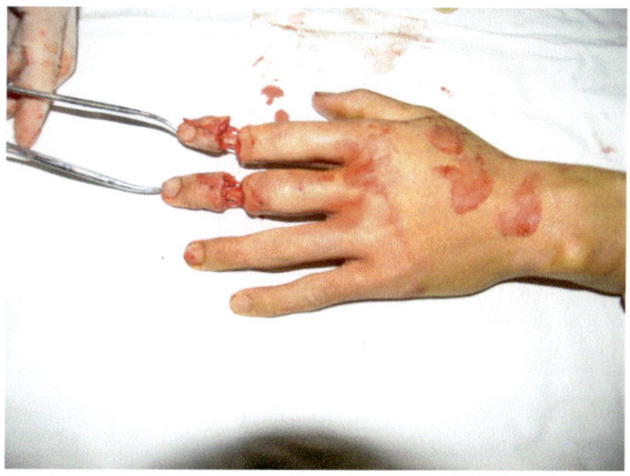

Fig. 12.28 The dorsal side of the severed fingers of the left hand

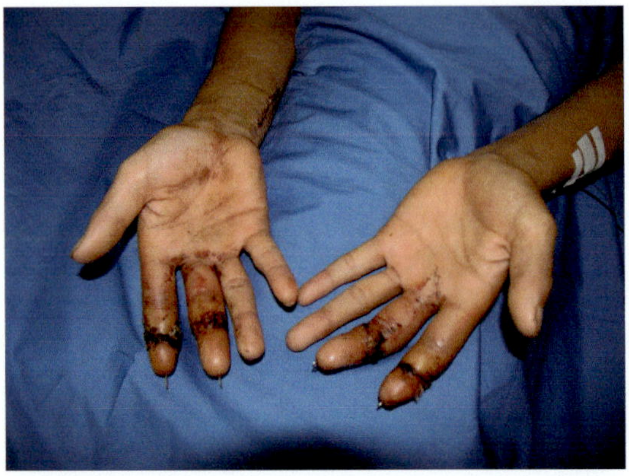

Fig. 12.29 The palm side of the severed fingers 2 weeks later

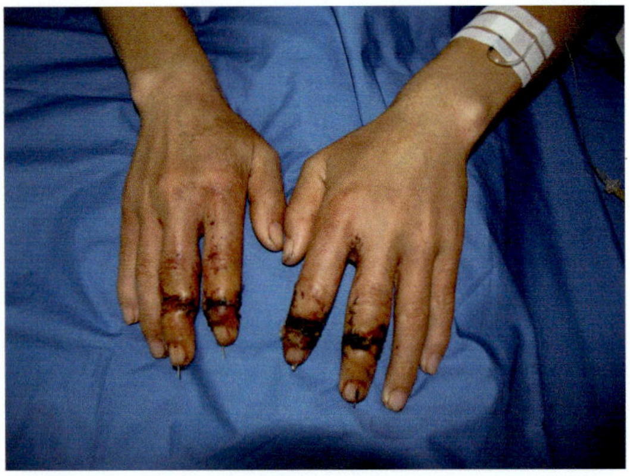

Fig. 12.30 The dorsal side of the severed fingers 2 weeks later

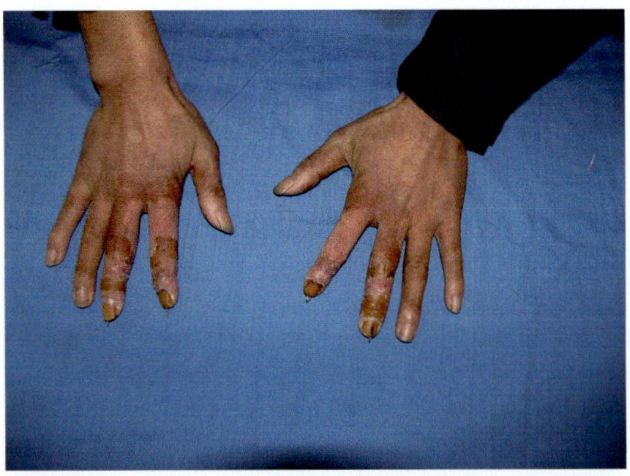

Fig. 12.31 The dorsal side of the severed fingers 6 months later

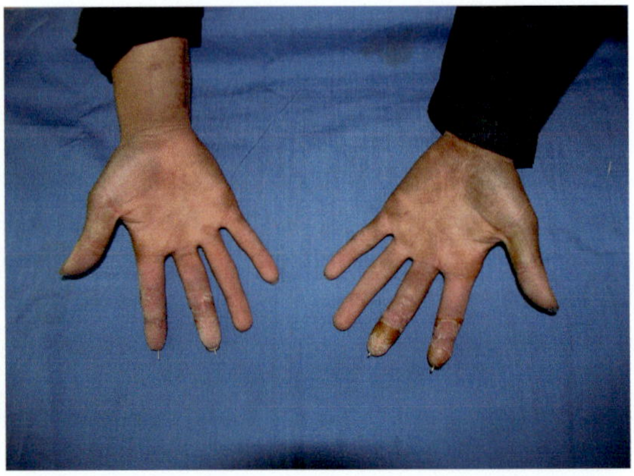

Fig. 12.32 The palm side of the severed fingers 6 months later

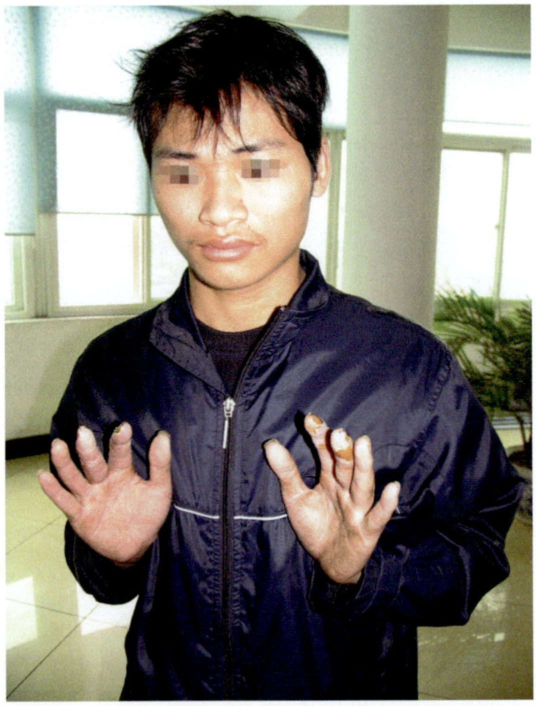

Fig. 12.33 Function 6 months later

12.3 Key Points in Surgery

(a) Elevate the transverse fiber mediastinum and the flap to expose the arch of the fingertips and its branches and the terminal portion of the finger nerves under a ×10 microscope.

Dissect the digital dorsum vein in the elevated flap. Then, dissect the finger artery, finger nerve, and digital dorsum vein microscopic line.

(b) Shorten the finger bone by 1–2 mm and fix it with a needle. Suture the finger artery, nerve, and vein with 11-0 or 12-0 nontraumatic suture and close the incision.

(c) Except for conventional blood vessel anastomosis, sometimes venous arterialization should be undertaken according to the different situations. The blood supply problem can be solved by nail bed bleeding, small incisions in the digital dorsum, enlarging the bone marrow cavity, etc.

(d) It is difficult to find the veins in the final section of the finger because they are very small. We can find them through these ways:
   - Move along the bleeding point to find the vein. Remember the rule: the veins are wider on the radial side of the thumb and index finger and they are wider on the ulnar side of the ring finger and little finger, but in the fingertips they are wider on the ulnar side of the thumb, index finger, middle finger, ring finger, and they are wider on the radial side of the little finger.
   - Use a tourniquet but without driving the blood to find the purple vein filled with blood.
   - We can loosen the tourniquet after the artery is anastomosed and find the vein along the bleeding point.

(e) The optimal spacing between the sutures should be accurate to ensure success first time. When free vascular transfer is needed, collateral blood vessels should be cut together because collateral blood vessel anastomosis may be safe, reliable, and convenient when vascular diameter differs three-fold.

(f) Preventing vascular crisis is of great significance in increase the survival rate of final-section replantation. We use heparin 100 mg + NS 500 mL and maintain for 24 h for anticoagulation when the severed finger is seriously injured.

12.4 Announcements

(a) The dorsal vein can be replaced by the palmar digital vein when it cannot be found or has too many defects.

(b) Vascular clamp should not be used as the wall of the palmar digital vein is weak, but it can be replaced by a rubber band at the root of the finger to control bleeding to reduce damage and maintain clear vision.

(c) Sometimes acupuncture bleeding is good after relaxing the tourniquet, but do not carry out bleeding if there is no problem with the anastomosis quality, vasospasm should be considered, and there is no need for vascular exploration, especially in fingertip replantation. Most patients take a turn for the better after keeping warm using a lamp and antispasmodic therapy.

(d) Pulling out the nail, making small incisions in the unmatched side, and a hydropathic heparin compress increases the survival rate.

(e) Active anticoagulant therapy and blood coagulation system monitoring should be applied after the operation if the patient was found to have high coagulation during surgery.

(f) Immobilization is important to the replanted finger without vein anastomosis to prevent vasospasm when bleeding therapy was being undertaken.

(g) The occurrence of hemorrhagic shock should be considered when bleeding therapy was undertaken in more than one finger.

(h) The surgery must have good psychological quality and endurance in multiple final-section finger replantation, and it is not advisable to reduce the time of operation by means of simplifying the performance technique.

(i) Increased incidence of postoperative vascular crisis occurs in the replantation of more than one section and one finger because of increased traumatic reaction and an increased number of vessels that need to be anastomosed. The key point is the survival of the middle section which is the basis for the survival of the other sections. Repair of nerve is also important, and can avoid postoperative contraction.

Suggested Reading

Chen YC, Chan FC, Hsu CC, Lin YT, Chen CT, Lin CH. Fingertip replantation without venous anastomosis. Ann Plast Surg. 2013;70(3):284–8.

Chengwu Z, Rui Z, Hang Z, et al. Application of different methods in fingertip replantation. Chin J Hand Surg. 2013;29(3):185–6.

Chunjiang L, Xiaona F, Wang B, et al. The application of arteriovenous shunt in replantation of amputation of fingertip. Chin J Hand Surg. 2009;25(2):125–6.

Guang C, Haifeng S, Yongjun R, et al. Clinical study of a reformed non-physiological method for fingertip replantation. Chin J Hand Surg. 2012;28(2):88–9.

Hui X, Jiewen L, Lijun X. The experience of replantation of fingertip distal to nail. Chin J Microsurg. 2005;28(1):73.

Huijiang S, Liang J, Jun Y, et al. Application of transferring branch of fingertip artery in replantation of amputated fingertip. J Beihua Univ (Nat Sci). 2005;6(3):236–7.

Imaizumi A, Ishida K, Arashiro K, Nishizeki O. Validity of exploration for suitable vessels for replantation in the distal fingertip amputation in early childhood: replantation or composite graft. J Plast Surg Hand Surg. 2013;47(4):258–62.

Mingrui C, Li T, Yan S, et al. Surgical anatomy of nerves and blood vessels of the finger distal phalanx and its clinical significance. Chin J Orthop Trauma. 2005;11:52–4.

Scheker LR, Becker GW. Distal finger replantation. J Hand Surg Am. 2011;36(3):521–8.

Shiming L, Changqing Z, Yanling Z, et al. Replantation of complete amputation of fingertip distal to nail semilunar line. Chin J Hand Surg. 2003;19(3):145–6.

Venkatramani H, Sabapathy SR. Fingertip replantation: technical considerations and outcome analysis of 24 consecutive fingertip replantations. Indian J Plast Surg. 2011;44(2):237–45.

Wang Q. Application of digital artery for recirculation in replantation of distal digits with venous defects. Chin J Orthop Trauma. 2006;6:583–4.

Wang Q, Qing X, Hua J, et al. 25 cases of replantation of fingertip with cross-anastomosis of digital artery. Chin J Trauma. 2007a;23(5):392–3.

Wang Q, Hua J, Yang D, et al. Replantation of fingertip in children with enlarging the medullary cavity. Chin J Pediatr Surg. 2007b;28(3):167–8.

Xiaofeng T, Hong C, Wang X, et al. Therapeutic analysis in 980 cases of digital replantation of distal segment. Chin J Pract Hand Surg. 2003;17(1):29–30.

Yoshimatsu H, Yamamoto T, Seki Y, Narushima M, Iida T, Koshima I. A new device expanding operability of fingertip replantation: subzone 1 fingertip replantation assisted by non-enhanced angiography in a 2-year-old boy. J Plast Reconstr Aesthet Surg. 2012;65(11):1592–4.

Zhongmei C, Liang S, Yuanzhuang C, et al. Simple artery anastomosis of finger distal segment replantation. Chin J Microsurg. 2002;25(4):306–7.

13 Replantation of Multi-section Severed Fingers

13.1 Summary

A finger severed with two or more planes on its vertical axis is called a multi-section severing or multi-plane severing. Replantation of a multi-section severed finger is one of the most serious types. There is more than one anastomotic stoma in the same finger and if an embolism occurred in any one of them, partial necrosis or total necrosis is inevitable, and the risk of a vascular crisis is greatly increased. It is by no means a simple accumulation of single-section replantation, it is uncommon clinically, and it is caused by cutting machines and punch failure. The different position of hand, the shape of the cutting tool, and the speed of the machine will cause different injuries. Multi-section replantation develops based on single-section replantation and it is of the difficulty of hand surgery because of the serious injury, complex conditions, multiple surgical sites, greater difficulty, higher technical requirements, and longer operation time. In most cases, such patients will accept stump revision, which greatly affects the appearance and function. However, in the highly developed microsurgery of today, if the severed tissue is relatively complete, replantation should be considered.

13.2 Case Description

Case 1: Multi-section Replantation of the Right Index Finger

Female patient, 35 years old, was admitted to hospital for a right index finger severing caused by a punch and bleeding for 2.5 h. Physical examination: The general situation was good; the vital signs were stable. The proximal close section and distal middle section were completely severed, with bones, vessels, nerves, and tendons revealed, uneven wounds, bleeding, and the blood supply to the rest of the fingers was good. There was no blood supply to the severed sections. Successful debridement and replantation were carried out under anesthesia under emergency conditions. The replanted finger was red and had moderate tension after relaxing the tourniquet. It was packed with sterile gauze and padded with broken cotton yarn, and the patient was brought back to the ward safely. The patient was given conventional treatments postoperatively, such as antibiotics, hormones, and antispasmodics. By 2 weeks later, the replanted severed finger had successfully survived. The appearance and function were good after regular follow-up and functional exercise guidance, and the needle was withdrawn after 8–10 weeks. The patient is satisfied with the appearance and function (Figs. 13.1, 13.2, 13.3, 13.4, 13.5, 13.6, 13.7, and 13.8).

J. Lin et al., *Special Type of Finger Replantation*, https://doi.org/10.1007/978-981-10-6229-2_13

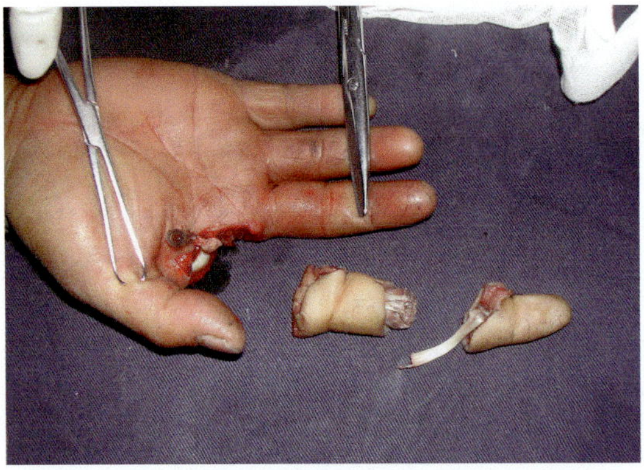

Fig. 13.1 The palm side of the severed finger

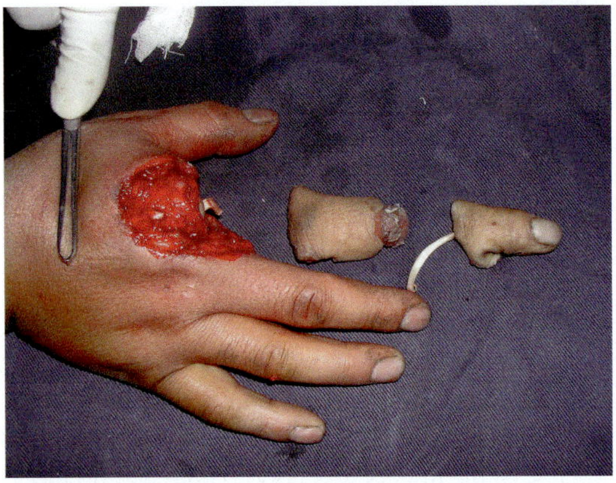

Fig. 13.2 The dorsal side of the severed finger

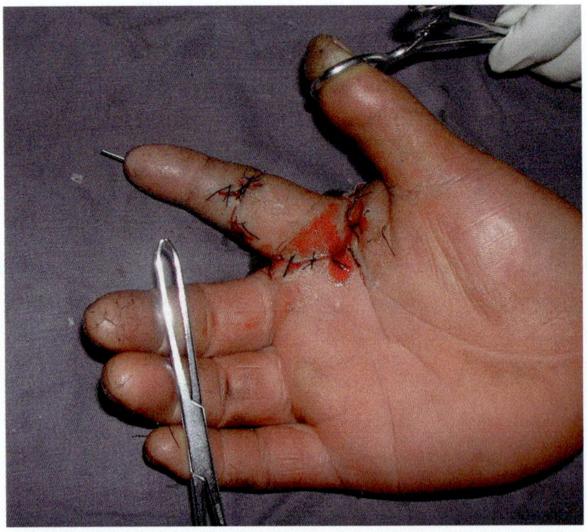

Fig. 13.3 The palm side after replantation

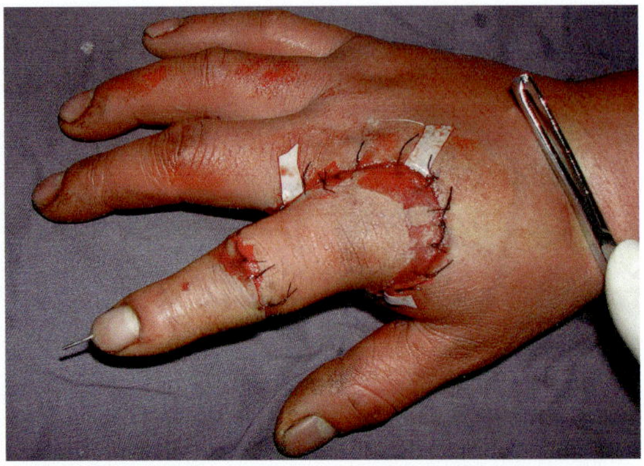

Fig. 13.4 The dorsal side after replantation

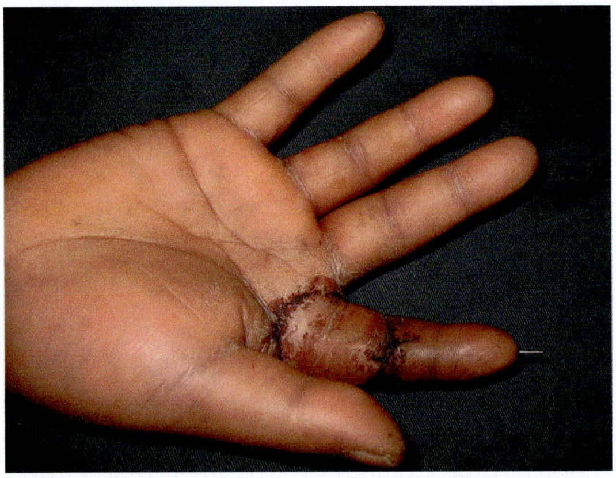

Fig. 13.5 The palm side 2 weeks later

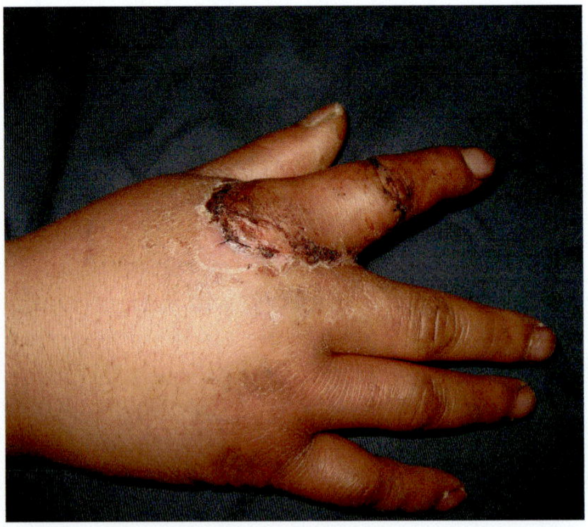

Fig. 13.6 The dorsal side 2 weeks later

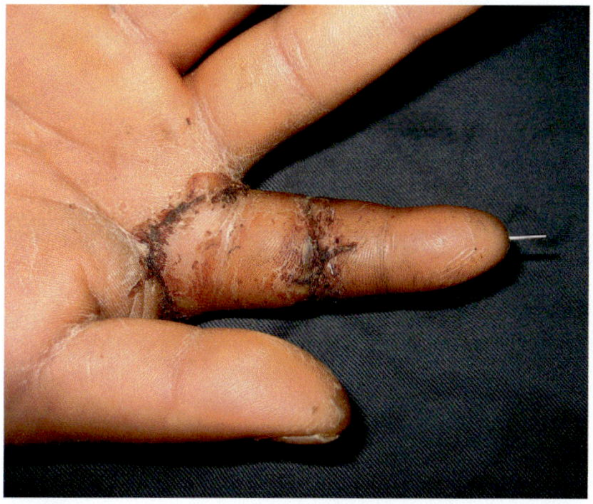

Fig. 13.7 The palm side 6 weeks later

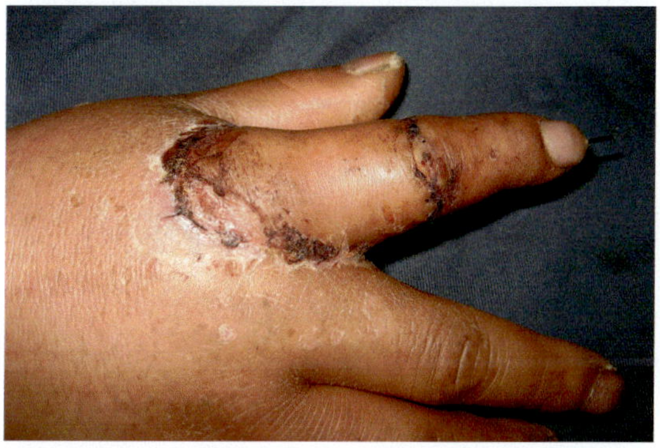

Fig. 13.8 The dorsal side 6 weeks later

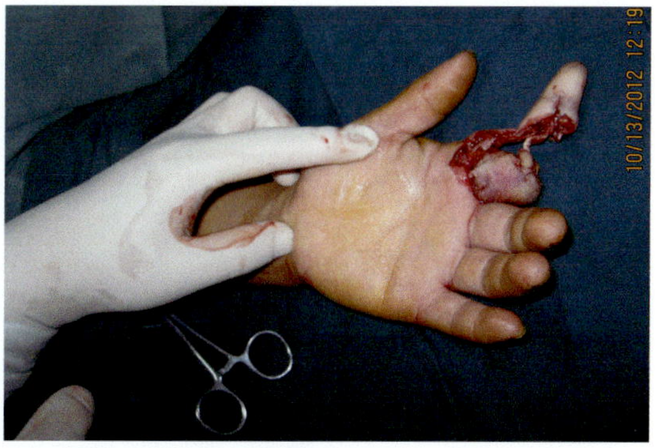

Fig. 13.9 The palm side of the severed finger

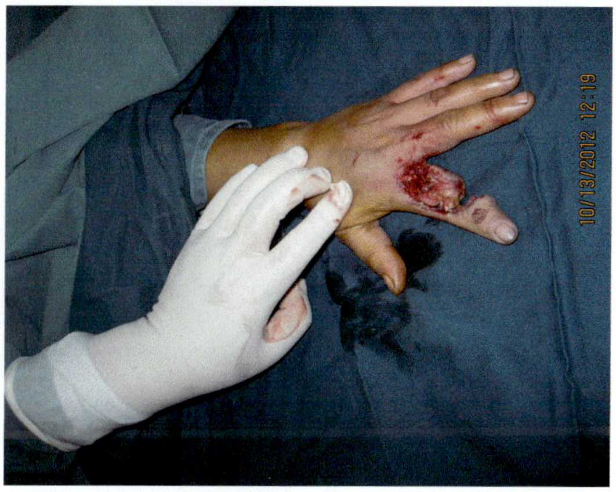

Fig. 13.10 The dorsal side of the severed finger

Case 2: Multi-section Replantation of the Right Index Finger

Male patient, 31 years old, was admitted to hospital for a severed left index finger caused by an injection molding machine and bleeding for 1.5 h. PE: The general situation was good; the vital signs were stable. The proximal close section and distal middle section were completely severed, with bones, vessels, nerves, and tendons revealed, uneven wounds, bleeding, and the blood supply to the rest of the fingers was good. There was no blood supply for the severed sections. Successful debridement and replantation were taken under anesthesia in emergency. The replanted finger was red with moderate tension after relaxing the tourniquet, and was packed with sterile gauze and padded with broken cotton yarn, with the patient brought back to the ward safely. He was given conventional treatments postoperatively, such as antibiotics, hormones, and antispasmodics. By 2 weeks later, the replanted severed finger had successfully survived. The appearance and function were good after regular follow-up and functional exercise guidance, and the needle was withdrawn after 8–10 weeks. The patient was satisfied with the appearance and function (Figs. 13.9, 13.10, 13.11, 13.12, 13.13, and 13.14).

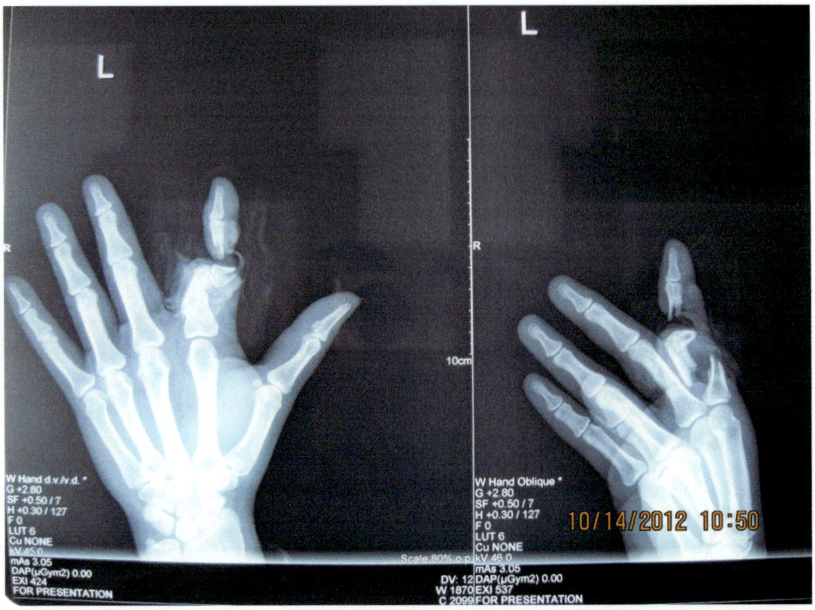

Fig. 13.11 Preoperative X-ray

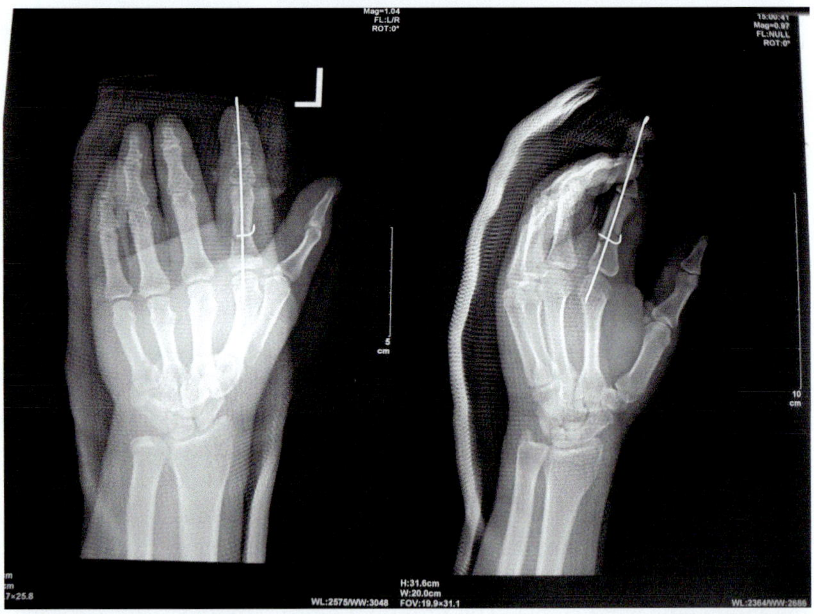

Fig. 13.12 Postoperative X-ray

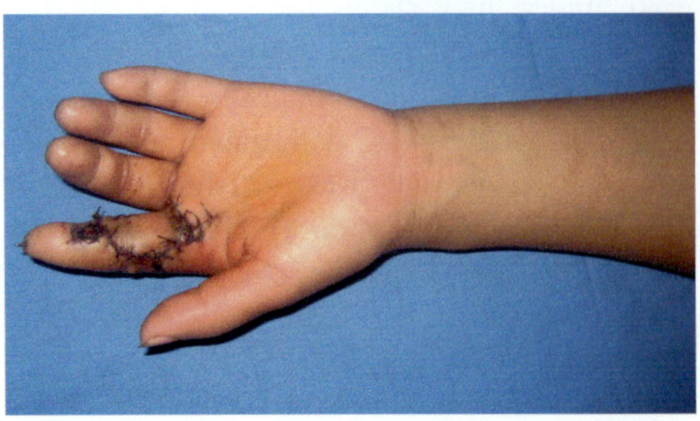

Fig. 13.13 The palm side 2 weeks later

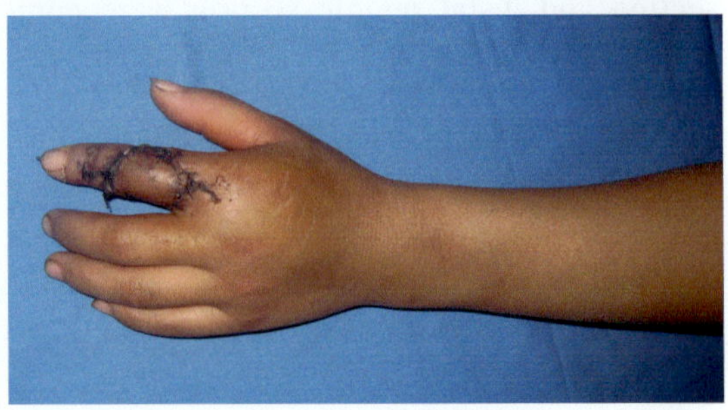

Fig. 13.14 The dorsal side 2 weeks later

Case 3: Replantation of Multiple-Planes and Multiple-Section Severed Fingers

The patient, female, 18 years old, knife cut that led to complicated injury of the right hand including 5 fingers, 6 planes and 17 sections. Admitted to hospital 3 hours after the injury. Physical examination: from the root of the right thumb, the distal part of the proximal section and the proximal three segments were completely broken off; the middle section of the index finger, the distal part of the proximal section and the proximal part were completely broken; the middle finger from the root, the middle section, the middle part and the proximal segment and the proximal part were completely broken; the ring finger from the root, the distal part to the proximal interphalangeal joint and the proximal part were completely broken; the small finger from the middle section, the middle section of the proximal part were completely broken off. The palms, 2–5 metacarpal, which were from the distal, middle and proximal were completely broken. Additionally, there was only a 2 cm wide connected area of skin in the middle part of the palm, the soft tissues of proximal dorsal lateral were cleft deep into the metacarpal, the margin of the wound was orderly. Under the brachial plexus anesthesia, we performed finger replantation. The operation was divided into 4groups, the first and the second group used the surgical microscope, dissected the index, middle and the served parts of the thumb, ring and small fingers of the bloodless state, then a complete debridement was also taken. The blood vessels, nerves and tendons were found and marked. According to the debridement situation of the vascular parts, some finger sections were chosen, and we did about 0.3–0.5 cm phalanx shortenin. Kirschner wire was used to fix through each section of the fingers, followed by suturing the stretched finger tendon, flexor deep tendon, anastomosing the 2–3 dorsal veins, 1–2 arteries of each segment. We used a 10–0 non-invasive suture for the proximal part, 12–0 non-invasive suture for the distal part of the thumb, middle, ring fingers, 9–0 non-invasive suture for the nerve and combination and replantation for 1–5 fingers; the third group replanted the multiple-planes and multiple-section severed palms. After the debridement, we used Kirschner wire to longitudinally fix 2–5 metacarpals, finding the "U" shape flexor tendon, connecting with the extension of the tendon by a "8" shape suturing. Under the microscope, we debrided and found the corresponding dorsal veins, anastomosing the common arteries and nerves of the fingers. The fourth group of doctors replanted the 1–5 fingers and the palms in the following order: the thumb → index finger → middle finger → ring finger → little finger. During the operation, there was a thrombosis after anastomosis of finger arteries of the proximal part of the index finger and middle part of the middle fingers. However, we found the defect of the finger arteries, so we grafted and anastomosed the forearm palmar superficial vein again. We found ruddy finger bodies and moderate tension in the replanted finger of the right hand. Blood circulation was established. The surgery lasted for 21 h, with a total of anastomosis of 3 common arteries and 10 inherent arteries, a total of 26 anastomosis; anastomosis of the 4 dorsal veins, 10 dorsal veins of the fingers, and 4 palm veins, a total of 33 anastomosis, and anastomosis of 27 nerves totally. After surgery, sterile shredded dressings were afixed, with gypsum external fixation, the regular "three anti" drug treatment was given, along with the special care and blood circulation monitoring. One week after the replantation, all replanted tissues survived and the patient was given some rehabilitation exercises. After a 5-year follow-up, the patient was satisfied with the hand shape and could engage in general work and daily activities (Figs. 13.15, 13.16, 13.17, 13.18, 13.19, 13.20, 13.21, 13.22, 13.23, 13.24, 13.25, and 13.26).

The cases are generally provided by Dr. Jianxi Hou.

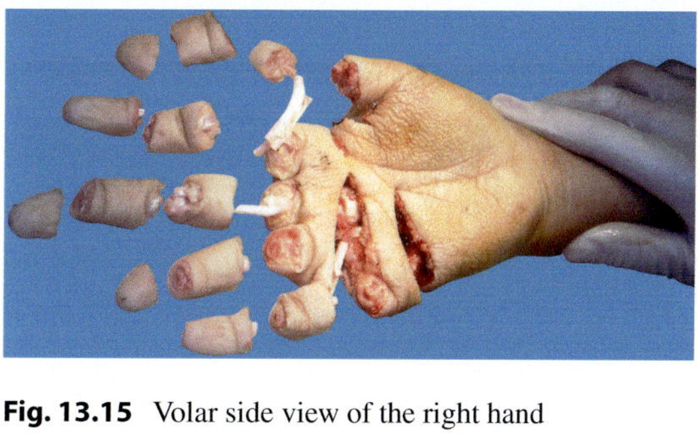

Fig. 13.15 Volar side view of the right hand

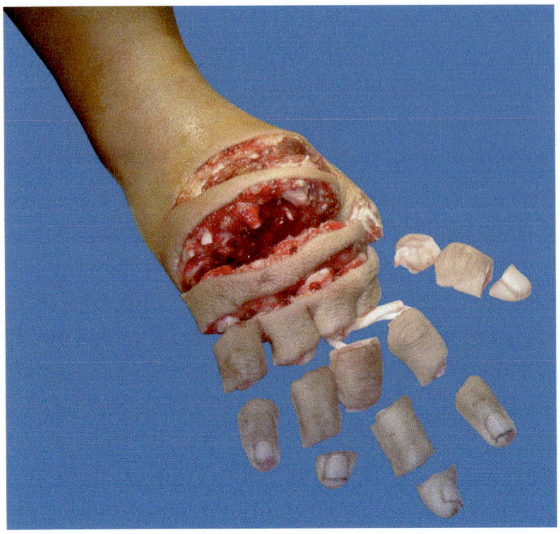

Fig. 13.16 Dorsal side view of the right hand

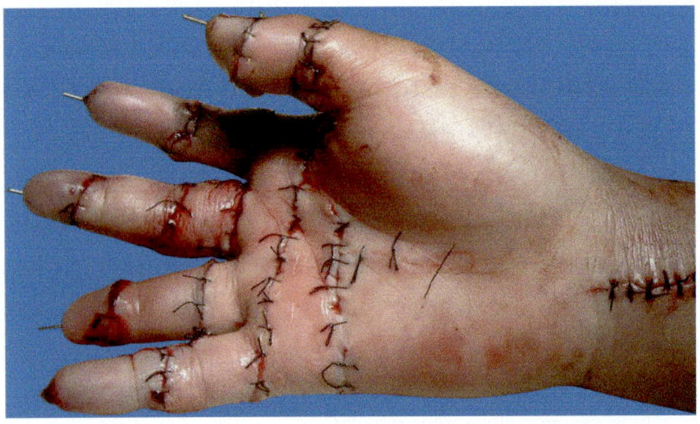

Fig. 13.17 Volar side view of the successfully replanted right hand

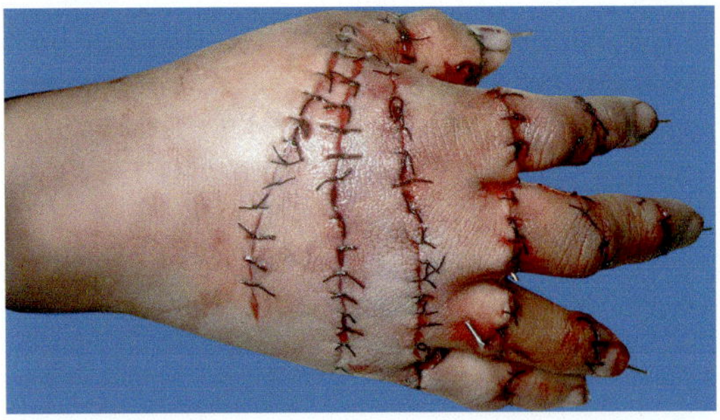

Fig. 13.18 Dorsal side view of the successfully replanted right hand

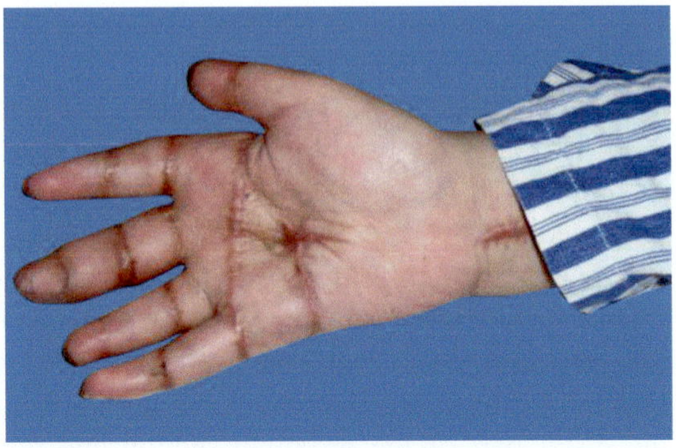

Fig. 13.19 3 months after the replantation

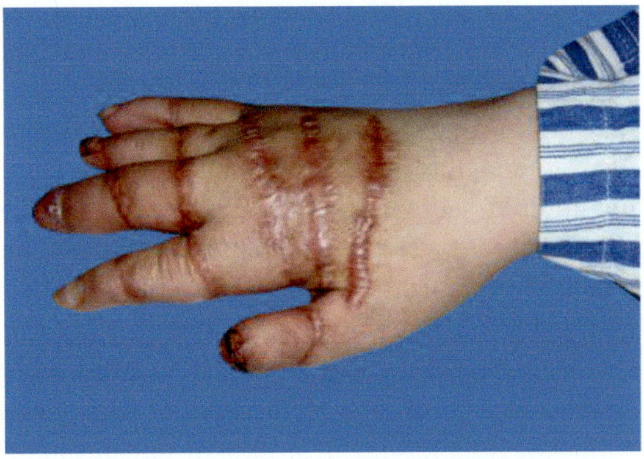

Fig. 13.20 3 months after the replantation

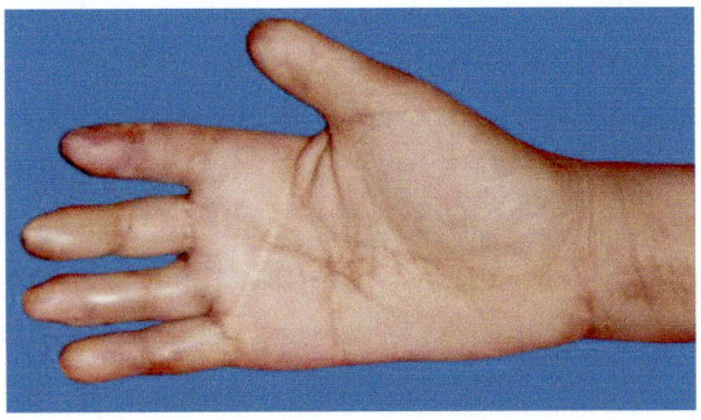

Fig. 13.21 12 months after the replantation

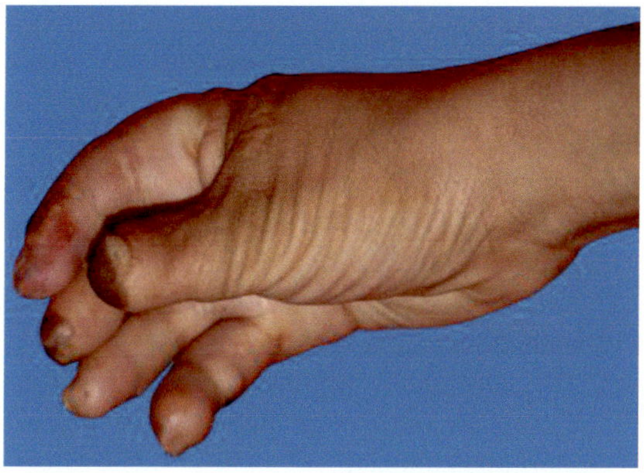

Fig. 13.22 24 months after the replantation

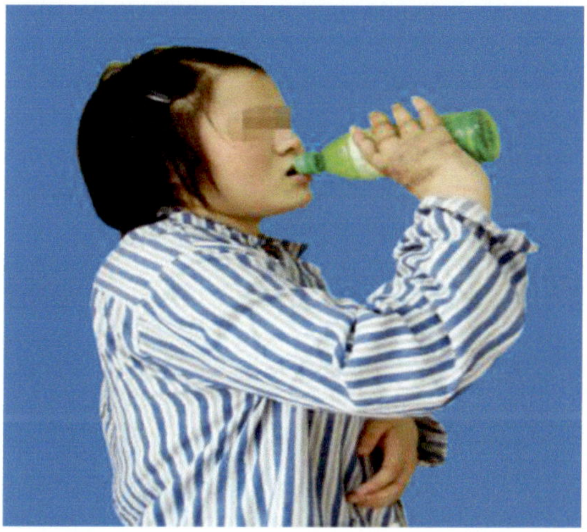

Fig. 13.23 Gripping function after the replantation

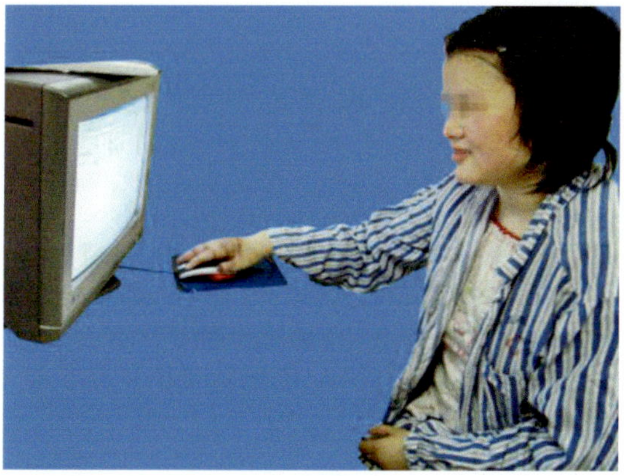

Fig. 13.24 Taking function after the replantation

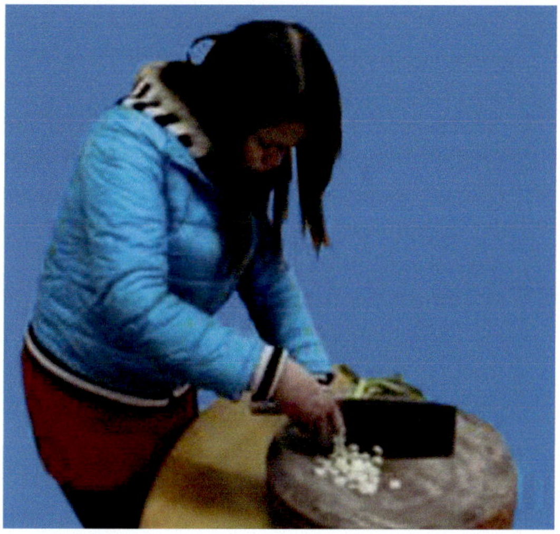

Fig. 13.25 Pinching function after the replantation

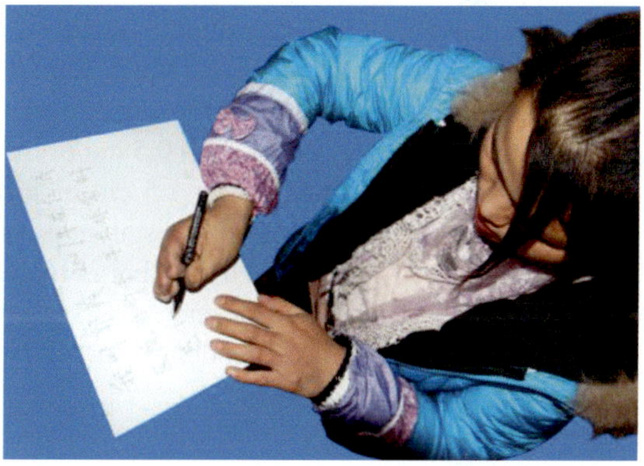

Fig. 13.26 Subtle gestures after the replantation

13.3 Key Points in Surgery

(a) Reasonably grouping of the operating room personnel is advantageous to shorten the ischemia time of the severed finger and keep the surgical staff energetic and vigorous.
(b) Anastomose vessels from proximal to distal. Relax the vascular clamp to let the blood flow to the proximal anastomotic stoma to prevent embolism before the distal anastomosis.
(c) Anastomose vessels from distal to proximal. All segments of the finger are synchronized

with blood together, as both approaches have advantages and disadvantages and there is no evidence-based medicine.

(d) Attach great importance to the choice of the section. If the middle section is shorter than 1.5 cm, it can be abandoned, which reduces the operating time.
(e) Take good care of the replanted sections.
(f) Pay attention to tendon tension, especially the lateral tendon bundle. Adjust the lines of force in time with external fixation of the postoperative dressing to prevent rotation and achieve good recovery.
(g) Professional microsurgical techniques and a good understanding of the anatomy and functioning of the fingers are the basis for successful multi-section replantation of severed fingers.
(h) If the tendon end of the middle section is smooth, it can be repaired in one stage. Tendon defects always occur in multi-section severed fingers. If the defect is less than 0.5 cm of the extensor tendon and less than 1.5 cm of the flexor tendon, the proximal and distal sections can be sutured directly. If the defect is more than 0.5 cm of the extensor tendon and more than 1.5 cm of the flexor tendon, it should be repaired in a second stage.

13.4 Announcements

(a) If there are too many sections, the distal sections can be saved in a 4 °C refrigerator. The bone end should be 2–3 mm shorter than the skin.
(b) Replant the severed multiple fingers in order of the index finger, the middle finger, the ring finger, and the little finger. Group operating room personnel to reduce operating time and save the fingers without debridement in a 4 °C refrigerator.
(c) The surgeon should understand the mechanism of injury and the condition of the wound. Observe the severed finger under a microscope before determining whether it is worth replanting.
(d) As a special type of replantation that has a serious injury and low success rate, which needs a detailed preoperative talk and communication.
(e) Attach great importance to the management of the middle section, which is the important part of the success.
(f) Make a mark before the operation to prevent replantation error.
(g) To control the using time and pressure of the tourniquet during the operation to prevent tourniquet damage.
(h) Postoperative close observation of the blood supply to prevent a vascular crisis, if there is more than one anastomotic stoma in the same finger and if an embolism occurred in any one of them, partial necrosis or total necrosis is inevitable.
(i) Postoperative close observation of the general situation and the vital signs of the patient and bleeding condition of the wound.
(j) The appearance of the hand is as important as the function of the hand to young adults, especially young women, whose fingers should be replanted as far as possible. On the contrary, in those patients who are in a poor general condition, those who are older, and those who have serious local wound damage, replantation is not allowed. Single multi-section severing of the ring finger and the little finger is a relative contraindication for replantation.

Suggested Reading

Arata J, Ishikawa K, Soeda H, Kitayama T. Replantation of multi-level fingertip amputation using the pocket principle (palmar pocket method). Br J Plast Surg. 2003;56(5):504–8.

Cheng G. Review and prospect of finger replantation of special types. Chin J Microsurg. 2000;23(1):19–20.

Cheng TJ, Cheng NC, Tang YB. Restoration of basic hand function by double transpositional digital replantation in five-digit amputations. J Reconstr Microsurg. 2004;20(3):201–5.

Dong H, Weichi W, Huiru Z, et al. A successful case of replantation of four severed fingers with eight segments. Chin J Microsurg. 2004;27(3):199.

Fei L. Nursing of 13 cases of replantation of multi-severed fingers in children. J Qilu Nurs. 2008;18:105–6.

Guo J, Baoshan L, Xuesong Z, et al. Replantation of final segment with multi parts. Chin J Pract Hand Surg. 2003;01:28.

Guoxian P, Kuanhai W. Replantation of multi-level hand severances. Chin J Mod Oper Surg. 2000;4(3):169–72.

Haitao S, Wancheng T, Quanzhong L, et al. Replantation of multiple digits and multiple segments. Chin J Orthop Trauma. 2003;1:41–4.

Jian H, Wang S, Mintao T, et al. Retrospective study of replantation of multi-planes severed finger. Mod Pract Med. 2012;11:1219–20.

Ma L, Liangyan L, Yanjun Y, et al. Discussion of methods for replantation of multi segments of severed finger. J Pract Med. 2008;16:2841–2.

Shen M, Wei Z, Duobao Q, et al. Replantation surgery of multiple amputated digital and phalanges by chaff cutter. Chin J Pract Hand Surg. 2011;25(1):10–1.

Xie Z, Liang M, Lie Y. A successful case of replantation of ten fingers. Chin J Microsurg. 1998;04:247.

Xie C, Jianxi H, Xie S, et al. A successful case of replantation of one hand with 17 segments. Chin J Microsurg. 2009;32(3):244–5.

Yanhua L. Nursing care of cases receiving replantation of severed fingers (limbs). J Fourth Military Med Univ. 2004;12:1146.

Yingxue Z. Nursing of replantation of multi-segments. Chin Med Cosmetol. 2015;1:180–1.

14 Replantation of Multiple Severed Fingers

14.1 Summary

Multiple severed fingers means two or more fingers severed, what is more complicated than would occur in one hand or both hands. Most cases are caused by mechanical damage and the rest are caused by knife cuts or other penetrating trauma. Multiple severed fingers are a common hand injury, compared with a single severed finger, it is characterized by:

(a) More serious trauma, a more complicated condition, more blood loss, which would cause changes in blood volume, blood components, and hemodynamics, and activate systemic compensatory vasoconstriction.
(b) Longer operating time, more difficulty, which requires not only more energy and stamina from the surgeon, but also a stricter anesthesia way and perioperative period treatment.
(c) Higher microtechnical requirements of racing against time to reduce the ischemia time of severed fingers.
(d) Close observation of the replanted fingers after the operation and maintaining general stability to prevent high coagulation, while preventing excessive bleeding.

With the development and improvement of microtechniques since the 1970s, which makes it possible to replant multiple severed fingers, children's severed fingers, and final segments of fingers. The techniques have become mature based on the successful replantation of multiple fingers severed from one hand, multiple fingers severed from both hands, and when all ten fingers are severed. There have been 29 cases of successful replantation of ten fingers since 2005. With the development of microtechniques and improvement of equipment, indications for replantation are expanding. There are increasing numbers of reports of successful replantations, which shows the maturity and development of replanting techniques and reaches a new high.

14.2 Case Description

Case 1: Replantation of Second to Fifth Fingers of the Left Hand

Male patient, 28 years old, was admitted to hospital for injury to the left hand caused by a molding machine and bleeding for 1 h. Physical examination: The general situation was good; the vital signs were stable. The distal metacarpophalangeal joints of the left hand were completely severed with bones, tendons, nerves, and vessels revealed, uneven wounds, and bleeding. The severed fingers were without blood supply. Successful debridement and replantation were performed under anesthesia under emergency conditions. The replanted fingers were red and had moderate tension after relaxing the tourniquet. They were

J. Lin et al., *Special Type of Finger Replantation*, https://doi.org/10.1007/978-981-10-6229-2_14

packed with sterile gauze and padded with broken cotton yarn, and the patient was brought back to the ward safely. He was given conventional treatments postoperatively, such as antibiotics, hormones, and antispasmodics. By 2 weeks later, the replanted severed finger had successfully survived. The appearance and function are good after regular follow-up and functional exercise guidance and the patient is satisfied (Figs. 14.1, 14.2, 14.3, 14.4, 14.5, and 14.6).

Case 2: Replantation of Multiple Final Segments of Both Hands

Male patient, 25 years old, was admitted to hospital for injury to both hands caused by a lathe and bleeding for 1 h. PE: The general situation was good; the vital signs were stable. The final segment of the middle and ring fingers of the left hand and the final segment of the middle, ring,

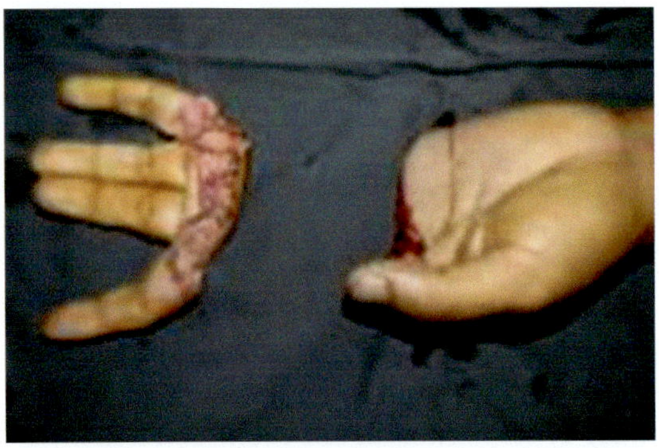

Fig. 14.1 The palm side of the severed fingers

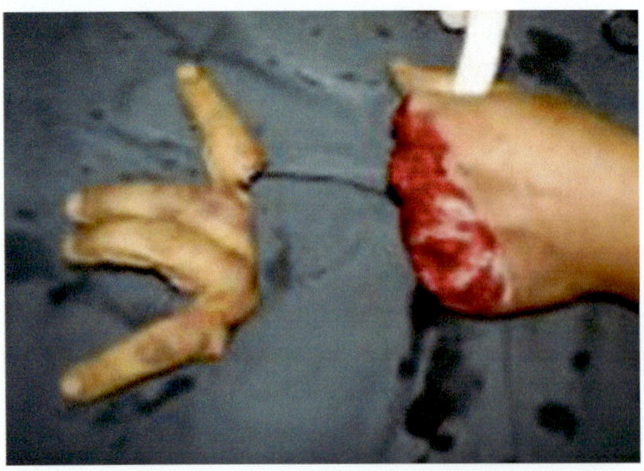

Fig. 14.2 The dorsal side of the severed fingers

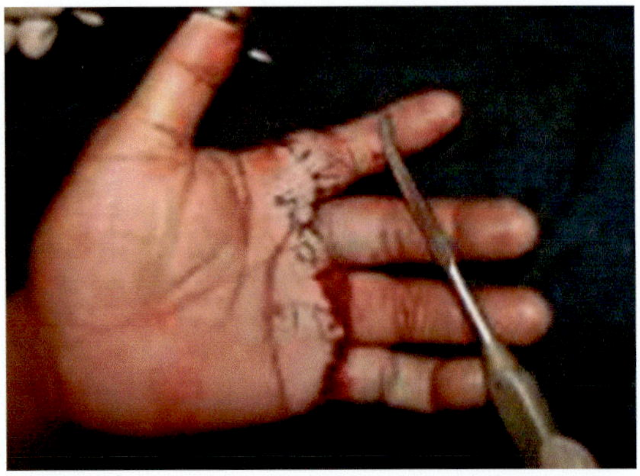

Fig. 14.3 Blood supply situation in the palm side during the operation

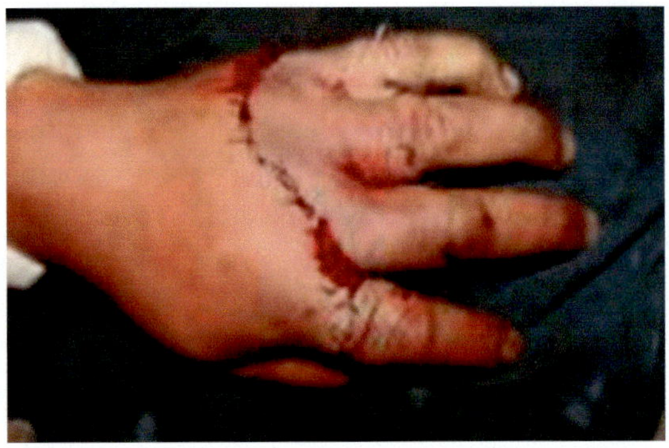

Fig. 14.4 Blood supply situation on the dorsal side during the operation

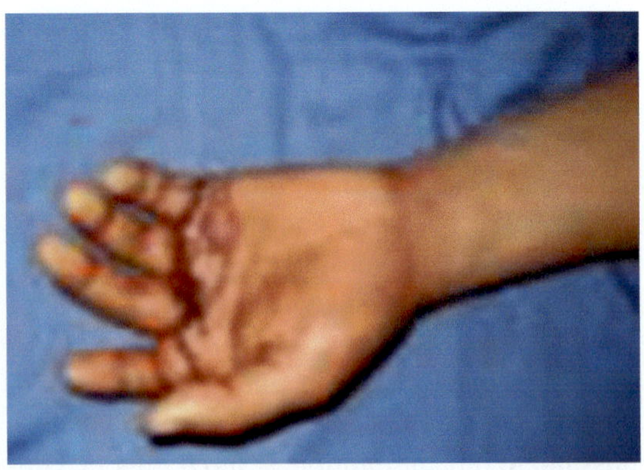

Fig. 14.5 The palm side of the severed fingers 4 weeks later

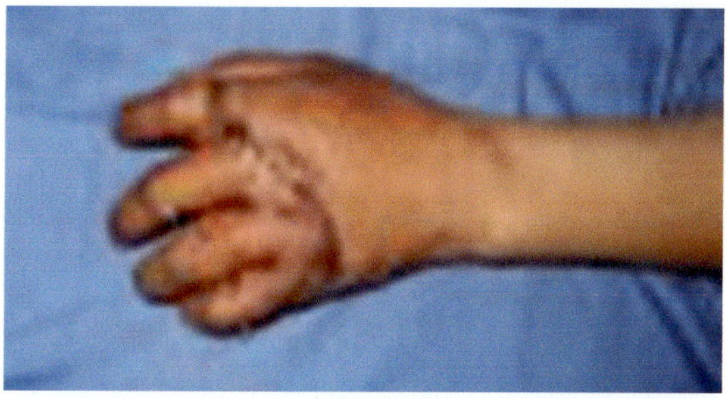

Fig. 14.6 The dorsal side of the severed fingers 4 weeks later

and little fingers of the right hand were completely severed, with bones, tendons, nerves, and vessels revealed, uneven wounds, and bleeding. The severed fingers were without blood supply, but the tissue was relatively complete except for the little finger which was severed from the fingertip without any vessels to be anastomosed. Successful debridement and replantation were carried out under anesthesia under emergency conditions. The replanted fingers were red and had moderate tension after relaxing the tourniquet. They were packed with sterile gauze and padded with broken cotton yarn, and the patient was brought back to ward safely. He was given conventional treatments after operation, such as antibiotics, hormones, and antispasmodics. By 2 weeks later, the replanted severed fingers had successfully survived. The appearance and function were good after regular follow-up and functional exercise guidance, and the patient was satisfied (Figs. 14.7, 14.8, 14.9, 14.10, 14.11, 14.12, 14.13, and 14.14).

Case 3: Replantation of Multiple Severed Fingers in Different Planes of the Right Hand
Male patient, 35 years old, admitted to hospital for injury to the right hand caused by a punch and bleeding for 2 h. PE: The general situation was good; the vital signs were stable. The first to fifth fingers were severed in different planes: the final segments of the thumb, the middle segment of the index finger, and the proximal segment of the ring finger were completely severed; only one flexor tendon was attached without blood supply. In the middle and little fingers, the middle segments were incompletely severed, with bones, tendons, nerves, and vessels revealed and the tendons and

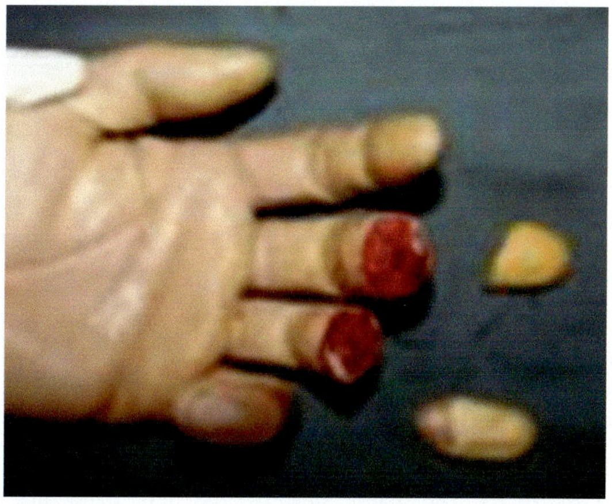

Fig. 14.7 The palm side of the severed fingers of the left hand

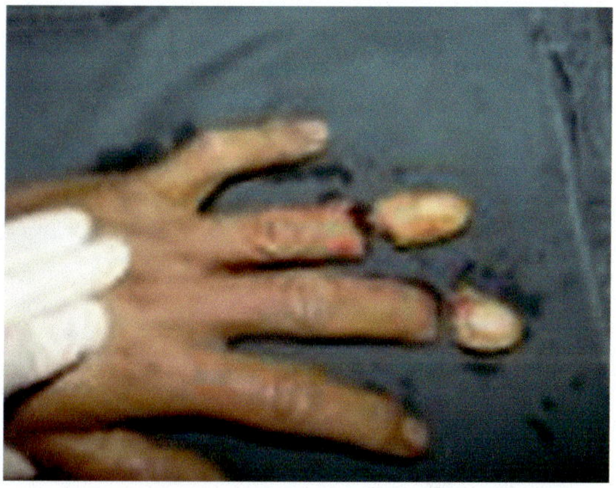

Fig. 14.8 The dorsal side of the severed fingers of the left hand

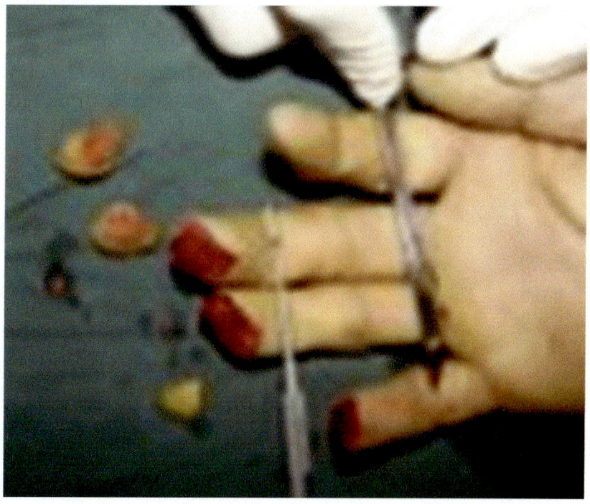

Fig. 14.9 The palm side of the severed fingers of the right hand

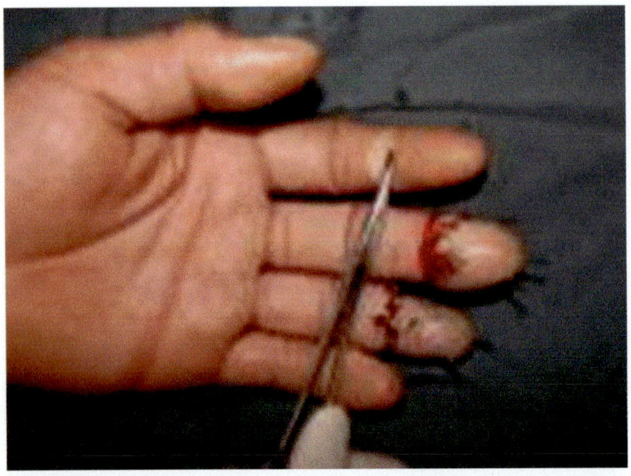

Fig. 14.10 The palm side of the left hand after replantation

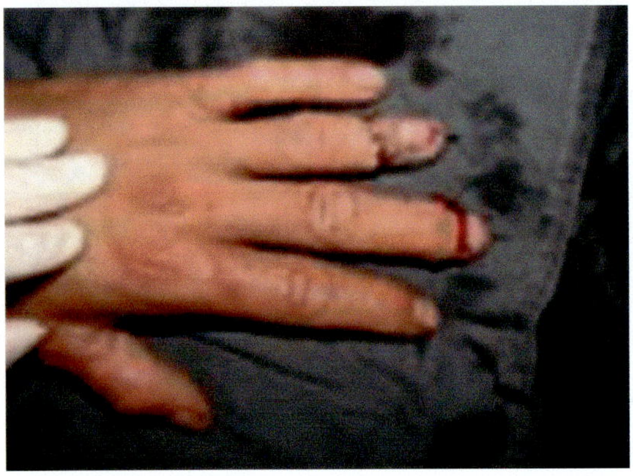

Fig. 14.11 The dorsal side of the left hand after replantation

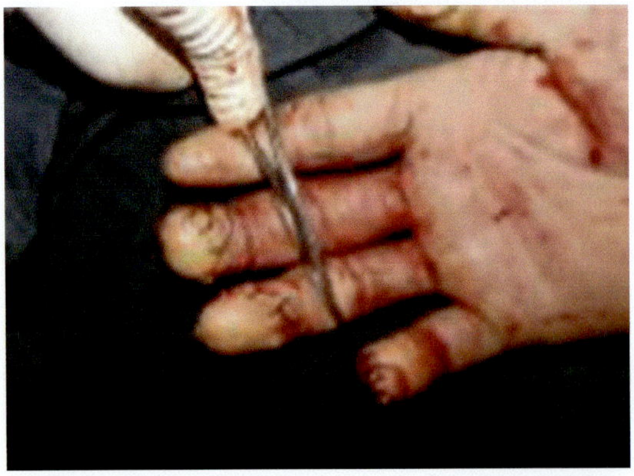

Fig. 14.12 The palm side of the right hand after replantation

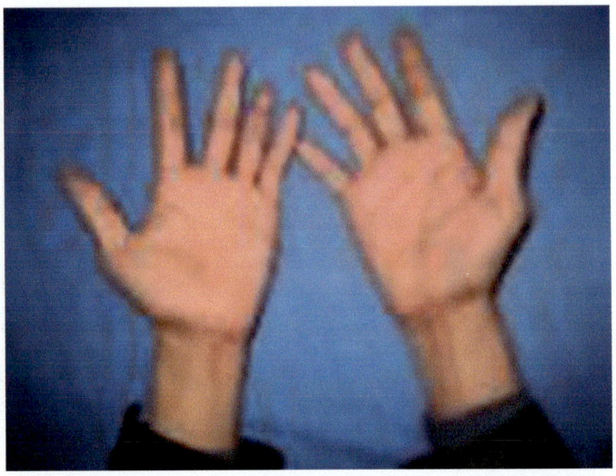

Fig. 14.13 The palm side of the severed fingers 18 months later

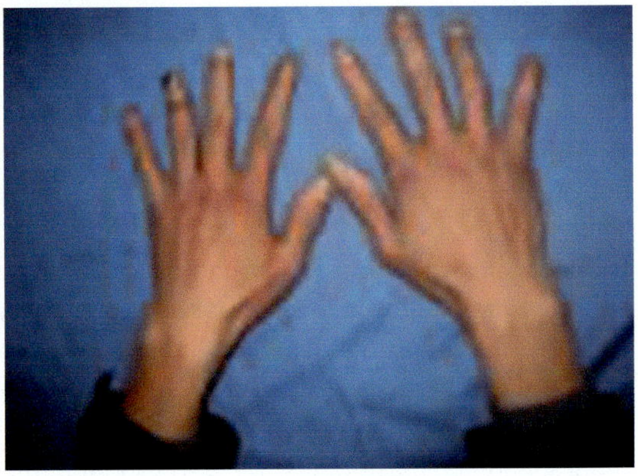

Fig. 14.14 The dorsal side of the severed fingers 18 months later

skin of the dorsal side complete. The severed fingers were relatively complete except for the little finger, which was severed from the fingertip without any vessels to be anastomosed. The wounds were uneven and seriously polluted. Successful debridement and replantation were performed under anesthesia under emergency conditions. The replanted fingers were red and had moderate tension after relaxing the tourniquet, and were packed with sterile gauze and padded with broken cotton yarn. The patient was brought back to the ward safely. He was given conventional treatments postoperatively such as antibiotics, hormones, and antispasmodics. The replanted severed finger successfully survived. The appearance and function were good after regular follow-up and functional exercise guidance, and the patient was satisfied (Figs. 14.15, 14.16, 14.17, 14.18, 14.19, 14.20, 14.21, 14.22, and 14.23).

Case 4: Replantation of Multiple Final Segments Severed from the Left Hand
Male patient, 41 years old, was admitted to hospital for injury to the left hand caused by a chainsaw and bleeding for 1.5 h. PE: The general situation was good; the vital signs were stable. The second to fifth fingers were severed in different planes: the final segments of the middle finger and the ring finger were completely severed, the index finger was severed at the fingertip with bones, tendons, nerves, and vessels revealed.

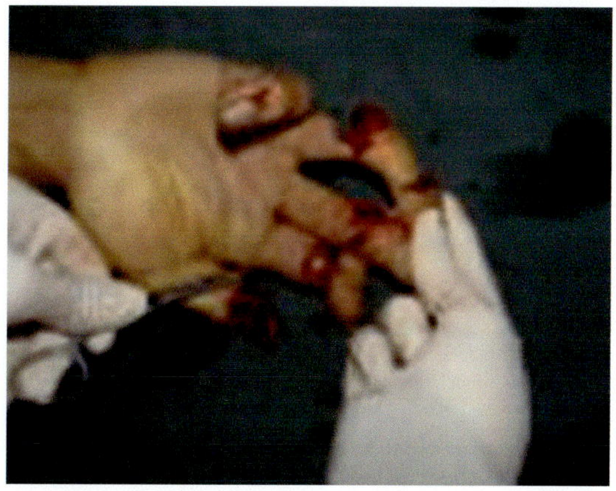

Fig. 14.16 The palm side of the severed fingers

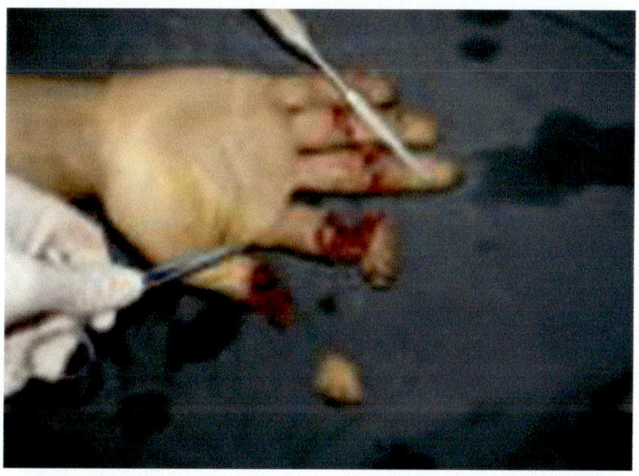

Fig. 14.15 The palm side of the severed fingers

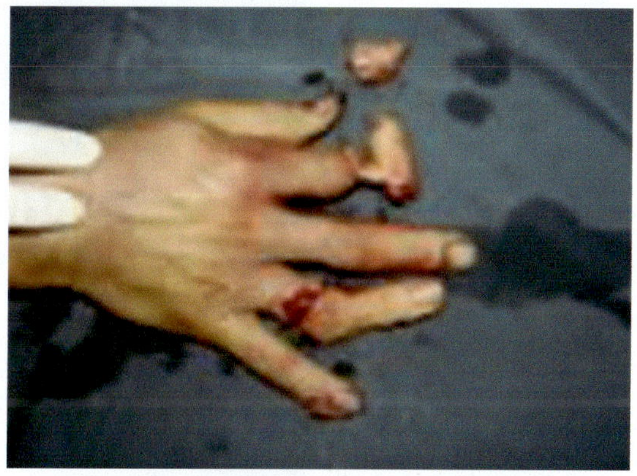

Fig. 14.17 The palm side of the severed fingers

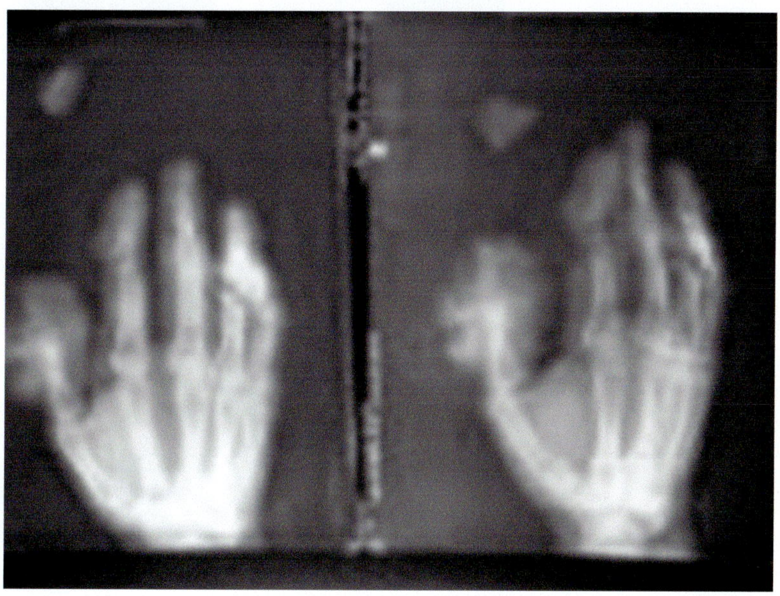

Fig. 14.18 Preoperative X-ray

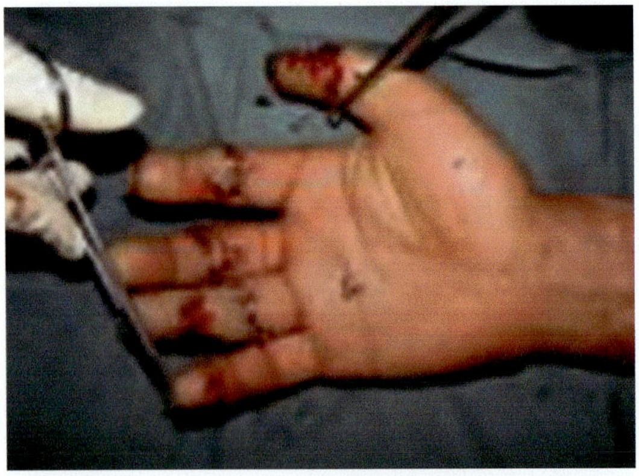

Fig. 14.19 The palm side after replantation

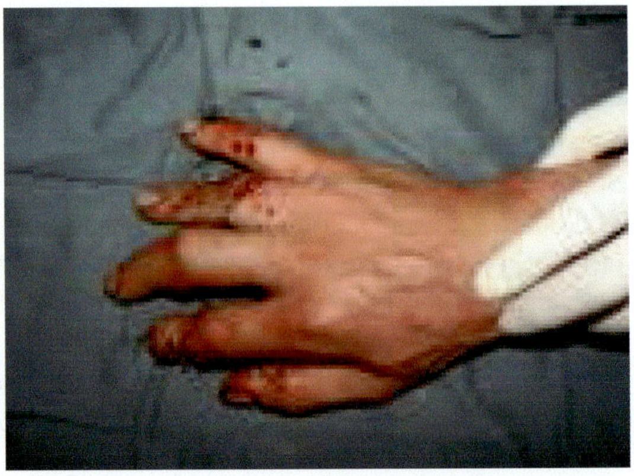

Fig. 14.20 The dorsal side after replantation

Fig. 14.21 Postoperative X-ray

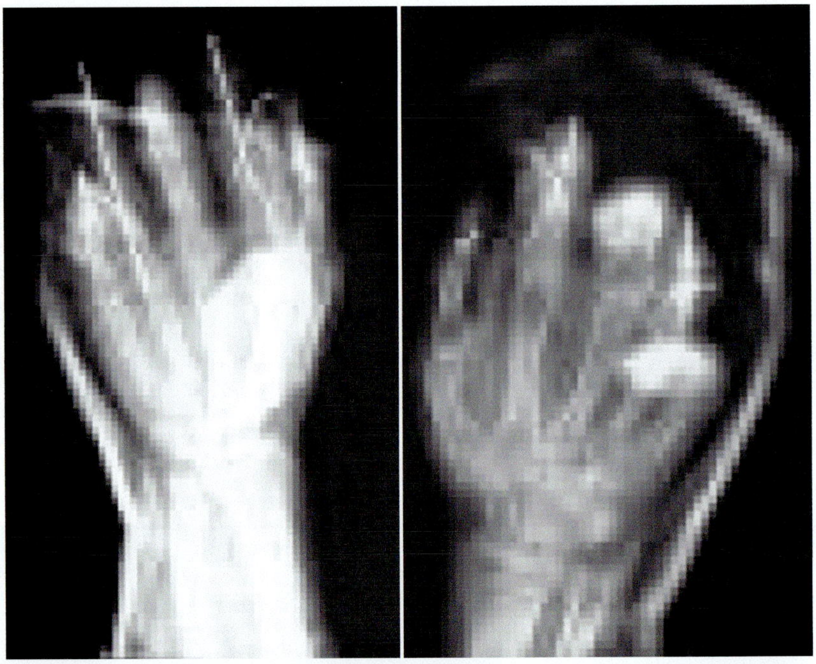

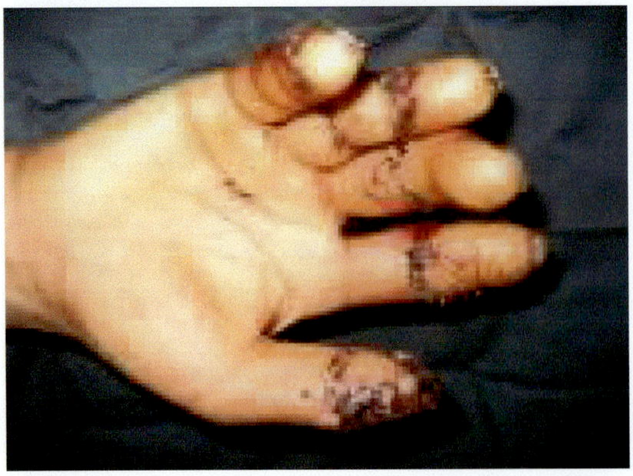

Fig. 14.22 Straight exercise 2 months later

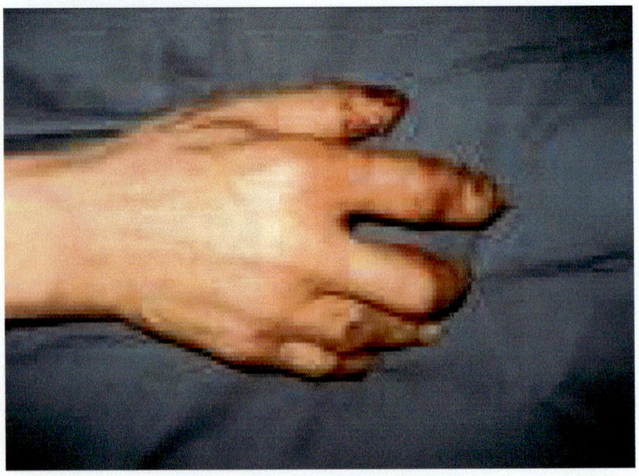

Fig. 14.23 Flexion exercise 2 months later

The severed tissues were relatively complete. Successful debridement and replantation were carried out under anesthesia under emergency conditions. The replanted fingers were red, had moderate tension after relaxing the tourniquet, and were packed with sterile gauze and padded with broken cotton yarn. The patient was brought back to the ward safely and was given conventional treatments postoperatively, such as antibiotics, hormones, and antispasmodic. The replanted severed finger successfully survived. The appearance and function were good after regular follow-up and functional exercise guidance and the patient was satisfied (Figs. 14.24, 14.25, 14.26, 14.27, 14.28, 14.29).

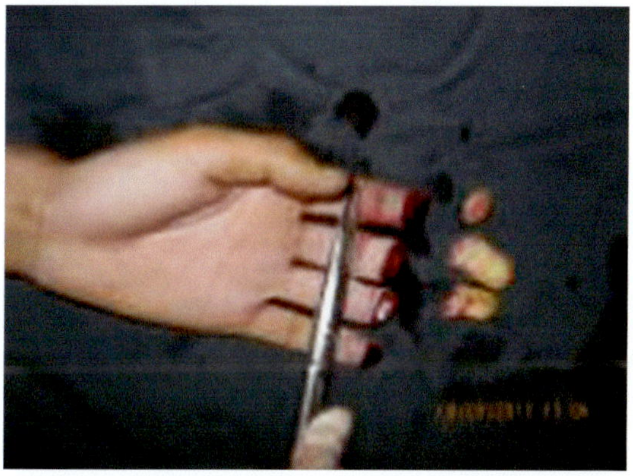

Fig. 14.24 The palm side of the severed fingers

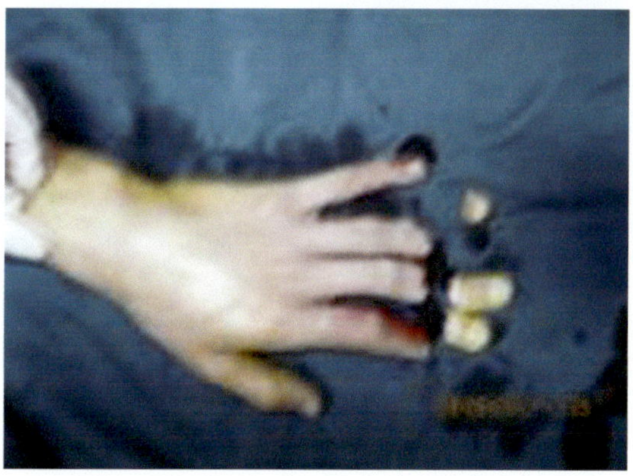

Fig. 14.25 The palm side of the severed fingers

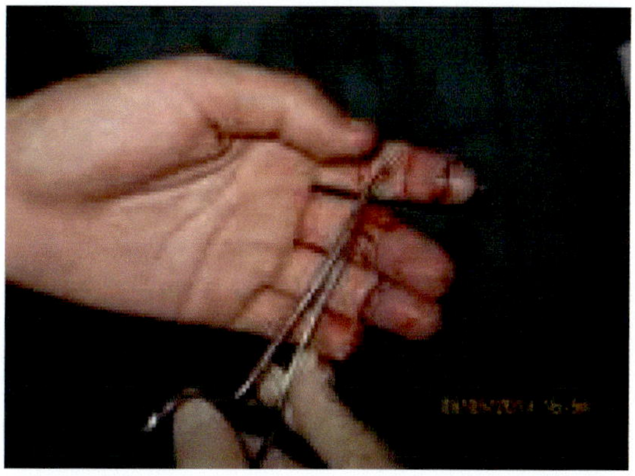

Fig. 14.26 The palm side after replantation

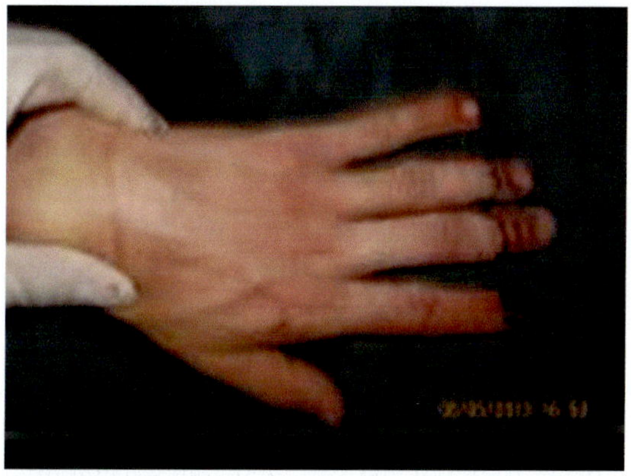

Fig. 14.27 The dorsal side after replantation

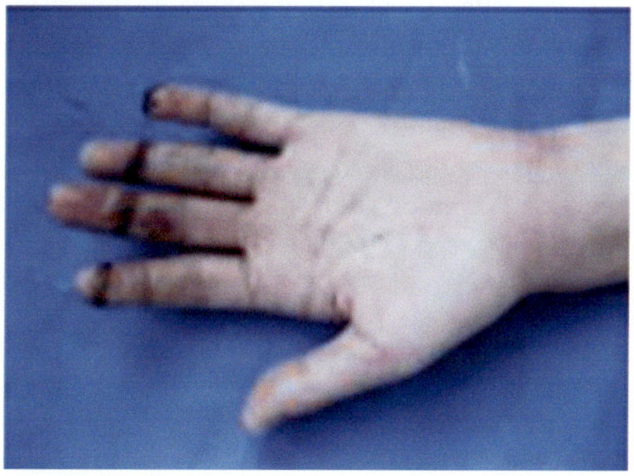

Fig. 14.28 The palm side 1 month later

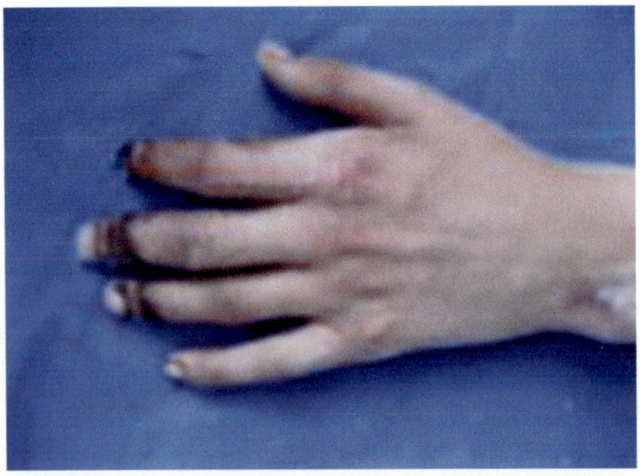

Fig. 14.29 The dorsal side 1 month later

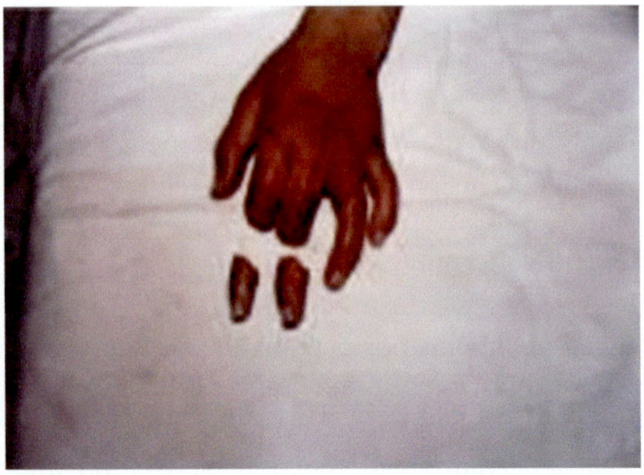

Fig. 14.30 The palm side of the severed fingers

Case 5: Replantation of the Severed Middle Segments of the Index and Middle Fingers

Male patient, 46 years old, admitted to hospital for injury to the left hand caused by a hot mold and bleeding for 1 h. PE: The general situation was good; the vital signs were stable. The middle segments of the index and middle fingers were completely severed with bones, tendons, nerves, and vessels revealed. Successful debridement and replantation were performed under anesthesia under emergency conditions. The replanted fingers were red and had moderate tension after relaxing the tourniquet. They were packed with sterile gauze and padded with broken cotton yarn and the patient was brought back to the ward safely. He was given conventional treatments postoperatively, such as antibiotics, hormones, and antispasmodics. The replanted severed fingers successfully survived. The appearance and function are good after regular follow-up and functional exercise guidance and the patient was satisfied (Figs. 14.30, 14.31, 14.32, 14.33, and 14.34).

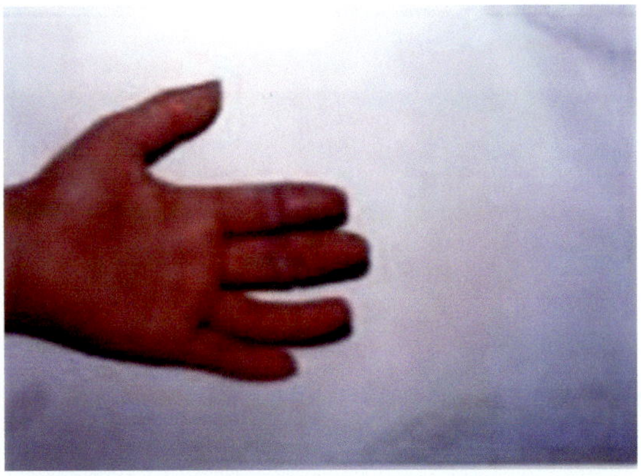

Fig. 14.31 The palm side 12 months later

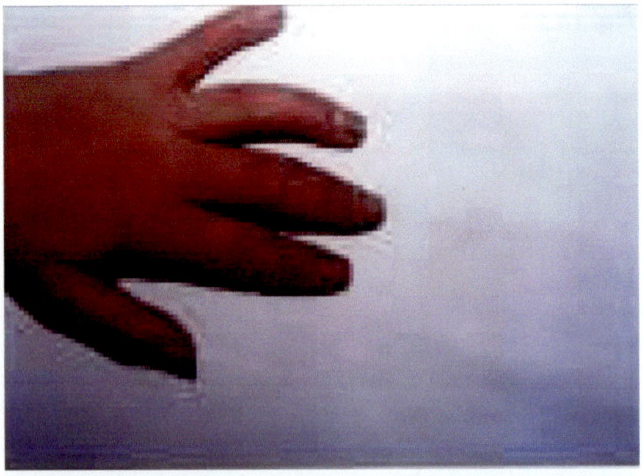

Fig. 14.32 The dorsal side 12 months later

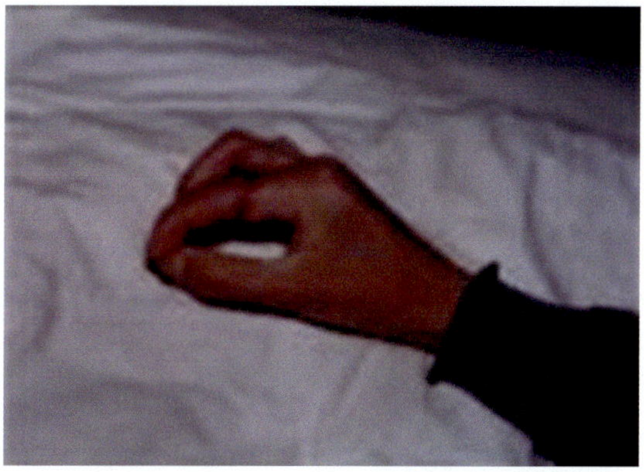

Fig. 14.33 The functioning of the replanted fingers

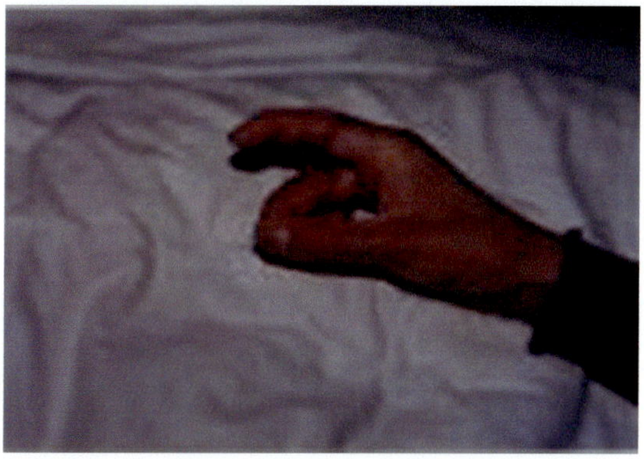

Fig. 14.34 The functioning of the replanted fingers

Case 6: Multi-severed Fingers Re-implantation (10 Severed Fingers)

Patient, male, 20 years old, hands were accidentally cut by a cutting machine, pain, admitted to hospital after 5 hours of bleeding. Physical examination: good general situation and vital signs, different sections of the proximal parts of the five fingers were completely broken off, the cross-section was homogeneous, the wound edge was irregular, the wound was bleeding while the off-body fingers didn't get any blood supply. With bilateral brachial plexus anesthesia, we made a re-implantation operation for 10 severed fingers, which was performed by 12 doctors in 5 groups for simultaneous replantation. In total, 34 veins, 18 arteries, 20 nerves were anastomosed. The replantation operation lasted for 21 h, with an intraoperative 1000 mL blood transfusion and 3000 mL infusion. The surgery went very well. When relaxing the tourniquet, we observed ruddy finger bodies and moderate tension. We used sterile cotton yarn banding to fix the fingers, bulkily packing the cotton yarn around the replanting incisors. When the patient returned to the ward, a post-operative routine "three-anti" treatment was given. An automatic blood circulation monitor was used to monitor the blood circulation of the replantation fingers. One week after the operation it was clear that all the replanted fingers had survived, and 4 weeks after the surgery the Kirschner wires were removed and the fingers began to receive active functional rehabilitation training. Six weeks after surgery the passive function of rehabilitation exercise was performed. After a 1-year follow-up, the feeling recovery went up to S3+, the distal pulp of two distinguishing points was to 9–10 mm. The patient could use chopsticks to eat, wear the clothing buckle and perform other daily activities, and was satisfied with the shape and function of the replanted fingers (Figs. 14.35, 14.36, 14.37, 14.38, 14.39, 14.40, 14.41, 14.42, and 14.43).

The cases are generally provided by Dr. JIan li jWang.

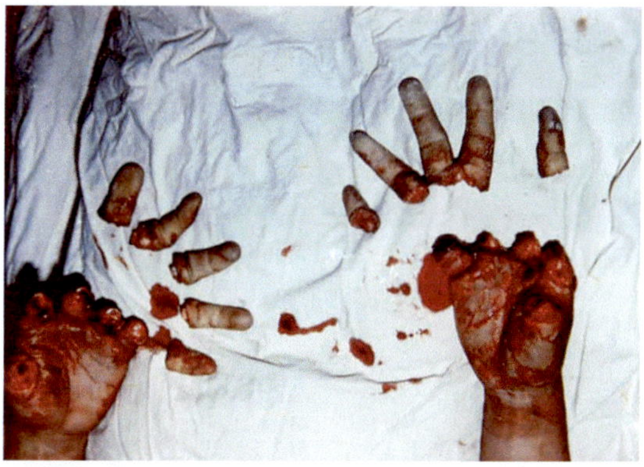

Fig. 14.35 The preoperative situation

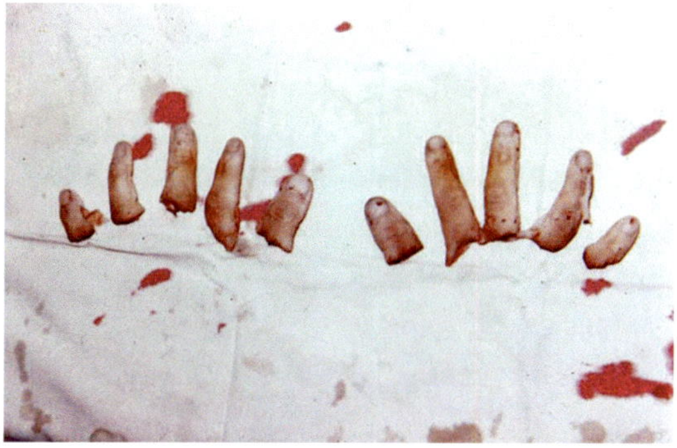

Fig. 14.36 The distal situation of the 10 severed fingers

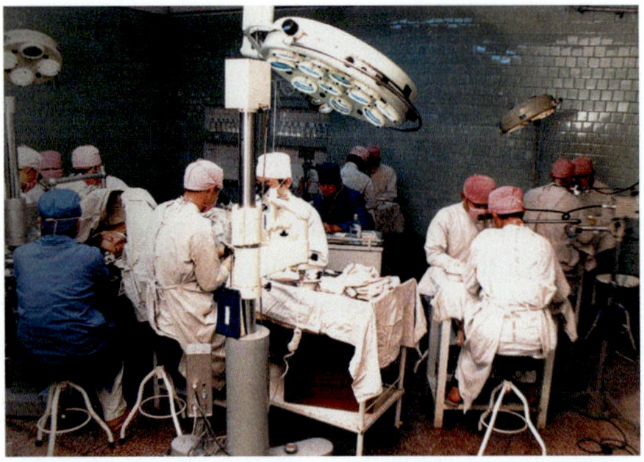

Fig. 14.37 The surgeons were divided into 5 groups

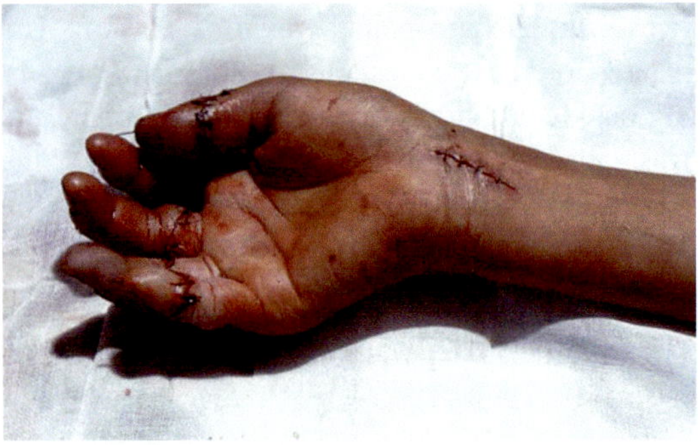

Fig. 14.38 All the replanted fingers of the left hand survived 10 days after surgery

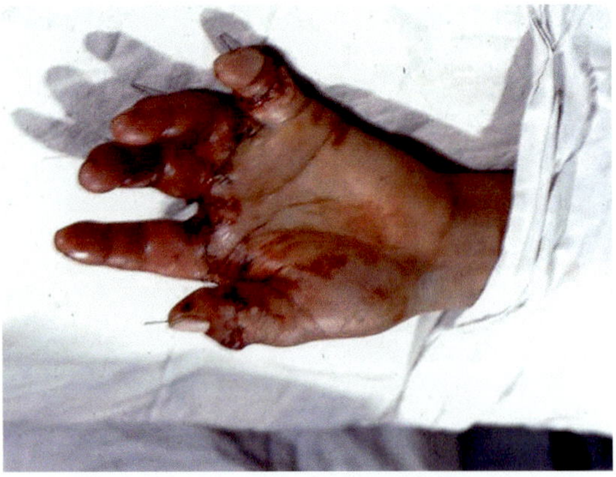

Fig. 14.39 All the replanted fingers of right hand survived 10 days after surgery

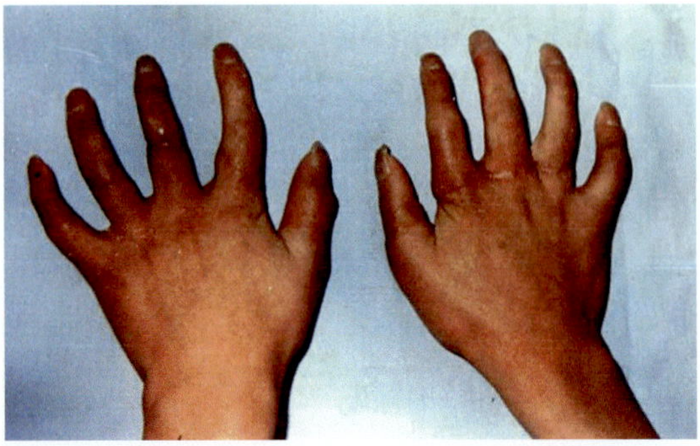

Fig. 14.40 Fingers' extensional function 1 year after surgery

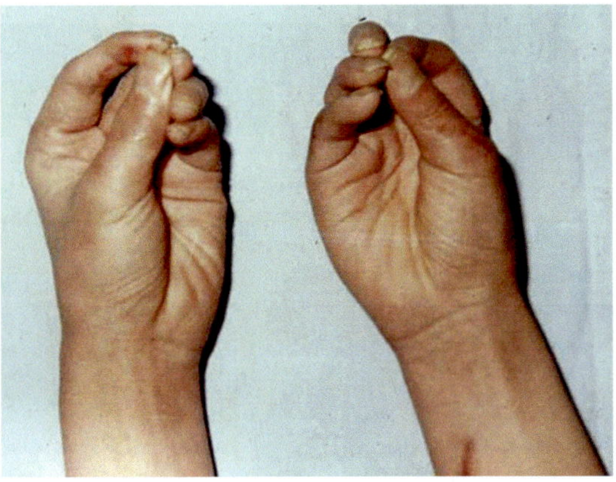

Fig. 14.41 The thumb opposing function 1 year after the surgery

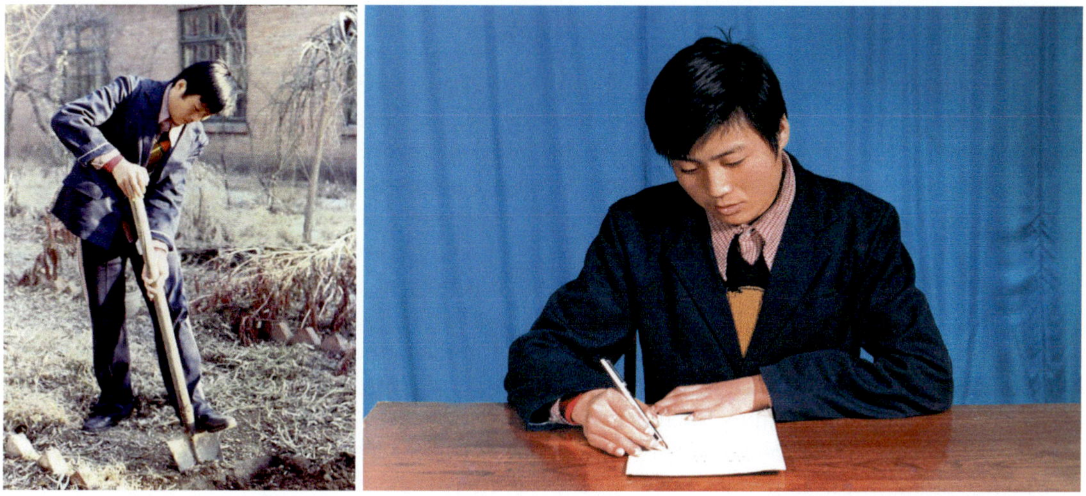

Fig. 14.42 Working and studying 3 years after the replantation surgery

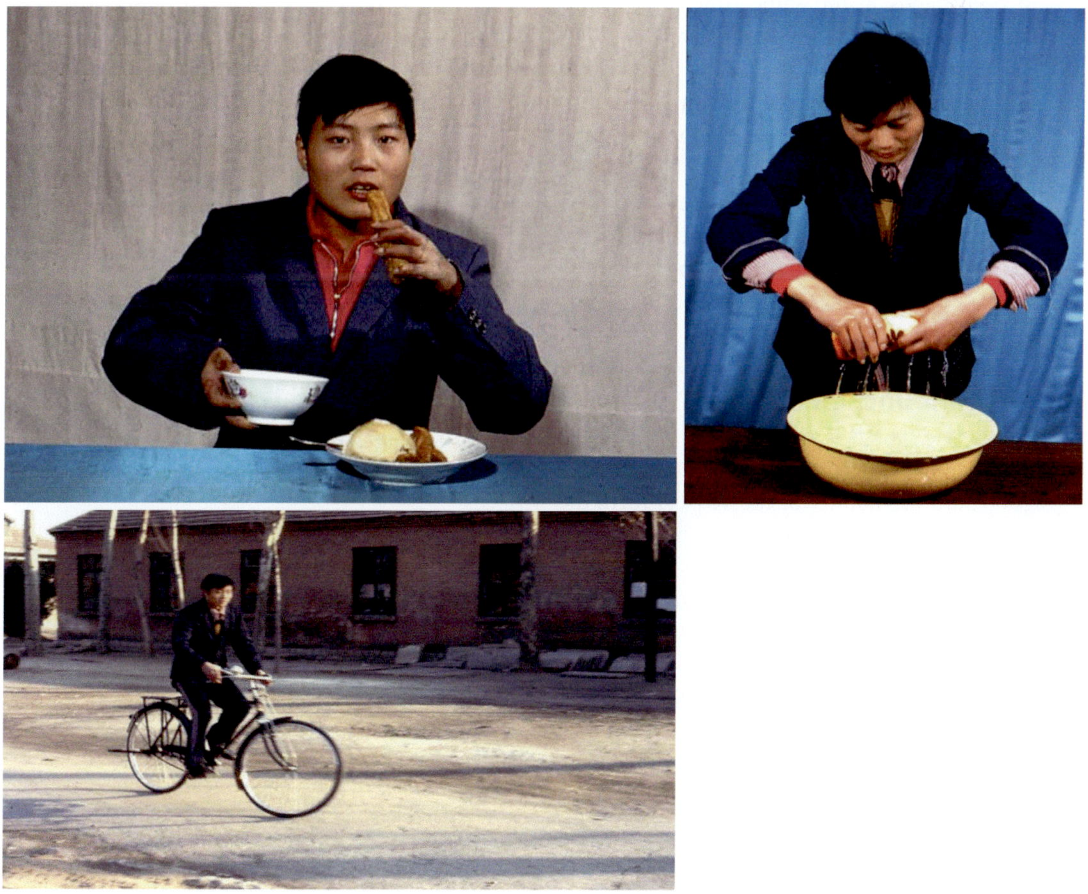

Fig. 14.43 Daily life 3 years after the replantation surgery

14.3 Key Points in Surgery

(a) Mark the severed fingers after assessment and save them in a 4 °C refrigerator with sterile gauze packed before replantation.
(b) Operating room personnel are grouped to carry out debridement on each hand under the guidance of a senior physician.
(c) In principle, the fingers should be replanted from the thumb to the little finger, one by one, and the priority finger should be chosen according to the importance of the function and the condition of the injury, such as restoring the function of the hand mostly by means of replanting a less important finger into a more important position.
(d) Two or more groups performing replantation in both hands at the same time is advantageous for increasing the success rate.
(e) Make one needle fixation as far as possible and suture the deep flexor tendon and extensor tendon in turn to shorten operating time significantly.
(f) When multiple fingers are severed in different planes, the amputated finger which is left less in proximal side should be replanted first.

14.4 Announcements

(a) Professional microsurgical techniques and good suturing quality of the vessels form the basis for the successful replantation of multiple severed fingers.
(b) We have to shorten the bones in serious multiple severed fingers and preserve the joints as far as possible, especially the metacarpophalangeal and proximal finger joints.
(c) Pay attention to preventing rotation, valgus–varus, and angulation in replanted fingers, and to adjusting the tension of the tendons.
(d) When more than five fingers have been severed, grouping operating room personnel to take it in turns to perform the replantation is advantageous in easing the burden on doctors and increasing the success rate.
(e) Multiple severed fingers are always combined with other damage that causes hemorrhagic shock, which should be corrected by supplementing the blood volume to increase the success rate.
(f) Compared with a single severed finger, the recovery of multiple severed fingers in multiple planes is worth it, because of the more serious condition and more time needed for fixation. We should withdraw the needles and guide the functional exercises.

Suggested Reading

Arata J, Ishikawa K, Soeda H, Kitayama T. Replantation of multi-level fingertip amputation using the pocket principle (palmar pocket method). Br J Plast Surg. 2003;56(5):504–8.

Arata J, Ishikawa K, Soeda H. Replantation of fingertip amputation by palmar pocket method in children. Plast Reconstr Surg. 2011;127(3):78e–80e.

Belsky MR, Ruby LK. Double level amputation: should it be replanted. J Reconstr Microsurg. 1986; 2(3):159.

Beris AE, Lykissas MG, Korompilias AV, et al. Digit and hand replantation. Arch Orthop Trauma Surg. 2010;130(9):1141–7.

Cai J, Cao X, Pan J, et al. Replantation of a multiple digit and circular palm amputation: a case report. Microsurgery. 1993;14:221–4.

Changqing Z, Jianing W, Guanglei T, et al. Clinical analysis of multi-fingers replantation of 207 fingers. Natl Med J China. 2001;81(3):182–3.

Changyue W, Qishen F, Deliang G. Replantation of multi-fingers severed. Chin J Reparative Reconstr Surg. 2000;1:55.

Cheng G. Review and outlook of special type replantation. Chin J Microsurg. 2000;23:19–20.

Cheng TJ, Cheng NC, Tang YB. Restoration of basic hand function by double transpositional digital replantation in five-digit amputations. J Reconstr Microsurg. 2004;20(3):201–5.

Davis Sears E, Chung KC. Replantation of finger avulsion injuries: a systematic review of survival and functional outcomes. J Hand Surg Am. 2011;36(4):686–94.

Dong H, Weichi W, Qingsong W, et al. Treatment outcome of multiple digital replantation. Chin J Microsurg. 2002;1:28–30.

Mingwu Z, Dongshen Z, Yang R, et al. 1 case of replantation of 11 segments of ten fingers. Chin J Microsurg. 2000;23(3):176.

Pei GX, Zhao DS, Xie CP, Wang ST. Replantation of multilevel hand severances. Injury. 1998;29(5):357–61.

Sebastin SJ, Chung KC. A systematic review of the outcomes of replantation of distal digital amputation. Plast Reconstr Surg. 2011;128(3):723–37.

Weiyan Z, Bingwan L, Yongsheng H, et al. Analysis of influencing factors of multi-fingers replantation. J Beihua Univ (Nat Sci). 2008;9(1):56–7.

Xiaoke S, Bin L, Dongping L, et al. Replantation of multi-fingers severed in multi-planes. Chin J Hand Surg. 2006;6:382–3.

Yang Z, Biguang Z, Zhengren P. Replantation of segmental destructive amputation of multiple fingers. Chin J Reparative Reconstr Surg. 2001;6:370–2.

Yousif NJ, Muoneke V, Sanger JR, Matloub HS. Hand replantation following three-level amputation: a case report. J Hand Surg Am. 1992;17(2):220–5.

Yu H, Wei L, Liang B, et al. Nonsurgical factors of digital replantation and survival rate: a metaanalysis. Indian J Orthop. 2015;49(3):265–71.

Zhuopeng W, Guojun X, Bilan Y, et al. The application of finger body of multi-fingers severed in reconstruct hand function. J Pract Hand Surg. 2005;19(1):45.

15 Replantation of Severed Fingers with Soft-Tissue Defects

15.1 Summary

With the development of industry and agriculture, and diversification of the automatic machine, there are and increasing number of types of severed fingers including those with soft-tissue defects. Soft-tissue defects include defect of the skin, vessels, and nerves, and there is a lack of a regular method for repair because of the complicated conditions, the variety of injuries, and variety of ways to repair them. Professional microsurgical techniques and a knowledge of flaps are required for surgeons so that they choose a suitable flap for repair according to the type of injury and the extent, position, and scope of the defect. Soft-tissue defect was listed as a contraindication for replantation in the 1980s. The replantation used to be applied by shortening bones that would survive, but without satisfactory appearance and function. Sometimes, to preserve the joints and length of the fingers, palliative debridement may cause infection, necrosis of the skin, and poor blood supply, which will affect finger survival or the finger survives, but the functioning is affected by the shortened finger, poor sensation, severe tendon adhesion, and stiff joints. With the development of microsurgery techniques and the maturity of flaps, vessels, tendons, flaps, and composite tissue flaps can be used to repair the soft-tissue defects of severed fingers to reduce postoperative vascular crisis, increase the survival rate, and expand the indications for replantation.

There are many methods of soft-tissue defect repair, and no uniform system of classification. According to the location of supply area, it can be divided into pedicle flaps and free flaps. Depending on the blood vessels in the tissue, these can be divided into artery flap and vein flap. A composite tissue flap can be composed of different tissues, such as tendons, nerves, deep fascia, plantar toe joints, and interphalangeal joints.

The flow-through flap was first introduced by Soutar et al. (1983) in 1983. Since then, it has become the ideal way to reconstruct the blood supply for soft tissue defects of severed fingers, which is believed to have the following advantages: convenient design, convenient gain, and constant vessel anatomy. Xu Yafei et al. (2011) then improved it and increased the survival rate of this flap, which created a new idea about how to treat such an injury.

15.2 Case Description

Case 1: Replantation of a Severed Left Thumb Severed with Soft Tissue and Flap Repair

Male patient, 27 years old, was admitted to hospital for injury to the left hand caused by a punch and bleeding for 1 h. Physical Examination. The general situation was good; the vital signs were stable. The soft tissue of the distal interphalangeal joint of the thumb had an avulsed defect, the structures and tissues of the proximal part had

J. Lin et al., *Special Type of Finger Replantation*, https://doi.org/10.1007/978-981-10-6229-2_15

changed and were polluted, with bones, tendons, nerves, and vessels revealed, an uneven wound, and bleeding. Successful debridement was performed, and an island flap of the dorsum of the index finger and the first dorsal metacarpal flap were carried out under anesthesia under emergency conditions. The replanted finger was red and had moderate tension after relaxing the tourniquet. It was packed with sterile gauze and padded with broken cotton yarn and the patient was brought back to the ward safely. He was given conventional treatments postoperatively, such as antibiotics, hormones, and antispasmodics. By 2 weeks later, the replanted severed finger and the flaps had successfully survived. The appearance and function were good after regular follow-up and functional exercise guidance, and the patient was satisfied (Figs. 15.1, 15.2, 15.3, 15.4, 15.5, 15.6, 15.7, and 15.8).

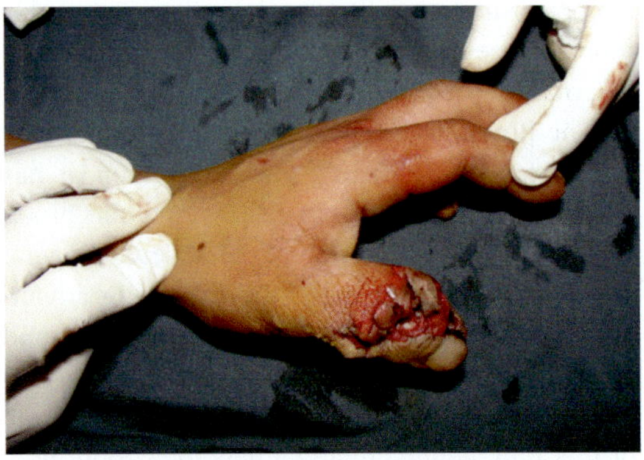

Fig. 15.1 The dorsal side

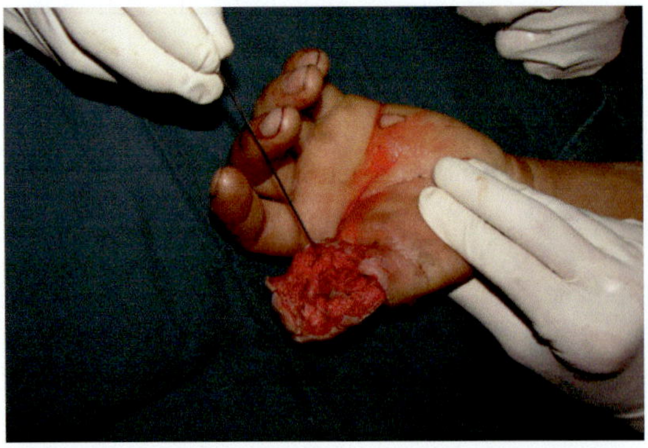

Fig. 15.2 The palm side

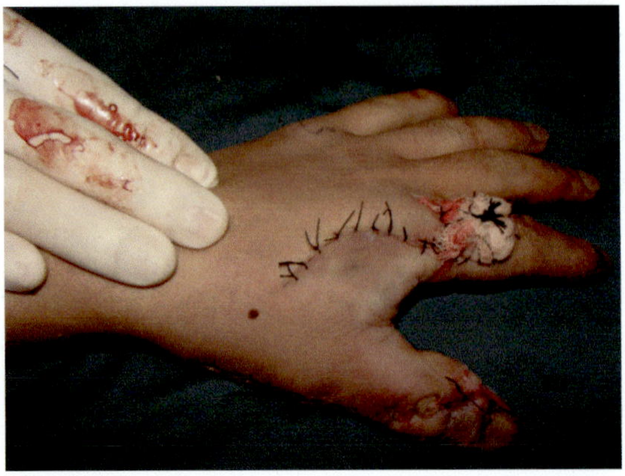

Fig. 15.3 During surgery

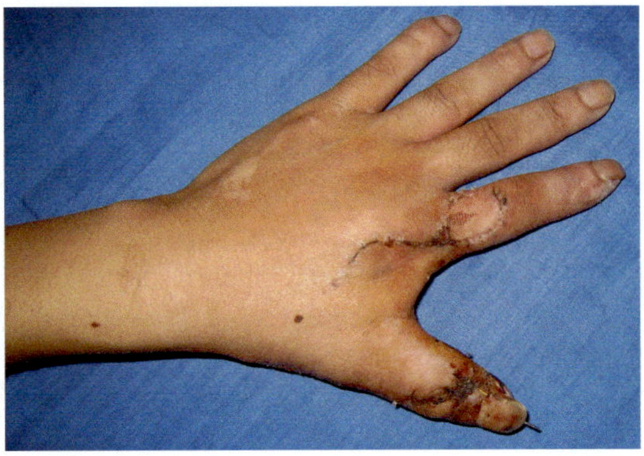

Fig. 15.4 Two weeks after the operation

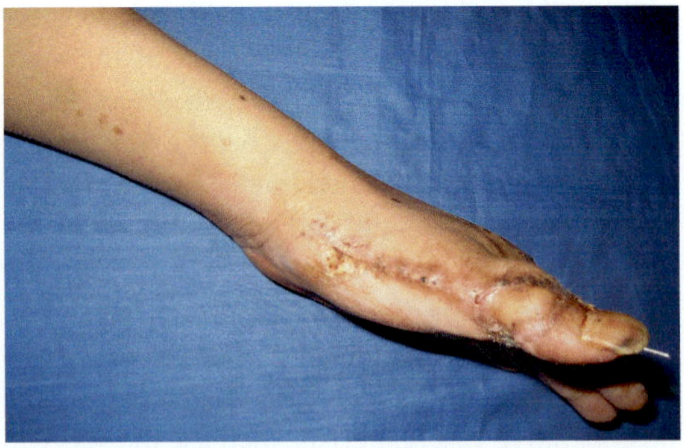

Fig. 15.5 Six weeks after the operation

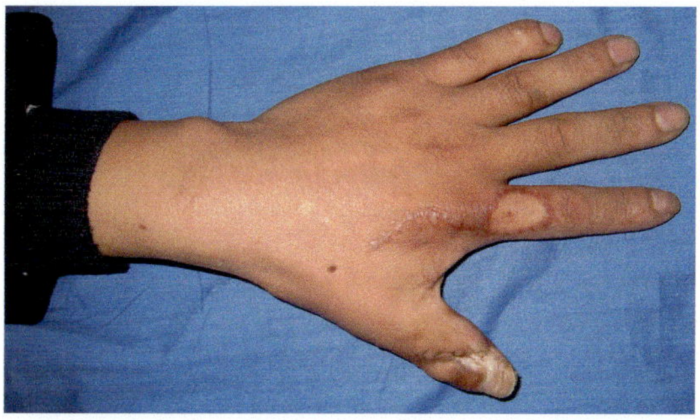

Fig. 15.6 The dorsal side 8 months later

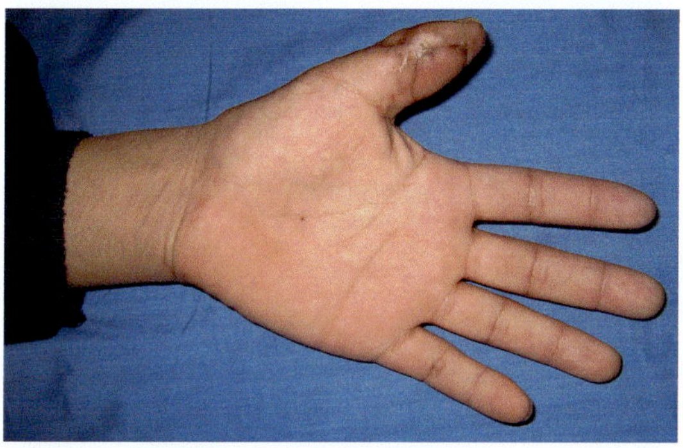

Fig. 15.7 The palm side 8 months later

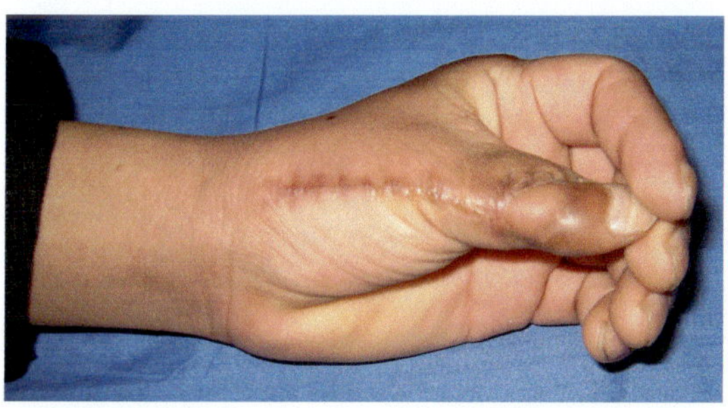

Fig. 15.8 The thumb opposing function 8 months later

Case 2: Replantation of the Right Hand with Destructive Fragmentation and Flap Repair
Male patient, 55 years old, was admitted to hospital for injury to the left hand caused by a punch and bleeding for 2 h. PE: The general situation was good; the vital signs were stable. The soft tissue of the distal wrist had an avulsed defect, the structures and tissues changed and were polluted, with bones, tendons, nerves, and vessels revealed, uneven wounds, and bleeding. Successful debridement was performed and a suprawrist cutaneous branch flap of the ulnar artery was made under anesthesia under emergency conditions. The replanted finger was red and had moderate tension after relaxing the tourniquet. It was packed with sterile gauze and padded with broken cotton yarn, and the patient was brought back to the ward safely. The patient was given conventional treatments postoperatively such as antibiotics, hormones, and antispasmodics. By 2 weeks later, the replanted severed finger and the flaps had successfully survived. The appearance and function were good after regular follow-up and functional exercise guidance, and the patient was satisfied (Figs. 15.9, 15.10, 15.11, 15.12, 15.13, 15.14, 15.15, 15.16, 15.17, 15.18, 15.19, and 15.20).

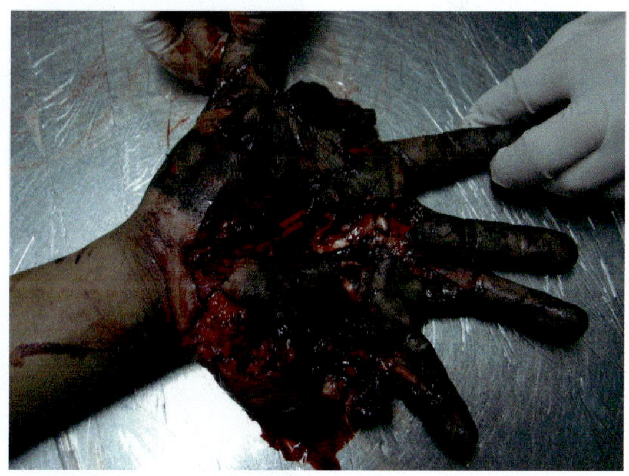

Fig. 15.9 The palm side

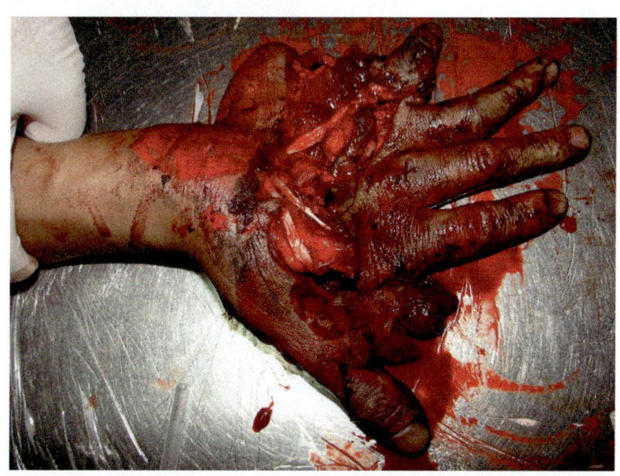

Fig. 15.10 The dorsal side

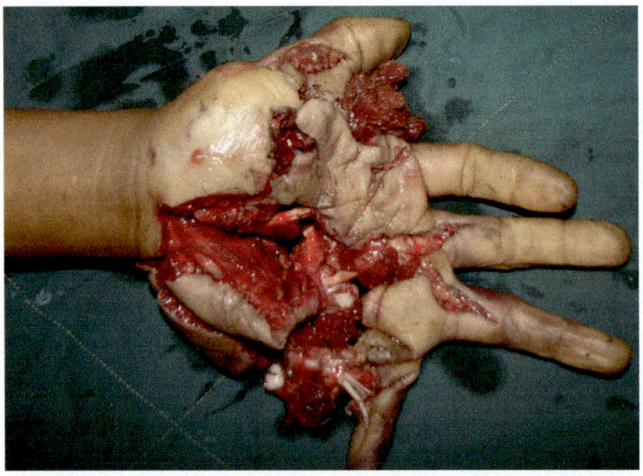

Fig. 15.11 The palm side after cleaning

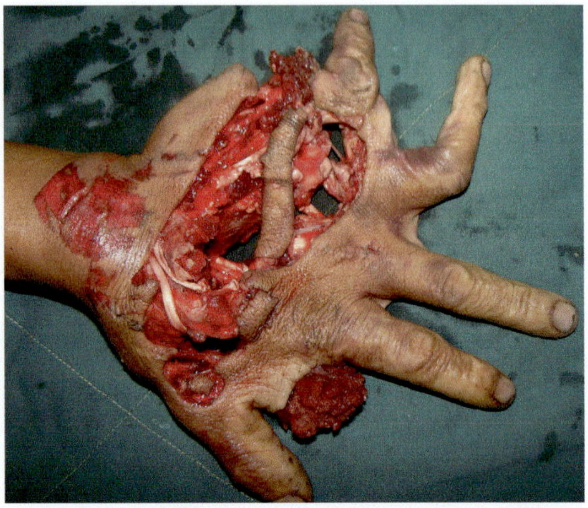

Fig. 15.12 The dorsal side after cleaning

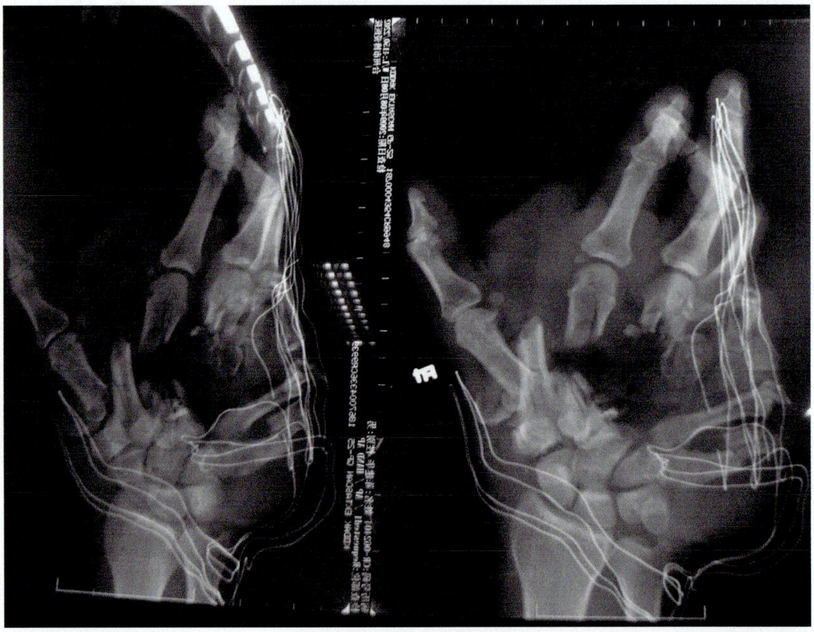

Fig. 15.13 Preoperative X-ray

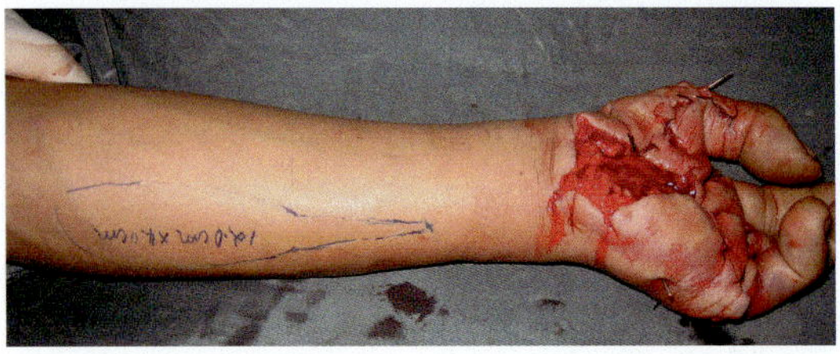

Fig. 15.14 The soft-tissue defect after replantation

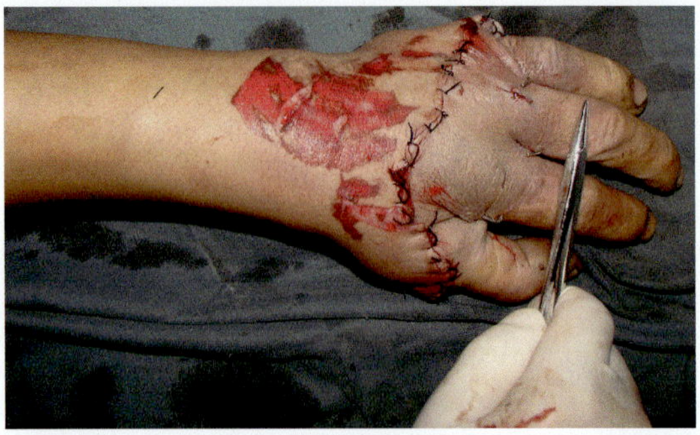

Fig. 15.15 The dorsal side after replantation

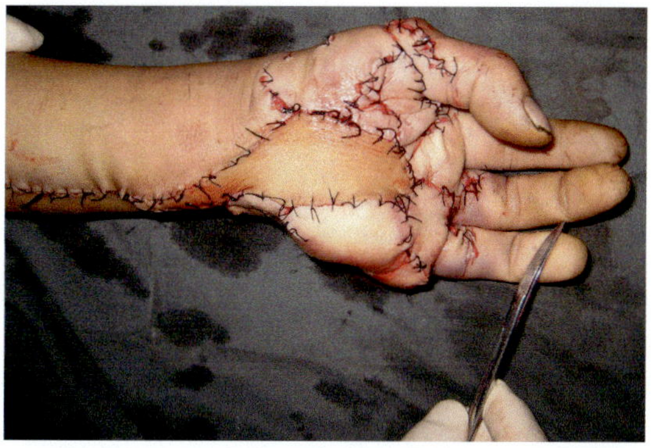

Fig. 15.16 After flap repair

Fig. 15.17 X-ray 6 weeks later

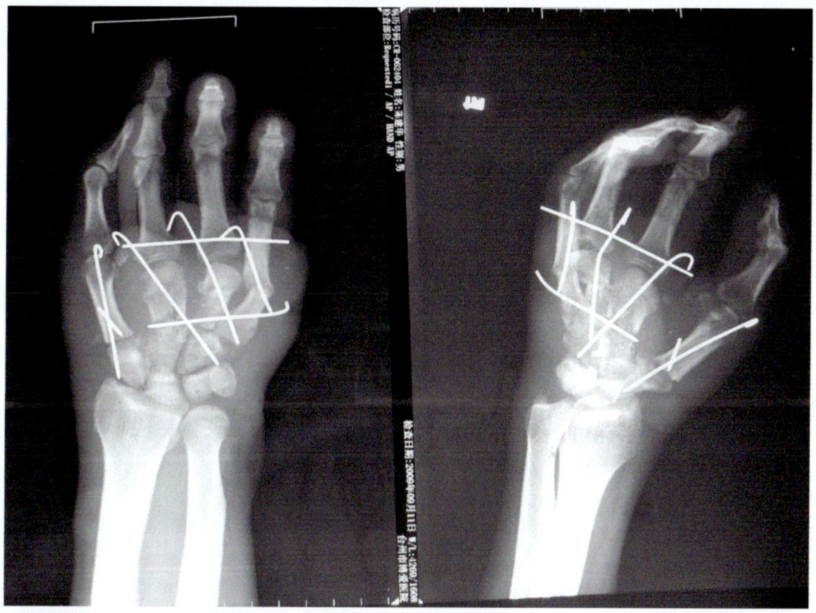

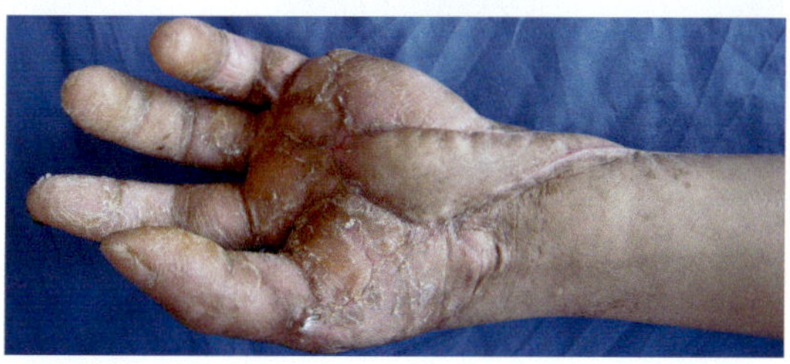

Fig. 15.18 The palm side 3 months later

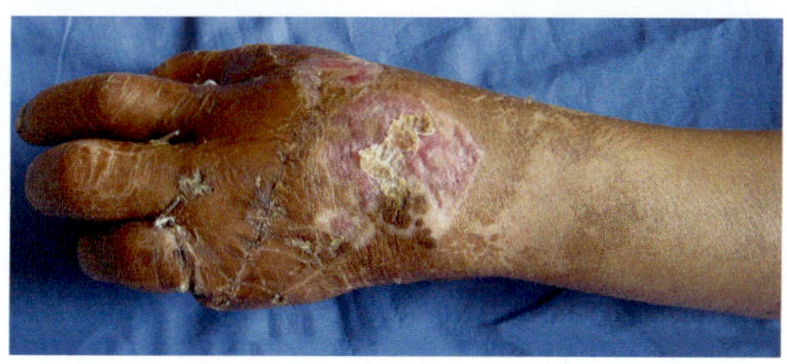

Fig. 15.19 The dorsal side 3 months later

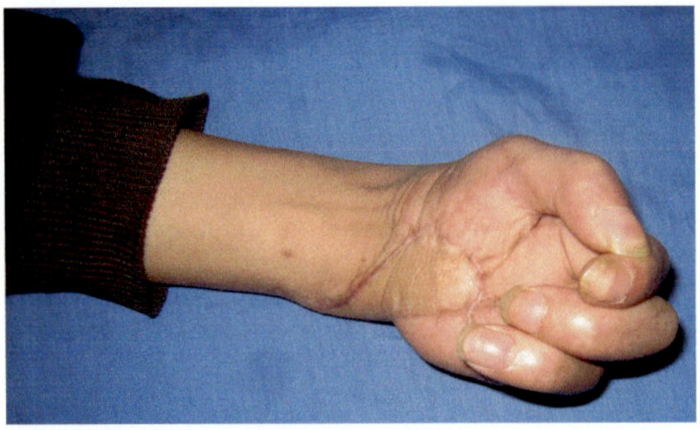

Fig. 15.20 Digital flexion function 7 months later

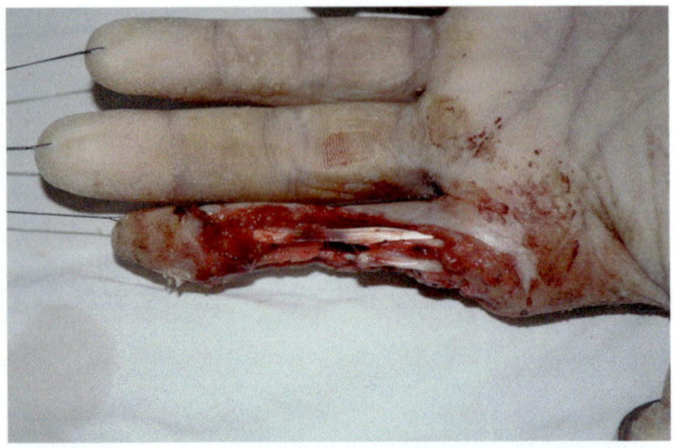

Fig. 15.21 Volar view of the right injured hand

Case 3: Replantation of Right Index Finger with Soft Tissue Defect

The patient, male, 41 years old, a machine crush led to severance of the right index finger, pain in the middle finger. He came to hospital after 2 hours bleeding. Physical examination: the general situation was good with stable vital signs. The right ring finger was broken from the interphalangeal joint, at the broken sites the soft tissue was seriously contused, while some skin and soft tissue were defected. Under anesthesia, we broke off the distal and the proximal part of the wound, the proximal part of the interphalangeal joint was missing; under the microscope we separated the distal and proximal end of the vascular nerves, and designed a composite tissue flap from the ipsilateral interphalangeal joint of the second toe, carrying joints and tibial toe inherent vascular nerve bundles combined with the dorsal skins to graft in the donor site, maintaining the fibular nerve bundles of the second toe. We fixed the severed finger and transplanted composite tissue flap with a 1.2 mm Kirschner wire, repaired the flexor tendon, anastomosed the radial nerve bundles and finger (toe) dorsal vein. After relaxing the tourniquet, the replanted finger and transplanted tissues showed a ruddy colour and moderate tension. The right second toe was partly shortened and fixed after suturing the skin margins. The replanted fingers and composite tissue flap survived well, with a good shape and satisfactory recovery function. The second toe of the donor site showed a good appearance plus a good function (Figs. 15.21, 15.22, 15.23, 15.24, 15.25, 15.26, 15.27, 15.28, and 15.29).

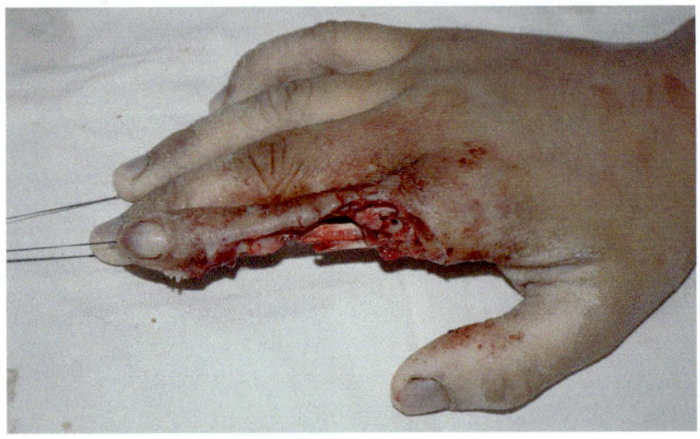

Fig. 15.22 Dorsal view of the right injured hand

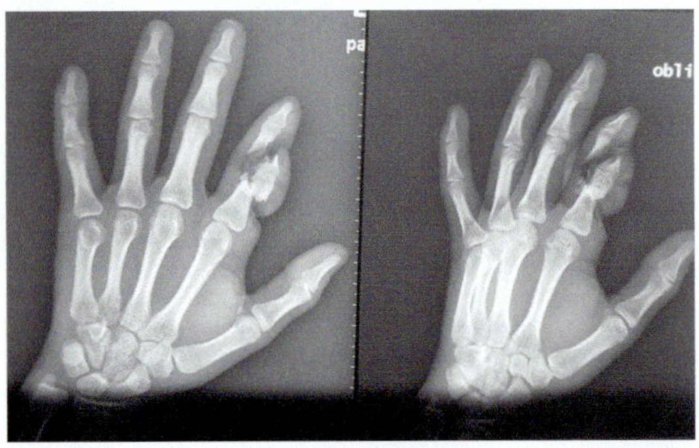

Fig. 15.23 X-ray before the operation

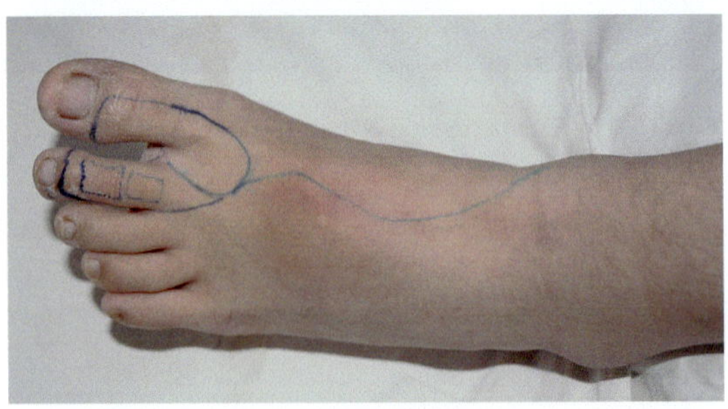

Fig. 15.24 Design of the composited tissue flap

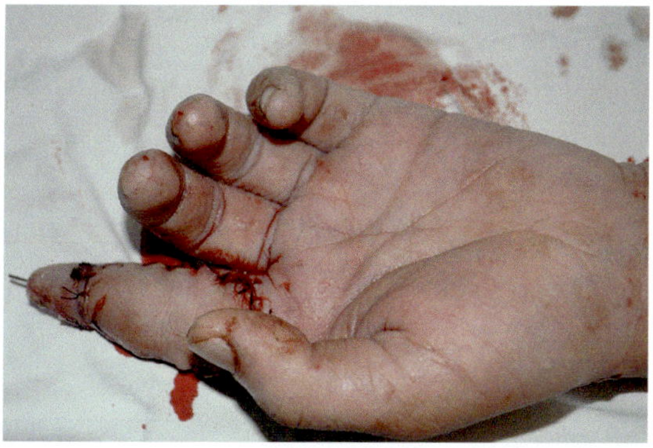

Fig. 15.25 Volar view of the flap in the operation

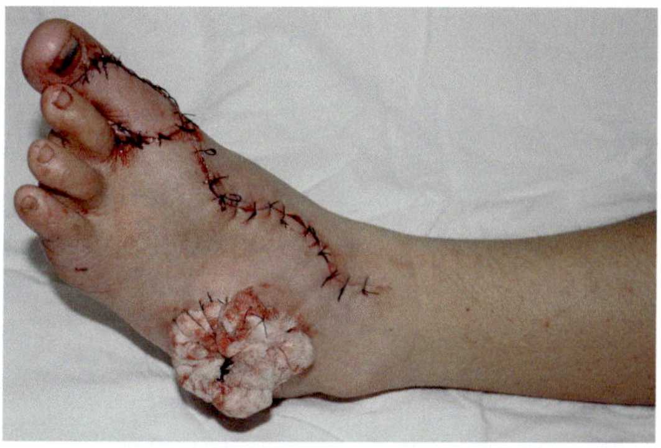

Fig. 15.26 The repair of the donor site

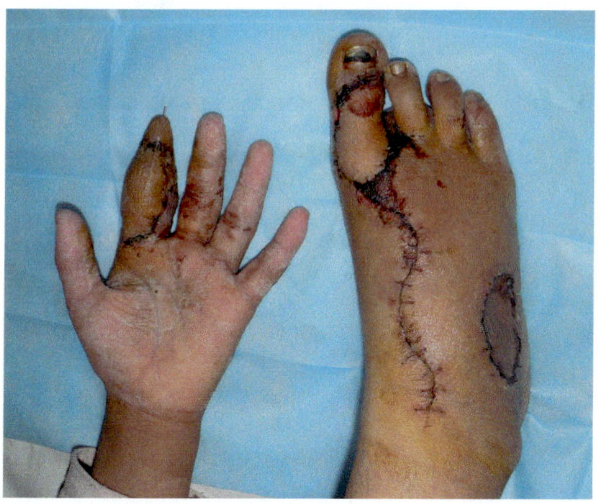

Fig. 15.27 The recipient and donor site 2 weeks post-operation

The cases are generally provided by Dr Ming wu Zhou.

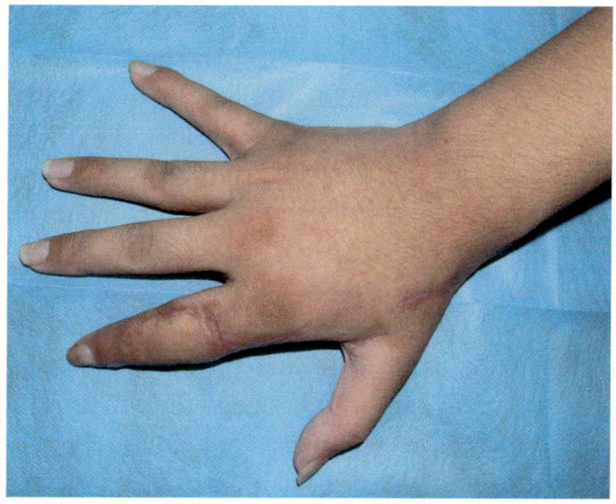

Fig. 15.28 Doral side view 12 months after surgery

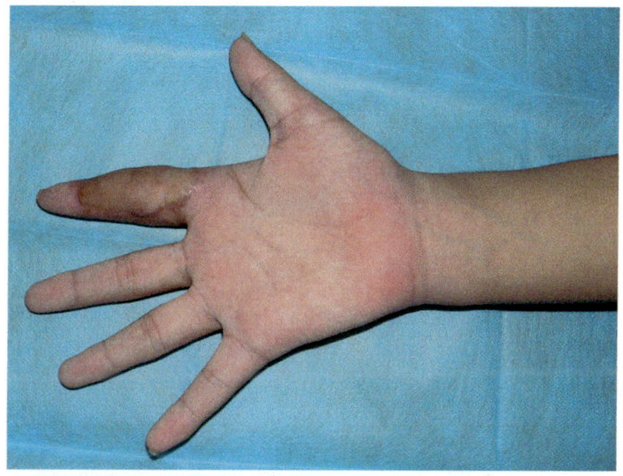

Fig. 15.29 Volar side view 12 months after surgery

Case 4: Free Intercostal Joint Tissue Flap Transplantation to Repair the Defect of Amputated Right Ring Finger with Complex Soft Tissue Defect

Patient, male, 41 years old, a machine crushed and severed the right fingers, pain, bleeding 2 hours before admission to hospital. Physical examination: the general situation was good, vital signs, the right ring finger was completely broken from the interphalangeal joint, the soft tissues were defected in the broken site and there was no blood supply in the distal part. The volar skins of the proximal part of right middle fingers were defected, the distal part got a little blood supply. Under brachial plexus anesthesia, we harvested the same side of the second toe interphalangeal joint complex tissue flap (including the joint, tibial toe inherent vascular nerve bundles) to repair the defected area and bridge the defective vascular. The surgery went very smoothly; after relaxing the tourniquet, we saw the replanted fingers along with the transplanted tissues showing ruddy colour and moderate tension, which indicated a good blood supply. We sutured the edge of the skin; and fixed the remaining and shortening the part of the second toe of the right foot. We did a postoperative follow-up; replantation and composite tissue flaps survived well, with an excellent shape and satisfactory function (Figs. 15.30, 15.31, 15.32, 15.33, 15.34, 15.35, 15.36, 15.37, and 15.38).

The cases are generally provided by Dr. Guang jun Liu.

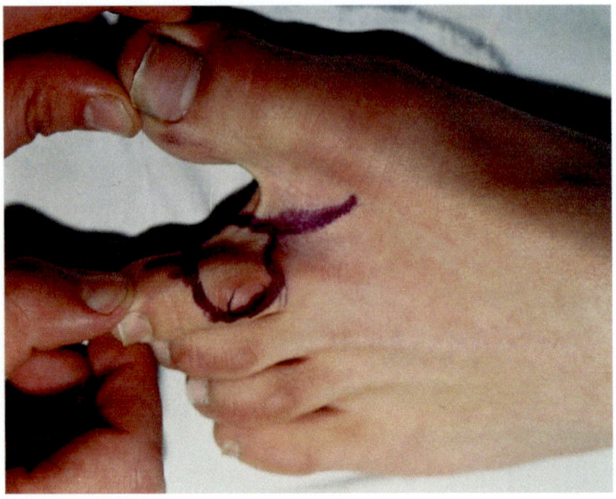

Fig. 15.32 The design of the composited tissue flap of the donor site

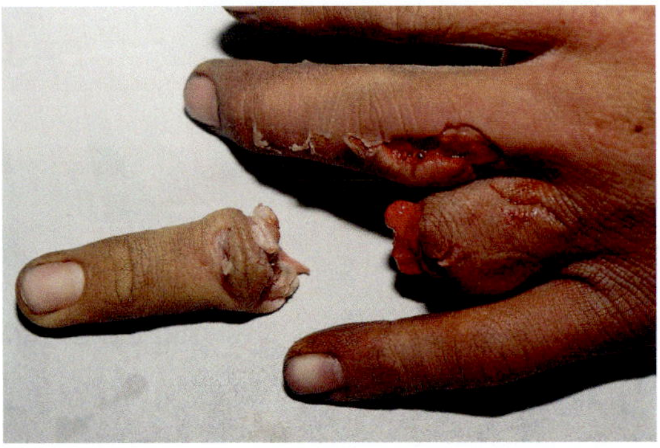

Fig. 15.30 Dorsal situation of the right hand

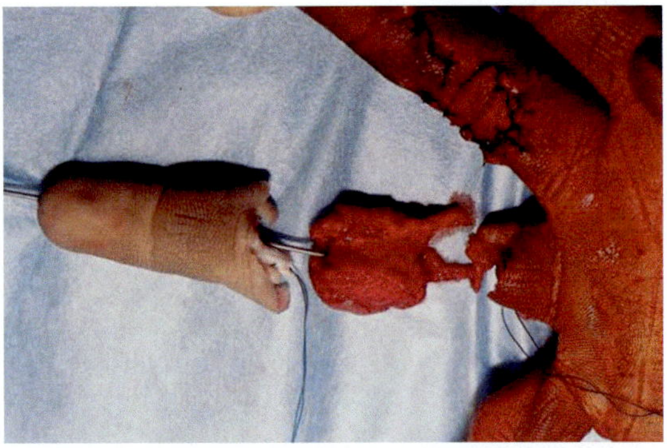

Fig. 15.33 Volar site of the transplanting tissues

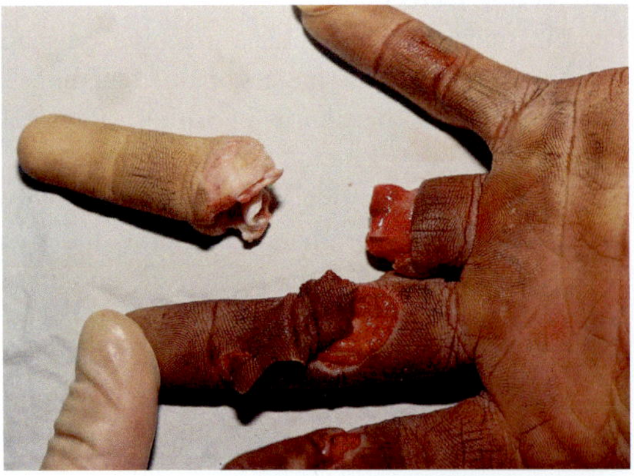

Fig. 15.31 Volar situation of the right hand

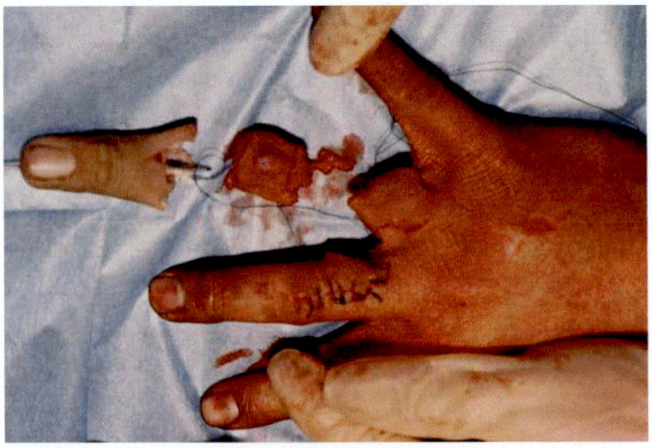

Fig. 15.34 Dosral site of the transplanting tissues

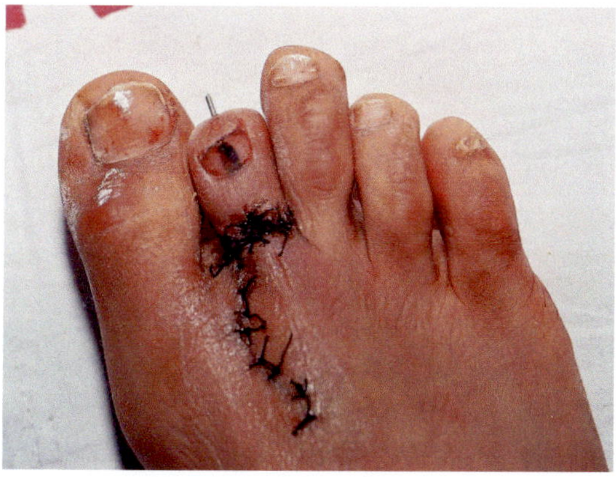

Fig. 15.35 The donor site situation after the operation

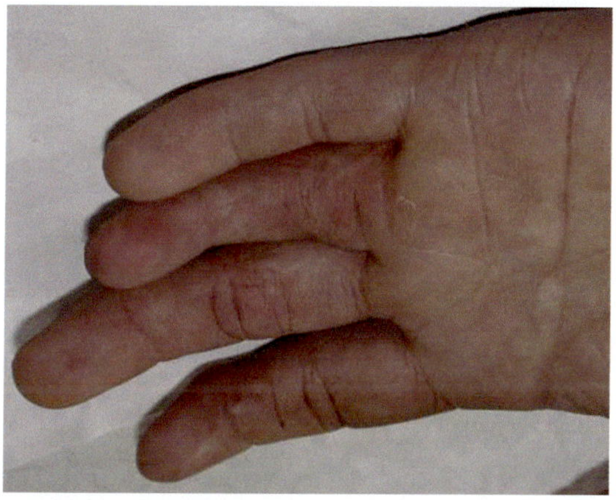

Fig. 15.36 Fingers extension function 18 months after surgery

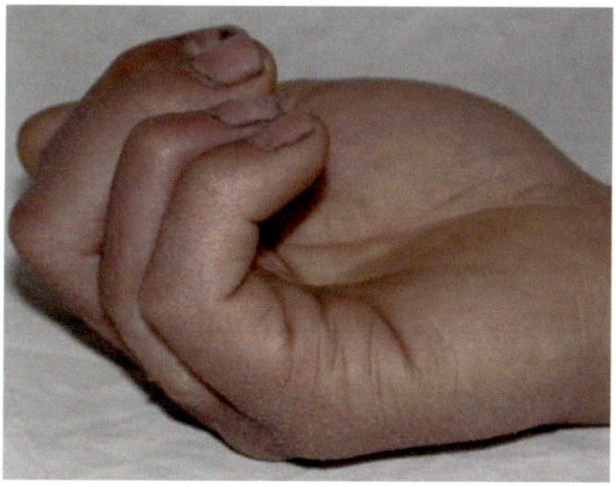

Fig. 15.37 Fingers flexing function 18 months after surgery

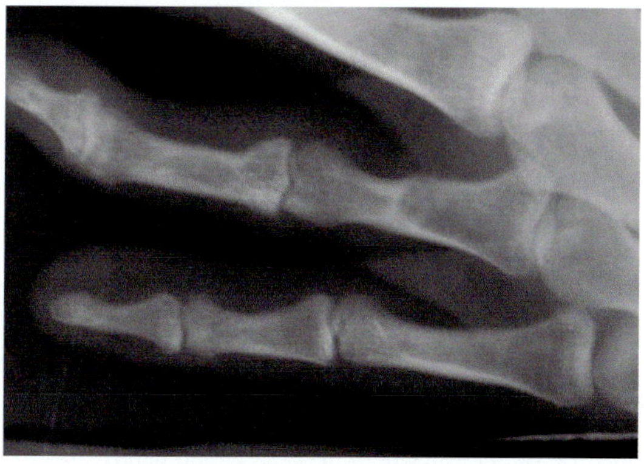

Fig. 15.38 X-ray situation 18 months after surgery

Case 5: Repair and Replantation of the Left Amputated Fingers with Soft Tissue Defect with Dorsal Pedis Flap

Patient, female, 35 years old, machine crush injury caused pain in the left hand, bleeding and a limited activity for 3 hours when coming to the hospital. Physical examination: the general situation was good, vital signs were stable, with the left index finger and the distal part of the second metacarpal completely defected, the middle finger was broken at the neck of the metacarpal, the structure of whole finger body was retained, the skin was defected in the area between the index finger and the thumb. During the emergency, under the brachial plexus anesthesia, we debrided and replanted the severed middle finger. Simultaneously, we harvested the same side of the dorsal pedis flap to repair the skin defects between the index finger and the thumb. After relaxing the tourniquet of the middle finger, we found the skin lustre ruddy and tension moderate. We then closed and drained the wound. Full thickness skins were grafted to cover the donor site. After the replantation, the flap and skin graft survived completely. After a 2-year follow-up, the shape and the function of both the donor and sites were very satisfying (Figs. 15.39, 15.40, 15.41, 15.42, 15.43, 15.44, 15.45, and 15.46).

The cases are generally provided by Dr. Guang jun Liu.

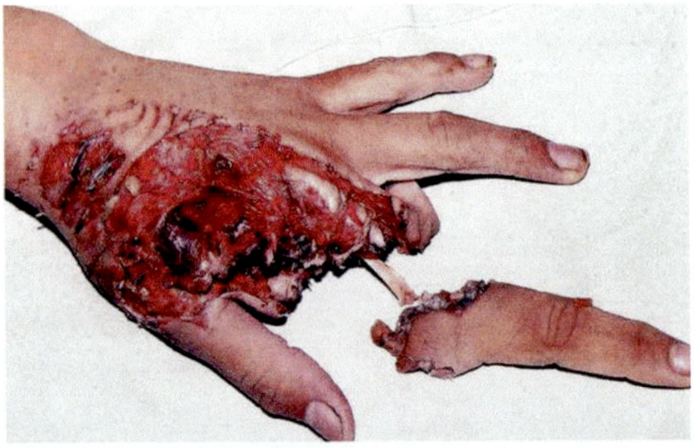

Fig. 15.39 Dorsal site of the severed left hand

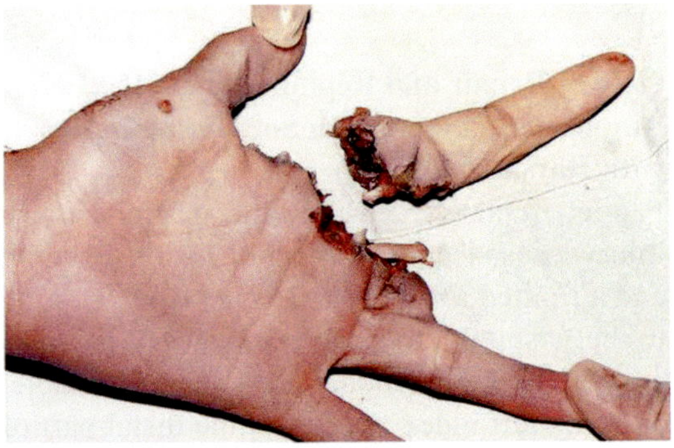

Fig. 15.40 Volar site of the severed left hand

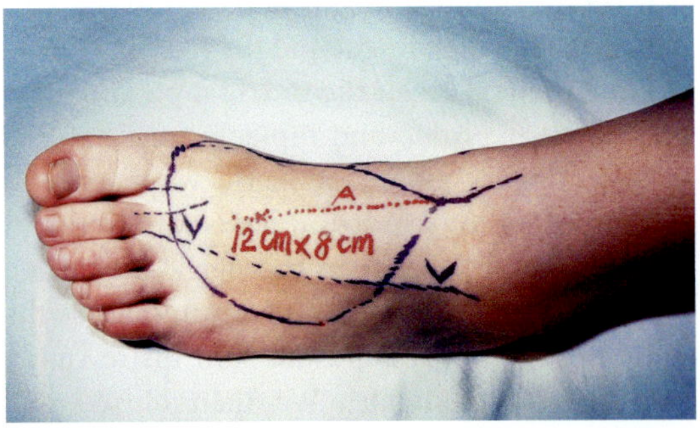

Fig. 15.41 Flap design

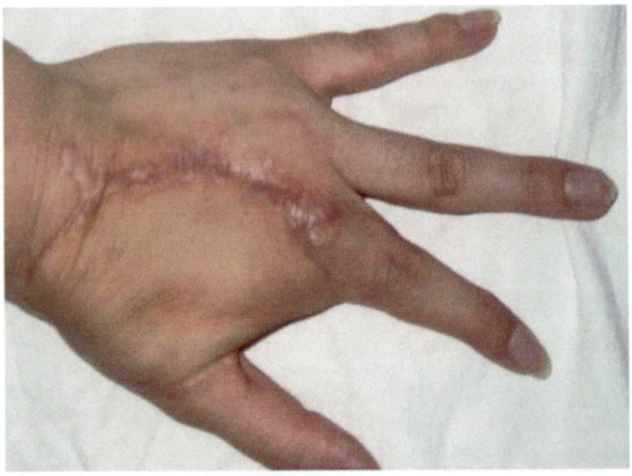

Fig. 15.42 Dorsal site after the surgery

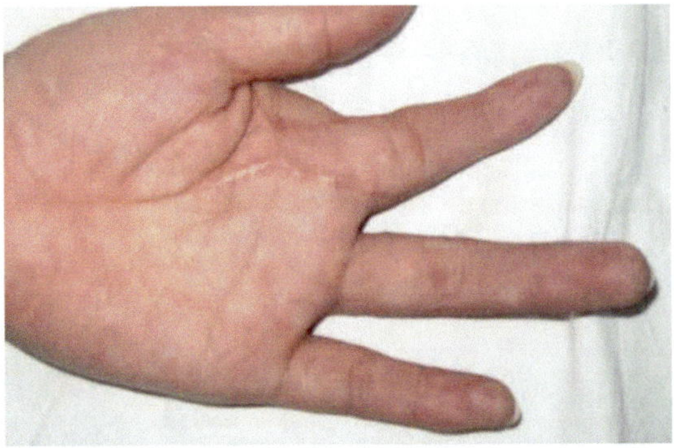

Fig. 15.43 Volar site after surgery

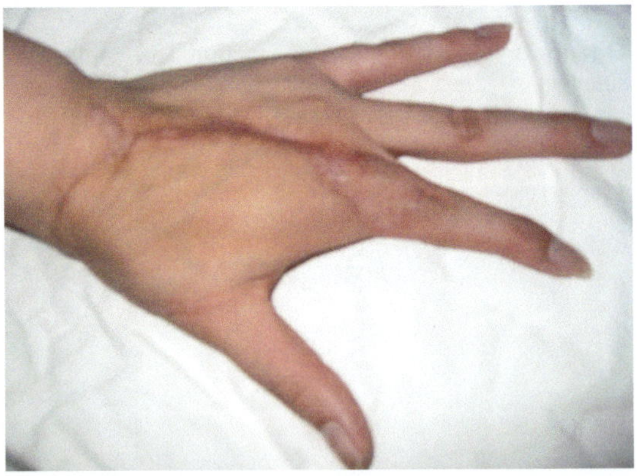

Fig. 15.44 Extension function of the fingers after surgery

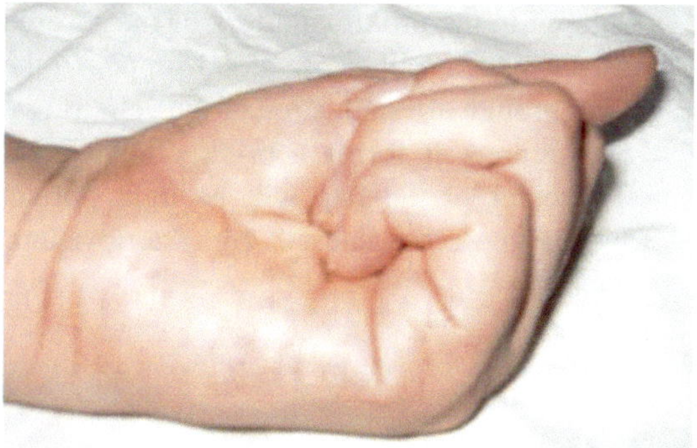

Fig. 15.45 Buckling function of the fingers after surgery

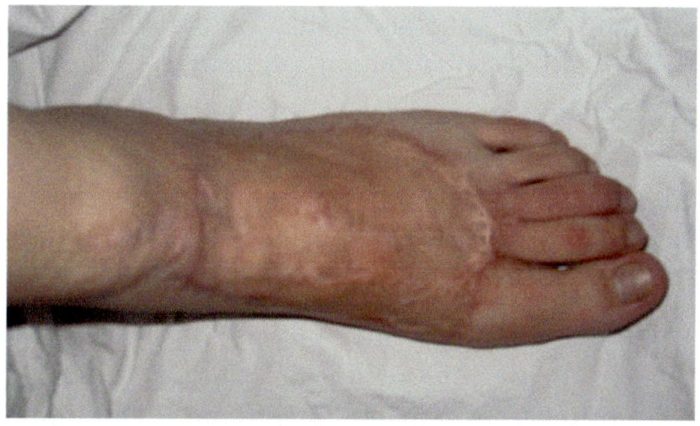

Fig. 15.46 Donor site view after surgery

15.3 Key Points in Surgery

(a) Choose the repair method according to the extent and location of the soft-tissue defect after regular replantation.
(b) In the situation of serious severing of multiple fingers, it is effective for the more important destroyed finger could be replanted by an abandoned finger to save the most function. A tendon defect could be repaired by the flexor superficial tendon of the severed finger or a vein flap with the palmar longus tendon. A nerve defect could be repaired by a superficial branch of the radial nerve or the dorsal branch of the proper digital nerve of the severed finger or the sural nerve.
(c) A digital artery island flap is mostly used to repair skin, artery, and nerve defects on the palm side of the severed finger nearby, which is easy to obtain, with a smaller anastomotic stoma that can cover the wound and bridge the arteries and nerves.
(d) A vein flap can be either an arterial nutrient flap or a venous nutrient flap. An arterial nutrient flap is mostly used to repair artery defects on the palm side, which would be swollen and purple after the operation. A venous nutrient flap is mostly used to repair vein defects on the dorsal side, which is arbitrary, easy to obtain, sacrificing no major blood vessels, and the donor site could be directly sutured, but with poor quality that could not be used to repair joints or in an active position.
(e) A ring tissue defect can be repaired using a big toe fibular skin flap and a second toe tibial skin flap.
(f) Large area defects that cannot be repaired using a regular flap could be repaired using a dorsalis pedis flap, which is highly required by surgeons.

15.4 Announcements

(a) Strictly control its indications and assess whether it is worth carrying out replantation before surgery.
(b) The digital artery island flap should be designed on the side as far as possible and in conformity with the principle of preventing scar contracture, which affects function.

(c) The subcutaneous tunnel of a pedicle flap should be wide enough going through that it prevents compression of the pedicle and cause surgical failure.
(d) Measure the length of the area of the tissue defect accurately, especially that combined with bone, joints, and skin defect.
(e) Venous nutrient flap is mostly used to repair a vein defect on the dorsal side, which is arbitrary, easy to obtain, with no major blood vessels sacrificed, and the donor site could be directly sutured. When it is used to repair the defect on the palm side, the flap should be upside-down.
(f) Internal fixation should not cross the joints, which should be good for fracture healing and facilitate functional exercises.
(g) The flap is inverted and transplanted to the affected area, the distal vein of the flap is sutured to the proximal artery of the severed finger, which will apply blood supply to the flap through arterialization of the vein. If two are sutured, it forms a bi-directional path. The color of the flap will be light purple, which may be caused by arteriovenous shunting.

References

Soutar DS, Scheker LR, Tanner NS, et al. The radial forearm flap: a versatile method for intraoral reconstruction. Br J Plast Surg. 1983;36:1–8.

Yafei X, Meiyi W, Dejun Z, et al. The application of arterialized venous flaps to the severed fingers with soft tissue defect. Chin J Microsurg. 2011;34(4):321–2.

16 Late Replantation of Severed Fingers

16.1 Summary

Severed tissues should be replanted within 6 h at room temperature (20–25 °C), as irreversible necrosis of the muscles occurs because of ischemia. The time can be increased to 12 h if refrigerated (4 °C). The ischemia time for fingers without muscles could be 8 h at room temperature and 12 h under refrigeration. The replantation of a finger whose warm ischemia time is over the time limit is called late replantation. There are very few successful reports of late replantation, and most of these are case reports.

The ischemia time of tissues is not clear. According to animal experiments, the changes in severed limbs include slight degeneration within 10 h and moderate to severe degeneration from 10 to 15 h, with significantly reduced glycogen and sharply increased lactic acid. Assumed that the time limit of refrigerated fingers and muscles would be 7 and 2 days, even 12 and 11 days for testing the activity of ALP, ATPase, and SDH in severed fingers and muscles. The longer the ischemia time, the lower survival rate. The capability of severed fingers to endure ischemia and lack of oxygen is relatively strong; thus, the best replantation time for severed fingers without muscles would be within 12 h at room temperature.

Seasonal changes have a great impact on the time limit of replantation. The warm ischemia time within 12 h should be a relative indication. There is a clinical report of successful replantation after 96 h. The time limit of replantation could be prolonged even further if the severed finger is kept properly, but we still think that the sooner replantation is undertaken, the better.

16.2 Case Description

Case 1: Replantation of Middle and Final Segments of the Right Index Finger After More Than 22 h

Female patient, 50 years old, was admitted to hospital for severing of the middle and final segments of the right index finger caused by a lathe and bleeding for 22 h (18 h after stump surgery in another hospital). Physical examination: The general situation was good; the vital signs were stable. After removing the dressing, we can see postoperative suturing with bleeding. The severed finger was kept in a disposable plastic bag without any other preservation measures. Successful debridement and replantation were performed under anesthesia under emergency conditions. The replanted finger was red and had moderate tension after relaxing the tourniquet, and it was packed with sterile gauze and padded with broken cotton yarn. The patient was brought back to the ward safely. She was given conventional treatments postoperatively, such as antibiotics, hormones, and antispasmodics. By 2 weeks later, the replanted severed finger had successfully survived. The appearance and function were

J. Lin et al., *Special Type of Finger Replantation*, https://doi.org/10.1007/978-981-10-6229-2_16

good after regular follow-up and functional exercise guidance and the patient was satisfied (Figs. 16.1, 16.2, 16.3, 16.4, 16.5, 16.6, and 16.7).

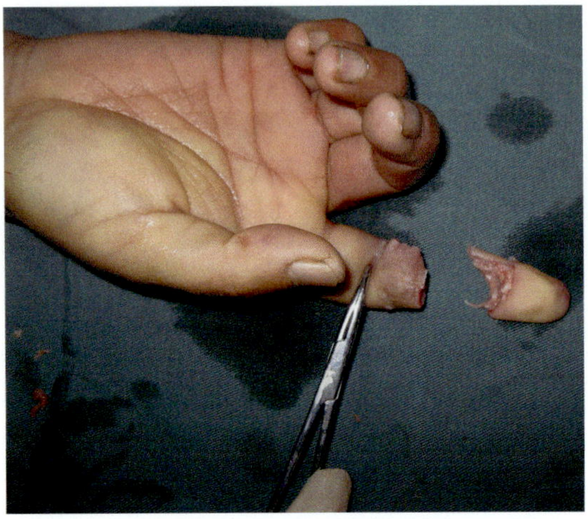

Fig. 16.1 The palm side of the severed finger

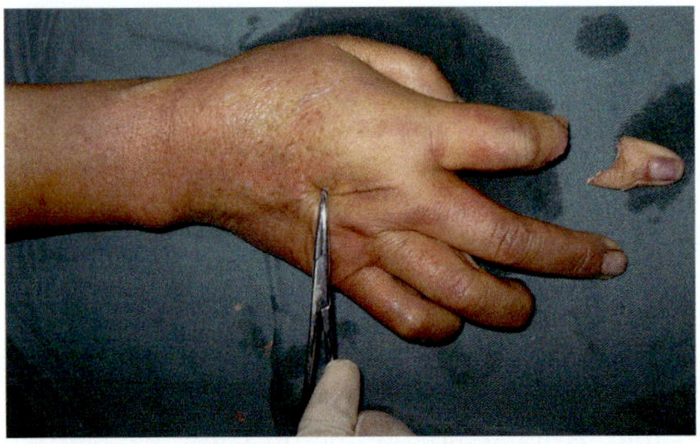

Fig. 16.2 The dorsal side of the severed finger

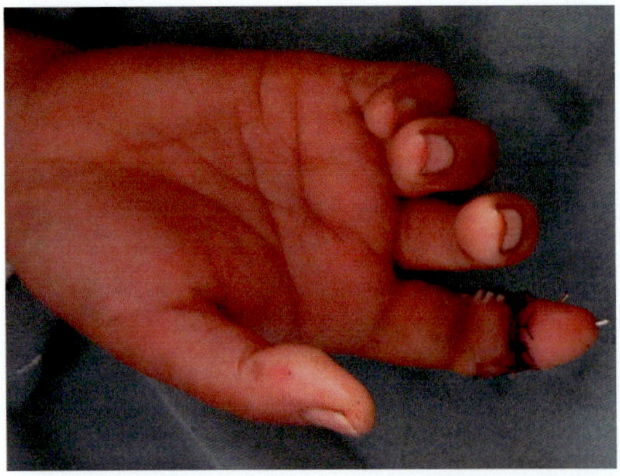

Fig. 16.3 The palm side after replantation

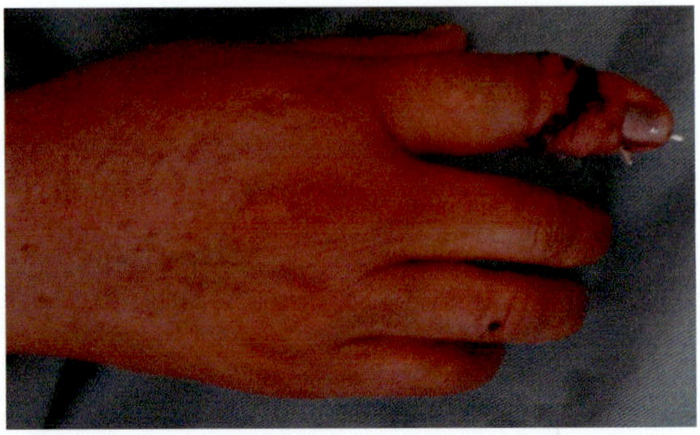

Fig. 16.4 The dorsal side after replantation

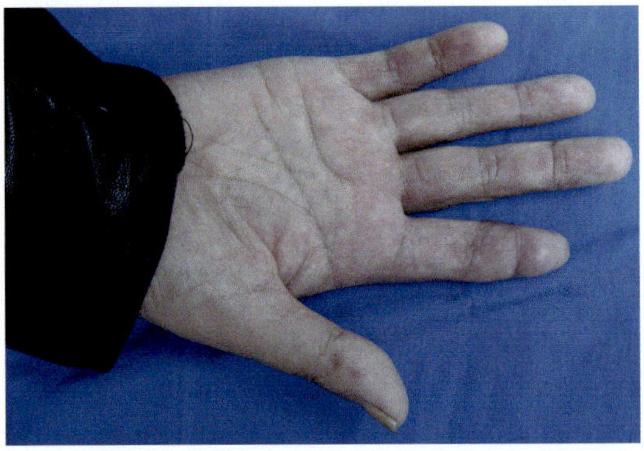

Fig. 16.5 The palm side 9 months later

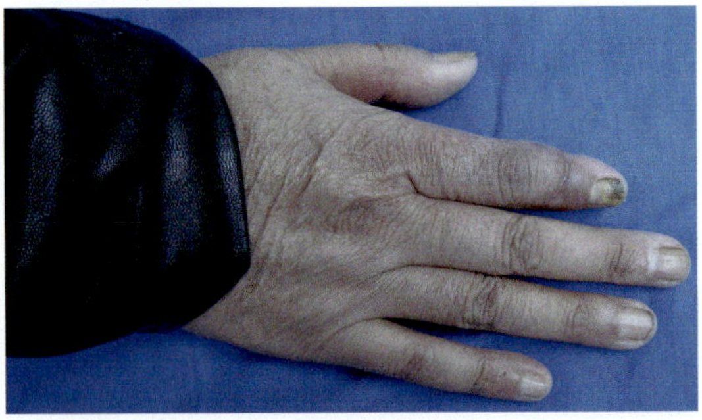

Fig. 16.6 The dorsal side 9 months later

Case 2: Replantation of the Final Segment of the Right Index Finger After More Than 16 h
Female patient, 23 years old, was admitted to hospital for a severed final segment of the right index finger caused by an incised wound and bleeding for 16 h. PE: The general situation was good; the vital signs were stable. The final segment was completely severed from the distal

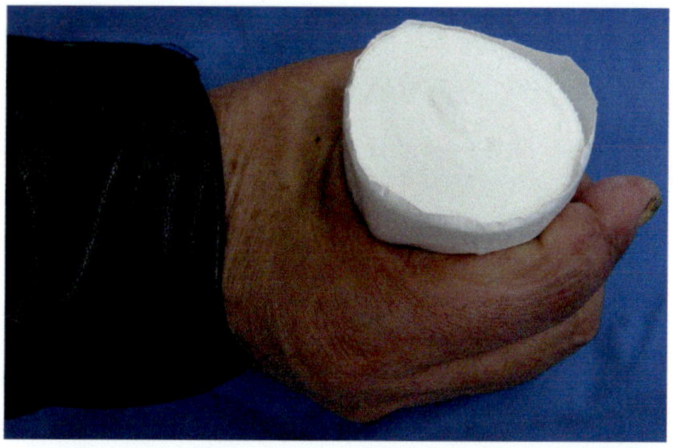

Fig. 16.7 Function 9 months later

interphalangeal joint of the right index finger with bone revealed, uneven wound, bleeding, and the blood supply to the rest of the fingers was good. Successful debridement and replantation were performed under anesthesia under emergency conditions. The distal finger joint was fused using a 1.0-mm needle. Two proper digital arteries on both sides and three palmar digital veins were anastomosed under the microscope. The replanted finger was red and had moderate tension after relaxing the tourniquet, and was packed with sterile gauze and padded with broken cotton yarn. The patient was brought back to the ward safely. She was given conventional treatments postoperatively, such as antibiotics, hormones, and antispasmodics. By 2 weeks later, the replanted severed finger had successfully survived. The appearance and function were good after regular follow-up and functional exercise guidance, and the patient was satisfied (Figs. 16.8, 16.9, 16.10, 16.11, 16.12, and 16.13).

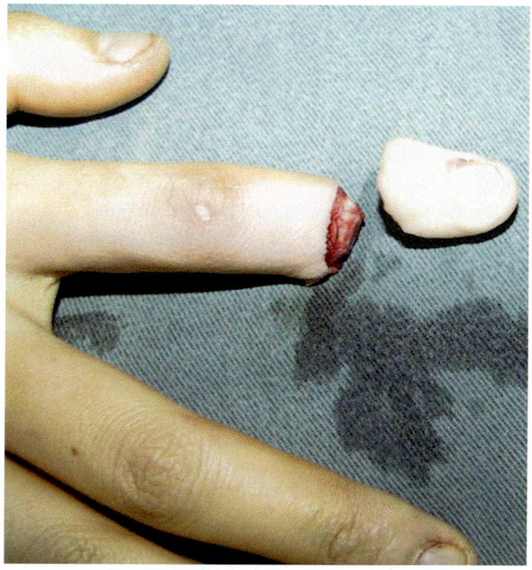

Fig. 16.8 The palm side of the severed finger

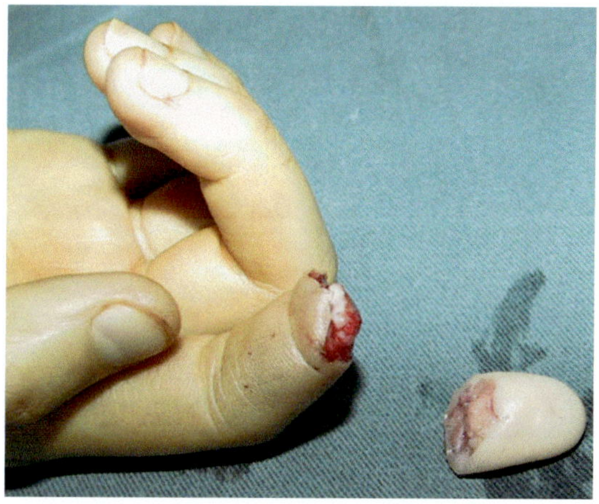

Fig. 16.9 The dorsal side of the severed finger

Case 3: Replantation of a Rotationally Avulsed Right Index Finger After More Than 25 h

The patient, a girl, 6 years old, was admitted to hospital for rotational avulsion of the right index finger caused by a grinding machine injury and bleeding for 25 h. PE: The general situation was good; the vital signs were stable. The proximal segment of the right index finger was completely severed. Stump surgery had been carried out locally, and we could see that about 13 mm of the flexor digitorum profundus tendon had been taken out. Successful debridement and replantation were performed under anesthesia under emergency conditions. The replanted finger was red and had moderate tension after relaxing the tourniquet, and it was packed with sterile gauze and padded with broken cotton yarn. The patient was safely brought back to the warm ward. Postoperative heat preservation, absolute non-smoking, and close observation of the blood supply were ensured. The patient was given conventional children's treatments postoperatively, such as antibiotics, hormones and antispasmodics. There were blisters 2 days later

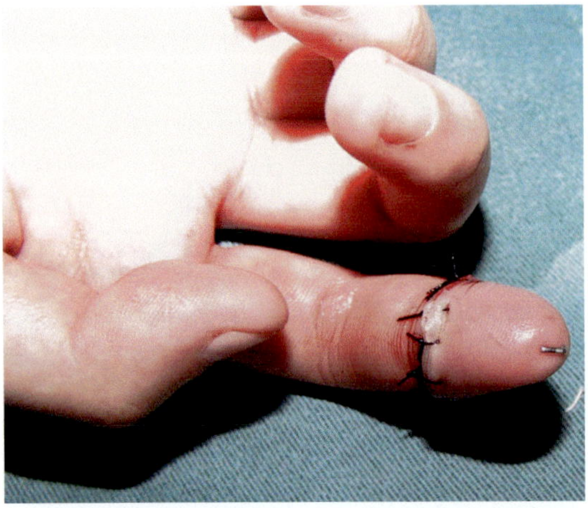

Fig. 16.10 The palm side after replantation

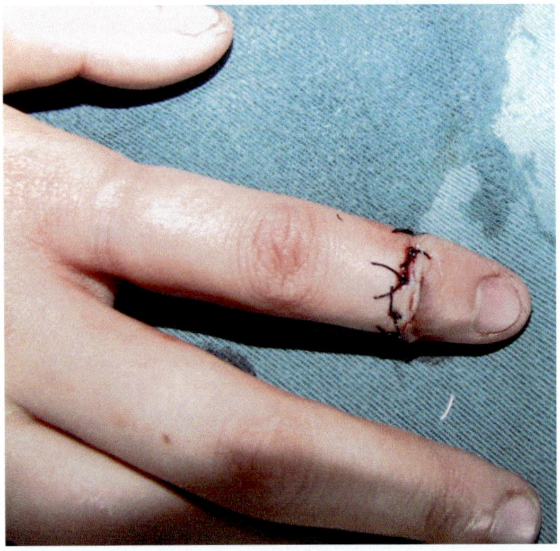

Fig. 16.11 The dorsal side after replantation

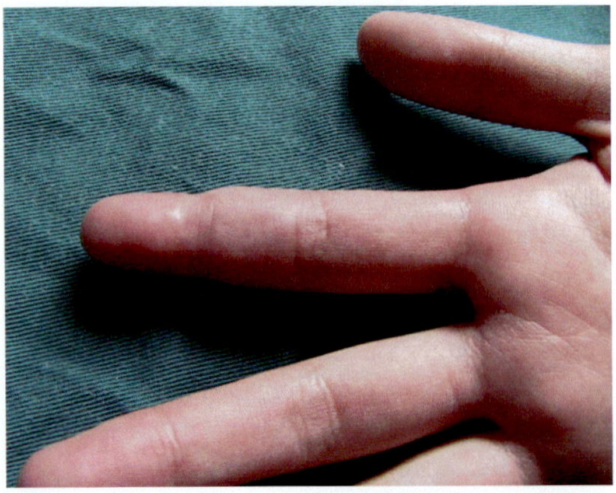

Fig. 16.12 The palm side 9 months later

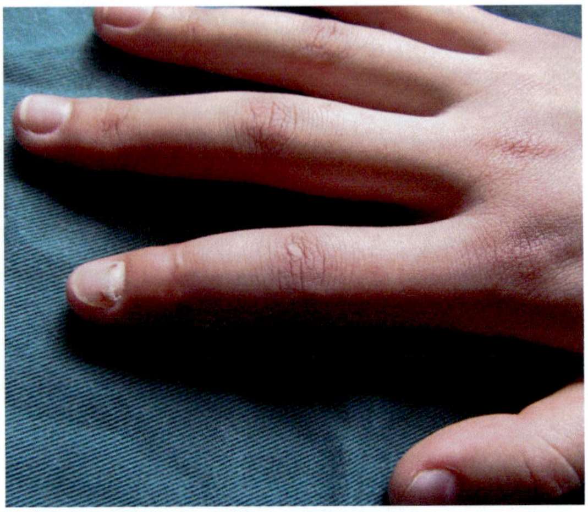

Fig. 16.13 The dorsal side 9 months later

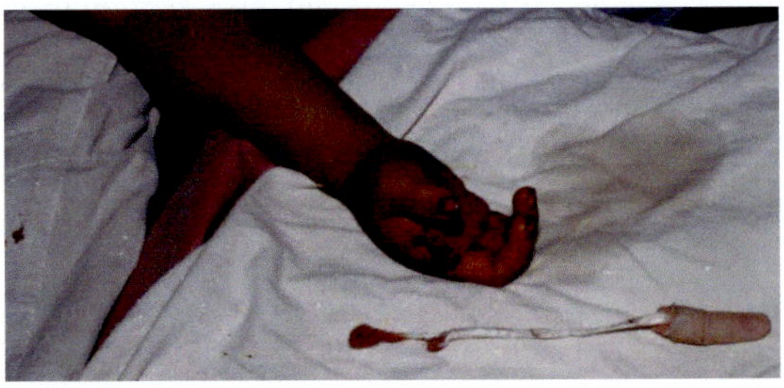

Fig. 16.14 The situation of the severed finger

and blood blisters 3 days later, which were pricked using a fine tip for drainage. By 7 days later, the replanted severed finger had successfully survived. The appearance and function were good after regular follow-up and functional exercise guidance, but a little shorter compared with the healthy side, and the parents were satisfied (Figs. 16.14, 16.15, 16.16, 16.17, 16.18, 16.19, 16.20, and 16.21).

16.3 Key Points in Surgery

(a) Quick action for debridement. For multiple severed fingers, the same operations should be processed simultaneously.
(b) Simple and quick fixation, which means that the fractures should be fixed using crossed needles. The surgical process could be simplified by shortening the phalanx with the general principle that the middle finger should not be shorter than

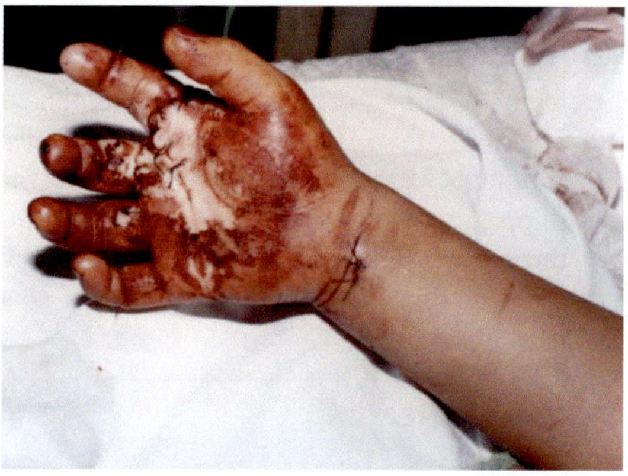

Fig. 16.15 The blood supply after replantation

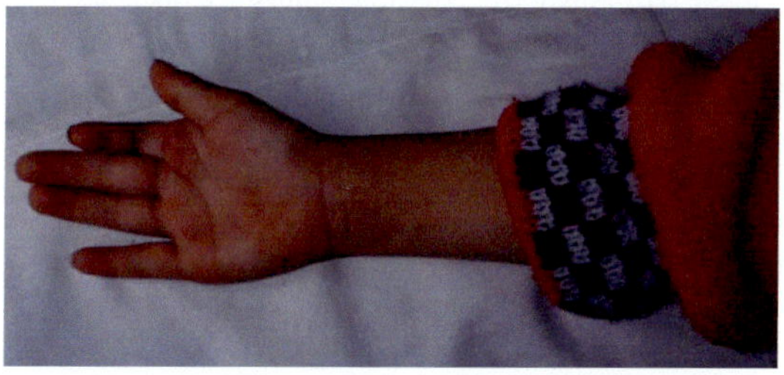

Fig. 16.16 The palm side 3 months later

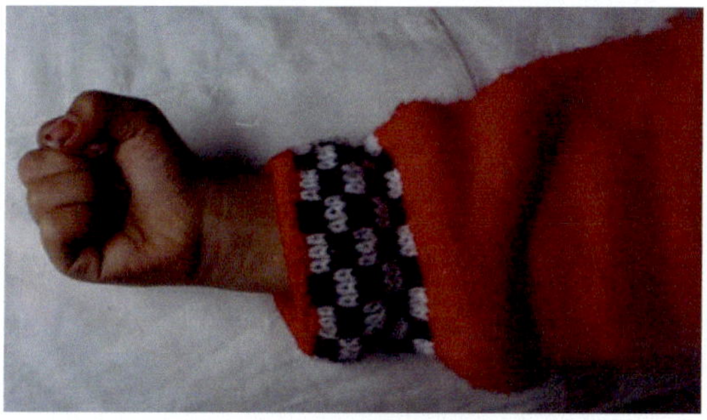

Fig. 16.17 The fist function 3 months later

the index finger and the ring finger should not be shorter than the little finger. Be careful to protect the epiphyseal line in children.

(c) First, anastomose the digital arteries, nerves, and superficial veins of the fronts of the finger on the dominant side to restore blood supply and reduce tissue necrosis after bone scaffold rebuild.

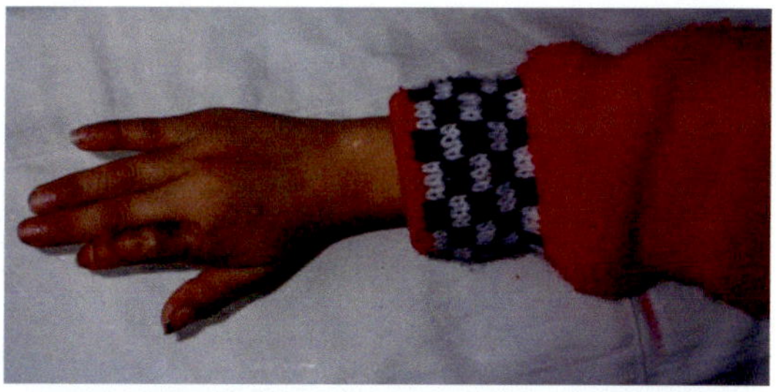

Fig. 16.18 The dorsal side 3 months later

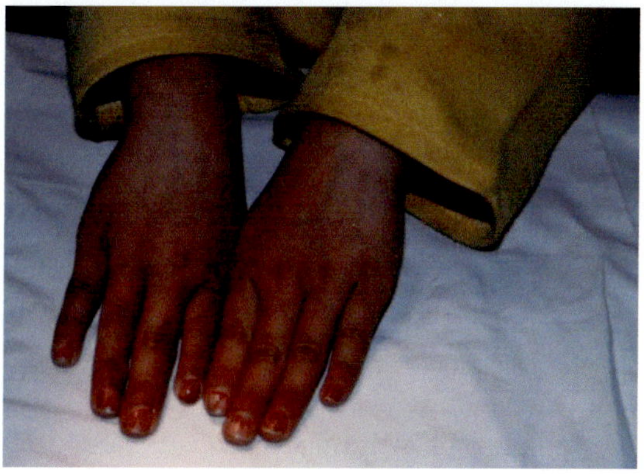

Fig. 16.19 The two hands compared 3 months later

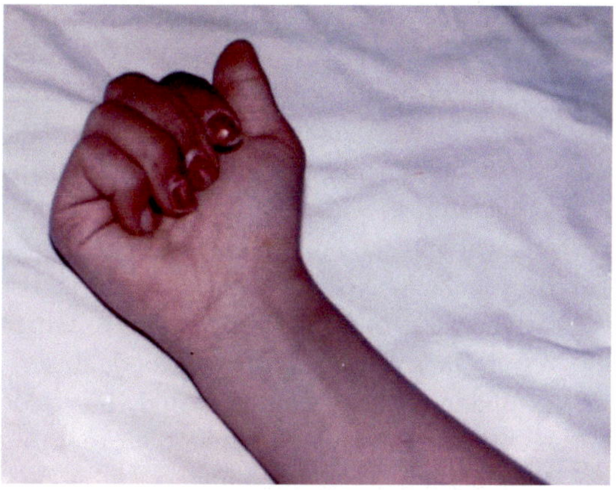

Fig. 16.20 The fist function 12 months later

(d) Strive for a successful revascularization in one attempt in those fingers severed for a long time.

(e) Inject a mixture of dexamethasone (10 mg) and heparin (12,500 U) in the severed proper digital arteries with a no-wound needle to reduce ischemia–reperfusion injury.

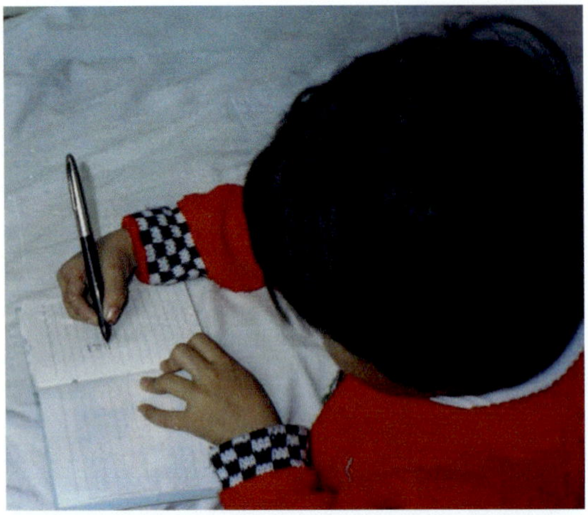

Fig. 16.21 The function 12 months later

16.4 Announcements

(a) Complete debridement is the basis for late replantation.
(b) Maintaining hypocoagulability with low molecular heparin and adequate blood volume with enough intravenous fluids before the operation can improve arterial spasm. Sufficient and effective antibiotics should be used to prevent infection postoperatively for late replantation.
(c) It is better to anastomose the proper digital arteries on both sides. This is beneficial to the blood supply and conducive to avoiding low temperatures, which affects recovery and renewal of distal bones, tendons, and nerves.
(d) Irreversible necrosis will occur in partial tissue because of prolonged ischemia, which results in swelling, blisters, blood blisters, exfoliation, etc., which should be close observed and handled in time to prevent ring compression in replanted fingers.
(e) Antispasmolysis should be given during the postoperative period. Small amounts of steroid drugs used during the first 3 days are available to reduce degeneration and necrosis reaction. For those severed fingers that are replanted within 16 h regular treatment is enough, but for those replanted after more than 16 h, heparin and hormones should be added to what is available for improving microcirculation to prevent thrombosis, but the clotting time should be monitored.

Suggested Reading

Feng Z, Yunshen T, Guo Y, et al. 15 cases of overtime replantation of severed fingers. Chin J Hand Surg. 2009;25(1):63.

Green NE, Allen BL. Vascular injuries associated with dislocation of the knee. J Bone Joint Surg Am. 1997;59(2):236–41.

He M, Meng Z, Yongxiang Y, et al. The rehabilitation effect of postoperative function exercises to overtime replantation of severed limbs (fingers). Chin J Clin Rehab. 2003;7(14):2114.

He Y, Wuxiang S, Yuxiong W, et al. Logistic regression analysis of the influencing factors of the survival rate of finger replantation. Chin J Hand Surg. 2015;31(5):369–72.

Ma L, Shen D. Replantation of severed fingers over 10 hours. Zhejiang Clin Med J. 2002;4(12):926.

Syrko M, Jablecki J. Quality of life-oriented evaluation of late functional results of hand replantation. Ortop Traumatol Rehabil. 2010;6(1):31–2.

VanderWilde RS, Wood MB, Zu ZG. Hand replantation after 54 hours of cold ischemia: a case report. J Hand Surg Am. 1992;17:217–20.

Wang Z, Wang C, Zhu L, et al. 1 case of replantation of cryopreserved severed finger over 81 days. Shandong Med J. 2004;44(3):29–3.

Wu H, Cheng T, Wang Z, et al. Observation of replantation of fingers over 12 hours. Shandong Med J. 2010;50(51):75–6.

Yabe T, Tsuda T, Hirose S, et al. Treatment of fingertip amputation: comparison of results between microsurgical replantation and pocket principle. J Reconstr Microsurg. 2012;9(3):149–50.

Yuke M, Bo S. A successful replantation of severed finger immersed with seawater over 10 hours. Chin J Reparative Reconstr Surg. 2001;15(2):85.

Zhang GL, Chen KM, Zhang JH, et al. Hand reconstruction using heterotopic replantation of amputated index and little fingers. Chin J Traumatol. 2011;5(3):25–6.

17 Replantation of Self-mutilated Severed Fingers

17.1 Summary

A self-mutilated severed finger is when the patient cuts his own finger off if he or she has an emotional disorder, depression or is intoxicated. It is characterized by the following:

(a) Most cases are young men with a bad temper.
(b) Most fingers severed in this way comprise the middle and final segments of the left little finger.
(c) The wound is smooth with no other injuries, which makes it easy to replant.
(d) The patient does not cooperate with treatment for a long time as he or she has so many negative emotions such as regret, angry, and guilt.
(e) The replantation is easier compared with other replantations, but postoperative nursing is more difficult because of the patients' noncompliance.

Psychological stress is the main reason for the lower survival rate of self-mutilated severed fingers, which may be caused by the following:

(a) Psychological and surgical trauma, especially amputation wounds, are intense stimulation to patients.
(b) Stress, which includes depression, anxiety, hostility, and low self-esteem, which reduce survival rate.
(c) The neuroendocrine axis increases the level of adrenaline and catecholamine, etc., in the blood, which leads to vasospasm or embolism.
(d) Anxiety lowers the pain threshold, which causes vascular crisis.

Although, as already stated, replantation of a self-mutilated severed finger is easier than other simple replantations, the survival rate is lower because of the postoperative pain, mood instability, and hypercoagulability. Postoperative sedation is effective in increasing the survival rate reported by Lin Jian and Yu Yunlan (2004), where 12 out of 14 cases were successful, and the survival rate was 85.7%. Su Xiaolei et al. (2013a) reported a survival rate of 83.3% of 30 cases in the postoperative sedation group, and 94% of 50 cases in the hibernation group. Wang Yufen et al. reported that postoperative psychological intervention could also be useful in increasing the survival rate.

17.2 Case Description

Case 1: Replantation of Self-mutilated Left Index Finger

Female patient, 28 years old, was admitted to hospital for the severed final segment of the left index finger, which she cut off herself when intoxicated and after a quarrel with her family.

J. Lin et al., *Special Type of Finger Replantation*, https://doi.org/10.1007/978-981-10-6229-2_17

She had been bleeding for 2 h. Physical examination: The general situation was good; the vital signs were stable. The distal part was completely severed from the base of the nail, with bone, vessels, tendons, and nerves revealed, a smooth wound, and bleeding. Successful debridement and replantation were performed under anesthesia under emergency conditions. The replanted finger was red and had moderate tension after relaxing the tourniquet. It was packed with sterile gauze and padded with broken cotton yarn and the patient was brought back to the ward safely. She was given conventional treatments postoperatively, such as antibiotics, hormones, and antispasmodics. By 2 weeks later, the replanted severed finger had successfully survived. The appearance and function were good after regular follow-up and functional exercise guidance, and the patient was satisfied (Figs. 17.1, 17.2, 17.3, 17.4, 17.5, 17.6, and 17.7).

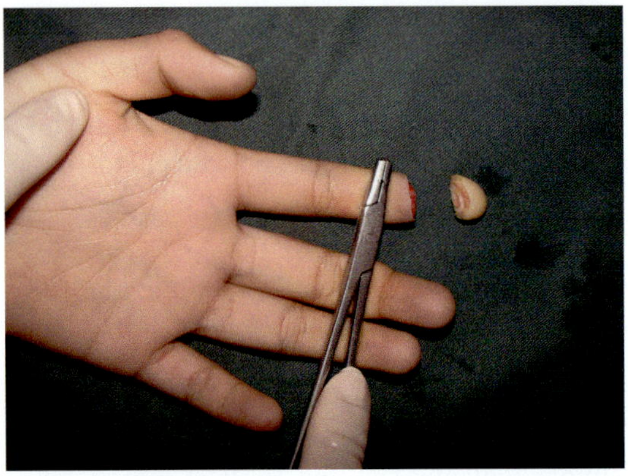

Fig. 17.1 The palm side of the severed finger

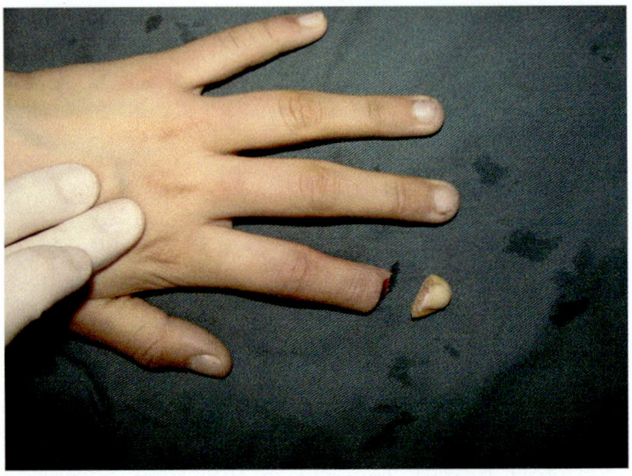

Fig. 17.2 The dorsal side of the severed finger

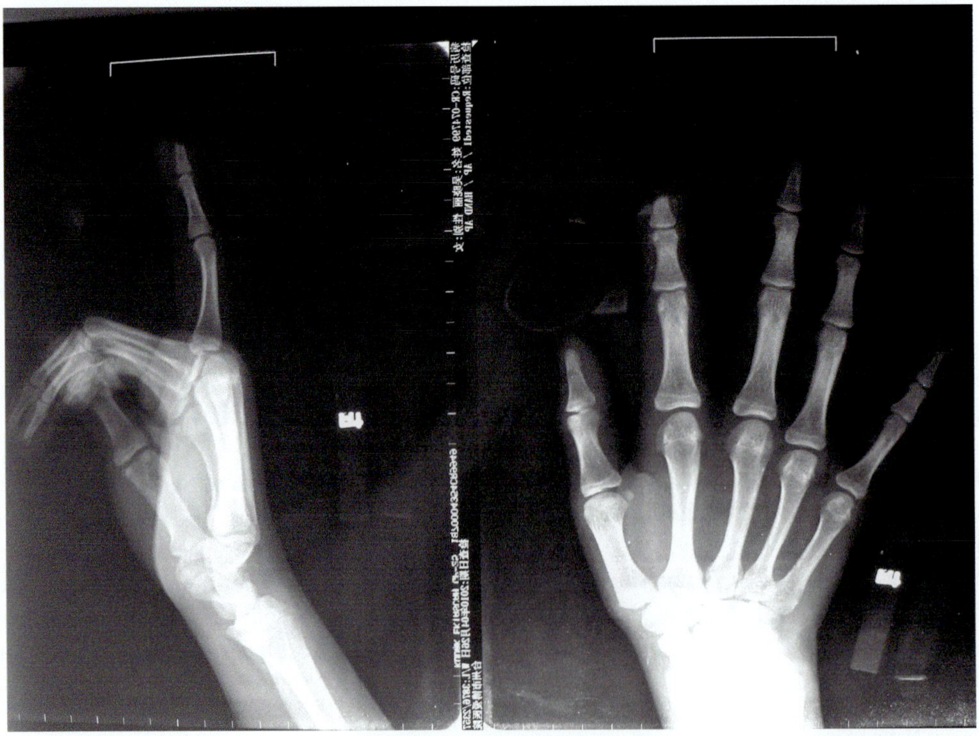

Fig. 17.3 Preoperative X-ray

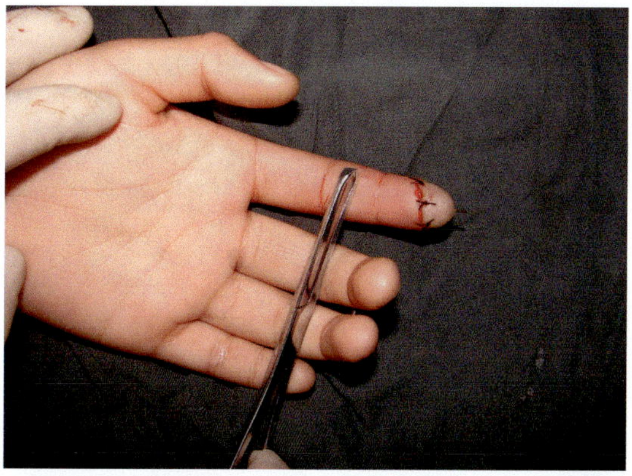

Fig. 17.4 The palm side after replantation

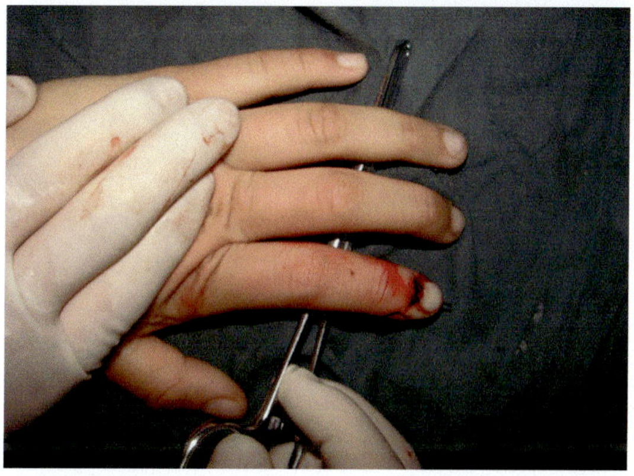

Fig. 17.5 The dorsal side after replantation

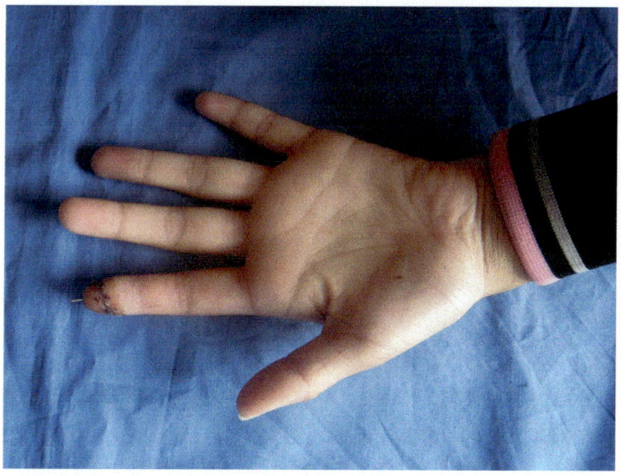

Fig. 17.6 The palm side 17 months later

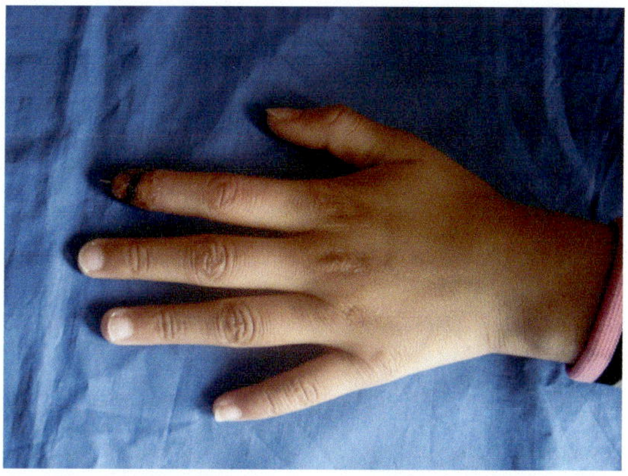

Fig. 17.7 The palm side 17 months later

Case 2: Replantation of Self-mutilated Left Little Finger

Male patient, 21 years old, was admitted to hospital for a severed final segment of the left little finger, which was cut off by himself after a quarrel with his lover, and he had been bleeding for 3 h. PE: The general situation was good; the vital signs were stable. The distal part was completely severed from the base of the nail, with bone, vessels, tendons, and nerves revealed, a smooth wound, and bleeding. Successful debridement and replantation were performed under anesthesia under emergency conditions. The replanted finger was red and had moderate tension after relaxing the tourniquet and was packed with sterile gauze and padded with broken cotton yarn. The patient was brought back to the ward safely and was given conventional treatments postoperatively, such as antibiotics, hormones, and antispasmodics. By 2 weeks later, the replanted severed finger had successfully survived. The appearance and function were good after regular follow-up and functional exercise guidance, and the patient was satisfied (Figs. 17.8, 17.9, 17.10, 17.11, and 17.12).

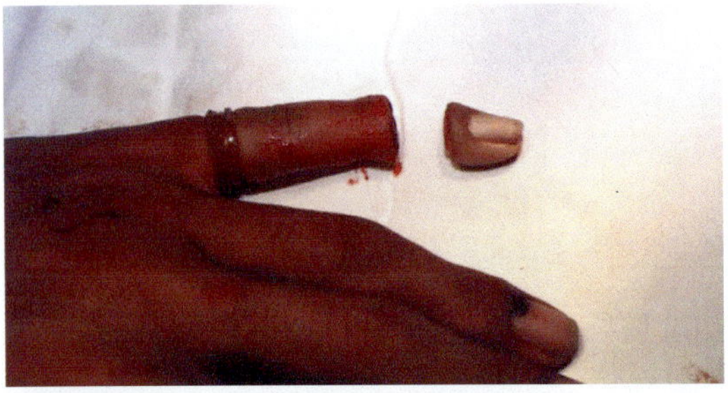

Fig. 17.8 The dorsal side of the severed finger

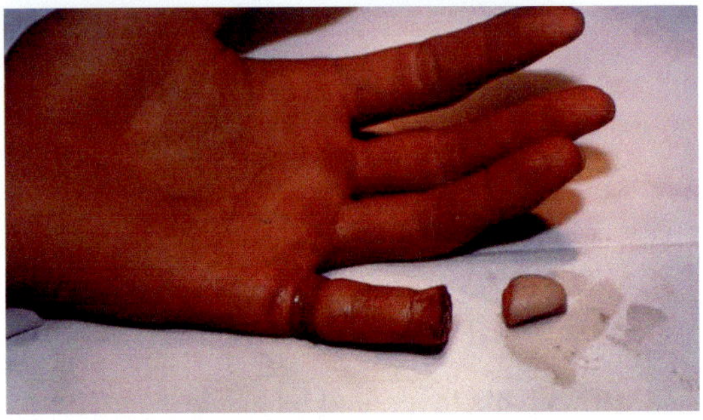

Fig. 17.9 The palm side of the severed finger

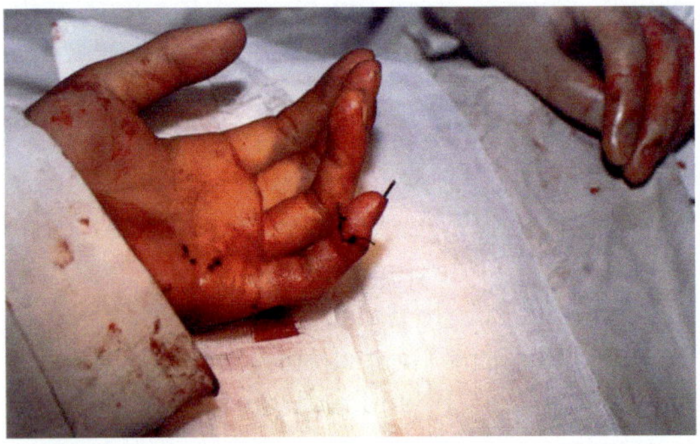

Fig. 17.10 After replantation

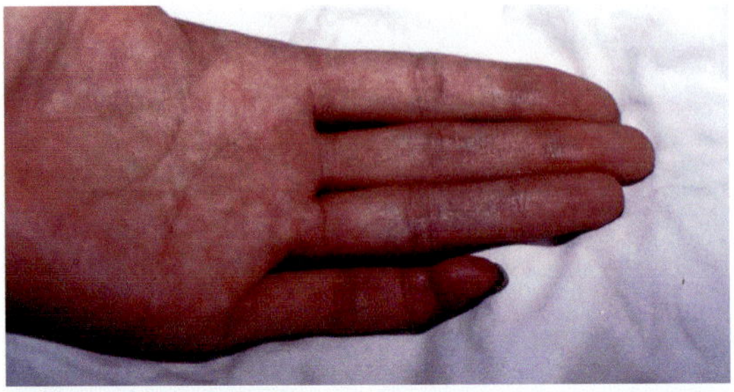

Fig. 17.11 The palm side 4 months later

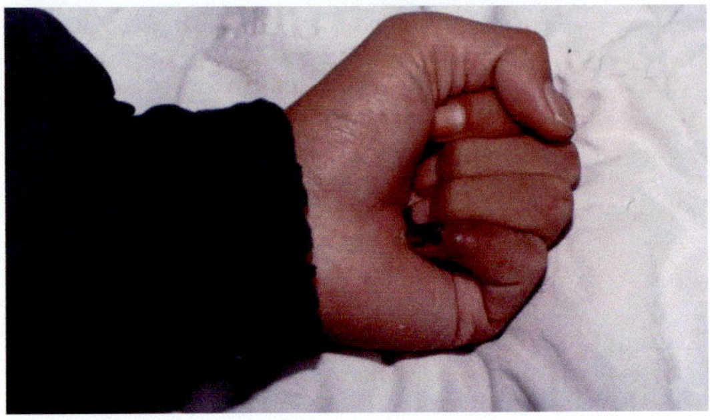

Fig. 17.12 Function 4 months later

Case 3: Replantation of Self-mutilated Left Index Finger

Male patient, 31 years old, was admitted to hospital for a severed final segment of the left index finger, which he cut off himself when intoxicated and after a quarrel with his girlfriend. He had been bleeding for 1.5 h. PE: The general situation was good; the vital signs were stable. The distal part was completely severed from the base of the nail, with bone, vessels, tendons, and nerves revealed, a smooth wound, and bleeding. Successful debridement and replantation were performed under anesthesia under emergency conditions. The replanted finger was red and moderate tension after relaxing the tourniquet. It was packed with sterile gauze and padded with broken cotton yarn and the patient was brought back to the ward safely. The patient was given conventional treatments postoperatively, such as antibiotics, hormones, and antispasmodics. By 2 weeks later, the replanted severed finger had successfully survived. The appearance and function were good after regular follow-up and functional exercise guidance and the patient was satisfied (Figs. 17.13, 17.14, 17.15, 17.16, 17.17, and 17.18).

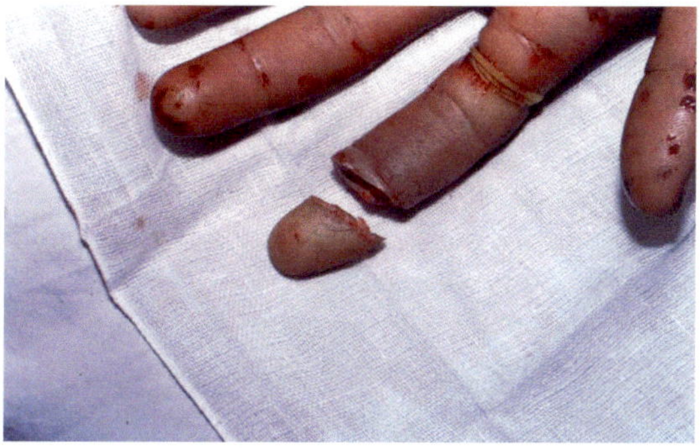

Fig. 17.13 The palm side of the severed finger

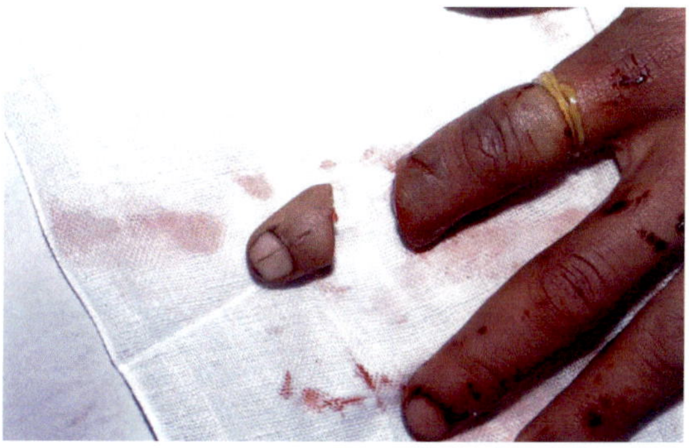

Fig. 17.14 The dorsal side of the severed finger

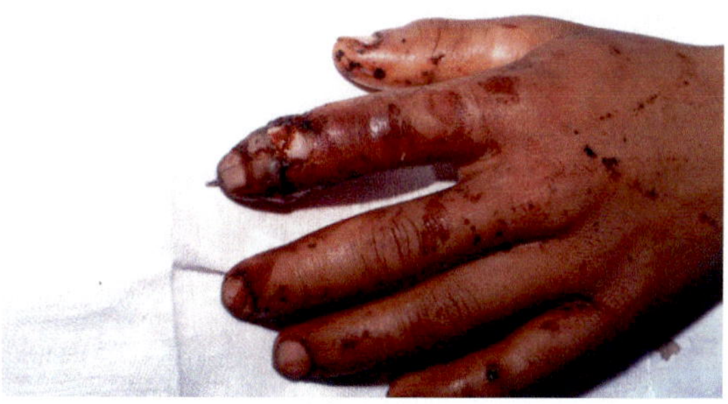

Fig. 17.15 After replantation

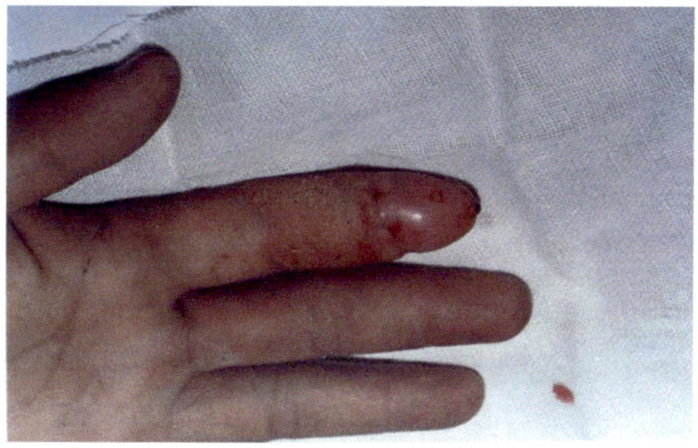

Fig. 17.16 The palm side 15 months later

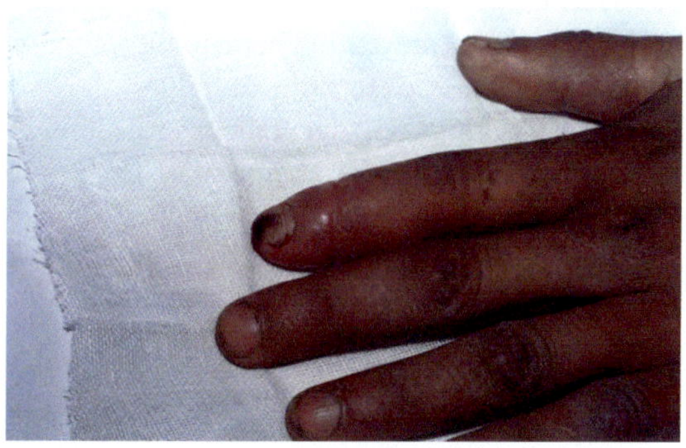

Fig. 17.17 The dorsal side 15 months later

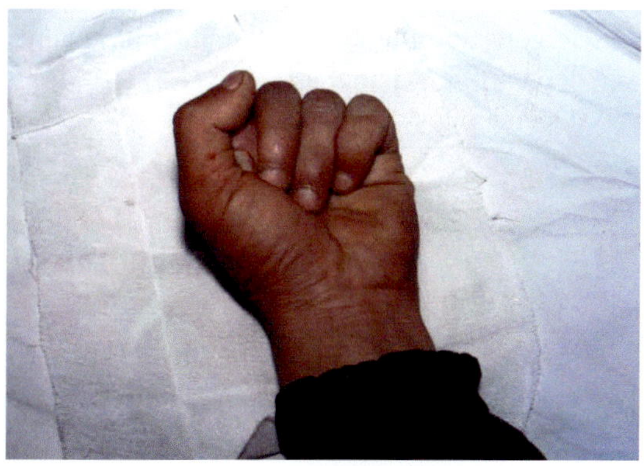

Fig. 17.18 The function 15 months later

17.3 Key Points in Surgery

(a) Replantation of a self-mutilated severed finger is relatively easy, but the severed part is usually the final segment or fingertip, which lacks veins to be anastomosed that can be replaced by palmar digital veins.
(b) Careful intraoperative dissection to avoid injuries of vessels and nerves, and anastomose vessels and nerves as far as possible, which is good for the recovery of appearance and function.
(c) During the operation, meticulous hemostasis is helpful for preventing hematoma compression, which leads to surgical failure.
(d) Do not administer subcutaneous injection of heparin, which causes hematoma, leading to surgical failure.

17.4 Announcements

(a) Replantation of self-mutilated severed fingers is suitable for patients who have a controlled transient mental disorder. Rigorous psychological assessment is required before surgery to rule out schizophrenia, mania, depression, paranoid psychosis, drug-dependent psychosis, etc.
(b) Pay more attention to the psychological nursing of patients.
(c) A second exploratory operation may be necessary if intractable vasospasm occurs. Effective treatment of mental disorders is useful for surgical success; ask a psychologist if it is necessary.
(d) Patients with poor psychological intervention could be treated with hibernation therapy.
(e) Hibernation therapy should last for 7 days, halved in the seventh day and stopped on the eighth day. Pay attention to drug-dependent phenomena, such as excitement and insomnia, and vascular crisis caused by drug withdrawal.
(f) The patient should be accommodated in a single room if conditions permit.
(g) If only the family requires the surgery, but not the patient, the replantation should not be undertaken.

References

Lin J, Yu Y. 14 cases report of replantation of self-destructive severed fingers. J Pract Hand Surg. 2004;18(3):176–7.

Xiaolei S, Zhiguo D, Mingbin D, et al. Observation of hibernation therapy used in replantation of self-destructive severed fingers. Chin J Hand Surg. 2013a;29(1):62.

18 Replantation of Severed Fingers in the Elderly

18.1 Summary

The replantation of severed fingers of old people relates to those whose over 60 years old. With the development of basic and clinical research, age is no longer a contraindication. If old people suffer severed fingers, their general condition should be assessed first to judge whether they can tolerate surgery, and then consideration should be given to whether or not they wish to undergo replantation and to ensure they understand the function of replanted finger. Any operative treatment should be considered on the assumption of a relatively good condition of the severed finger, short ischemia, good general condition, controlled internal diseases and expected good function recovery. The replantation of severed fingers of old people is always a challenge in clinical practice because of its specificity, but the age range of successful replantation is growing. There was successful case reported for a 72-year-old at No 153 Central Hospital of the People's Liberation Army in 1990, and for a 74-year-old at No 89 Hospital of the People' Liberation Army. Another successful case, for a 79-year-old, was described in *Hand Surgery*, edited by Gu Yudong, Wang Shuhuan and Shi De in 2000.

Physiological functions and morphology structure change in varying degrees when people enter old age, and these factors should be borne in mind in finger replantation. Successful surgery requires not only good surgical techniques but also relies on close observation and intensive care after surgery. The elastin of vessels in the elderly reduces and collagen increases with calcium deposition, which can cause hardening, lumen narrowing, decreased elasticity and increased resistance, especially in arteries.

18.2 Case Description

Case 1: Replantation of Final Segments of the Right Middle and Ring Finger of an Old Man
The patient, male, 66 years old, admitted to hospital for final segments of the right middle and ring fingers that had been severed by a cutting machine and bled for 1 hour. Physical Examination: The general situation was good and the vital signs were stable. The final segments were completely severed with bone, vessels and nerves revealed, uneven wound, bleeding and without blood supply. Successful debridement and replantation were undertaken under anesthesia in the hospital emergency department. The replanted fingers were red and moderate tension was observed after relaxing the tourniquet; the wound was packed with sterile gauze and padded with broken cotton yam and the patient taken back to the ward where he was given

J. Lin et al., *Special Type of Finger Replantation*, https://doi.org/10.1007/978-981-10-6229-2_18

conventional postoperative treatments such as antibiotics, hormone and antispasmodic. Some 2 weeks later, it was evident that the replanted fingers had successfully survived. The appearance and function were good after regular follow-ups and functional exercise guidance, and the patient was satisfied (Figs. 18.1, 18.2, 18.3, 18.4, 18.5, and 18.6).

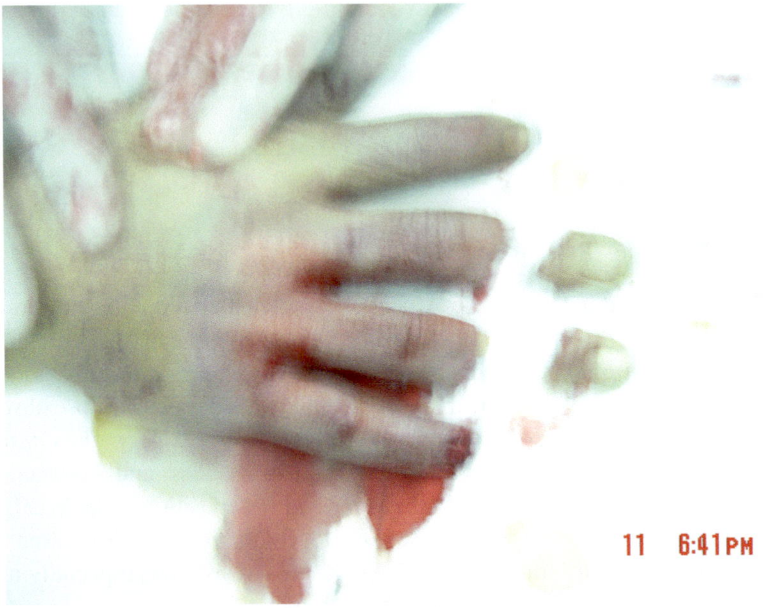

Fig. 18.1 Condition of the severed fingers

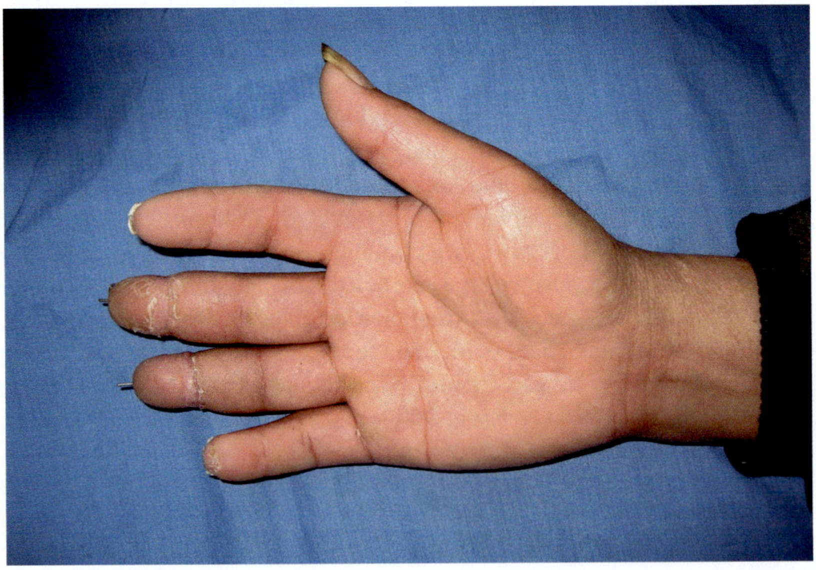

Fig. 18.2 The palm side 6 weeks after surgery

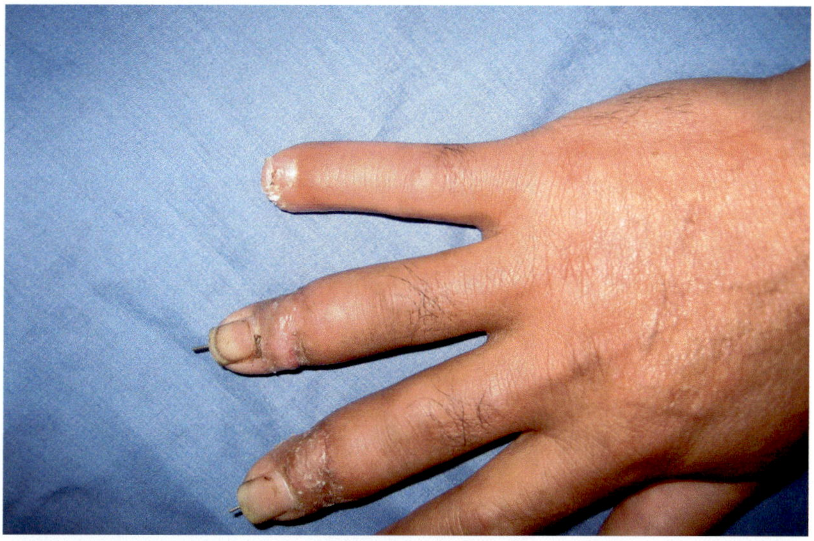

Fig. 18.3 The dorsal side 6 weeks after surgery

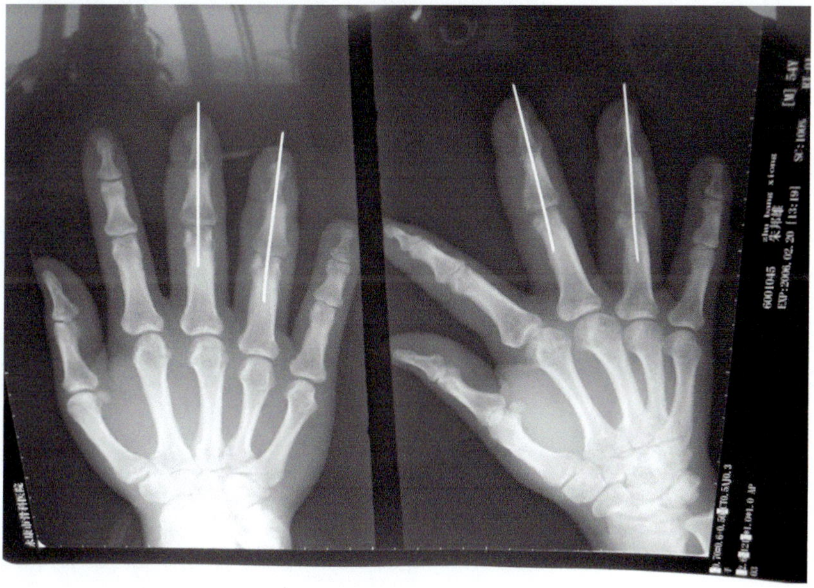

Fig. 18.4 X-rays 4 weeks after surgery

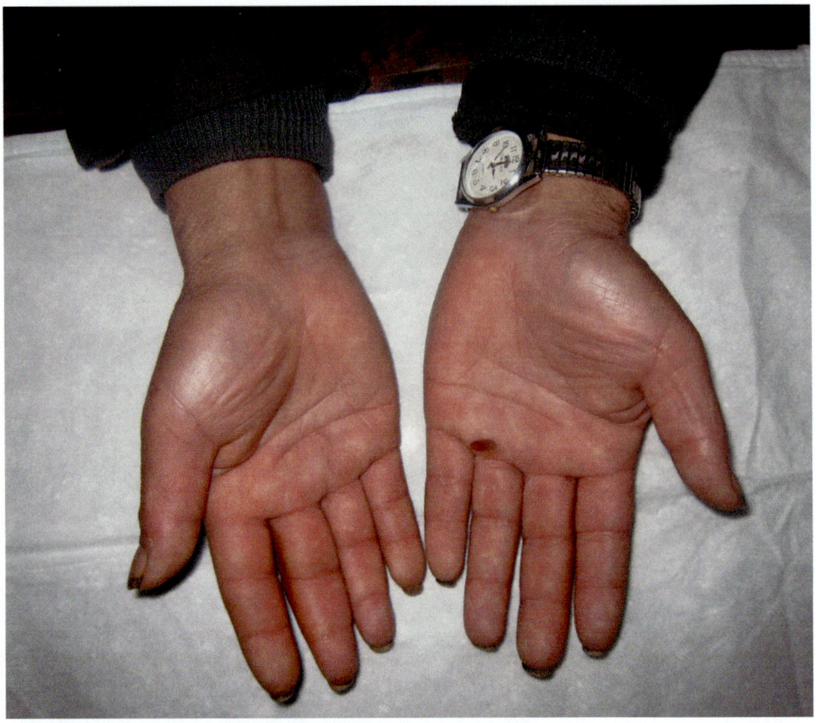

Fig. 18.5 The palm side 13 months and 6 weeks after surgery

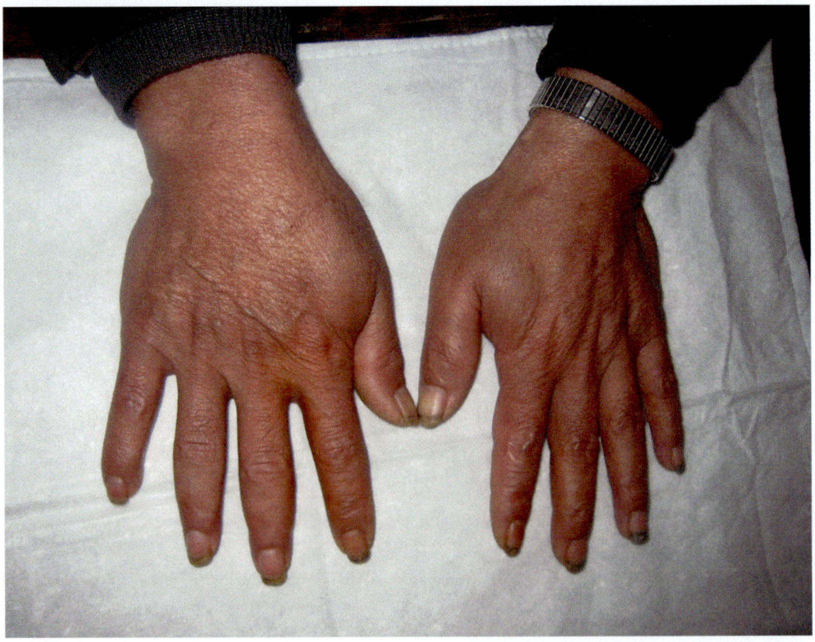

Fig. 18.6 The dorsal side 13 months and 6 weeks after surgery

Case 2: Replantation of Multi-fingers Severed of Old Man

The patient, male, 67 years old, admitted to hospital with both thumbs and index fingers severed by a shearing machine, having bled for 1.5 hours. Physical examination: the general situation was good and the vital signs were stable. The proximal segments of the thumbs were severed but only the flexor tendons attached to the bones, vessels and nerves were revealed, uneven wound, bleeding and without blood supply. The moderate segments of the index fingers were rotational avulsed with bones, vessels and nerves revealed, uneven wound, bleeding and with poor blood supply. Successful debridement and replantation were undertaken under anesthesia in the hospital emergency department. The replanted fingers were red with moderate tension after relaxing the tourniquet and packed with sterile gauze and padded with broken cotton yarn. The patient was taken back to the ward and given conventional postoperative treatments such as antibiotics, hormone and antispasmodic. And 2 weeks later, it was evident that the replanted fingers had successfully survived. The appearance and function was good after regular follow-up and functional exercise guidance and the patient was satisfied (Figs. 18.7, 18.8, 18.9, 18.10, 18.11, 18.12, 18.13, 18.14, 18.15, and 18.16).

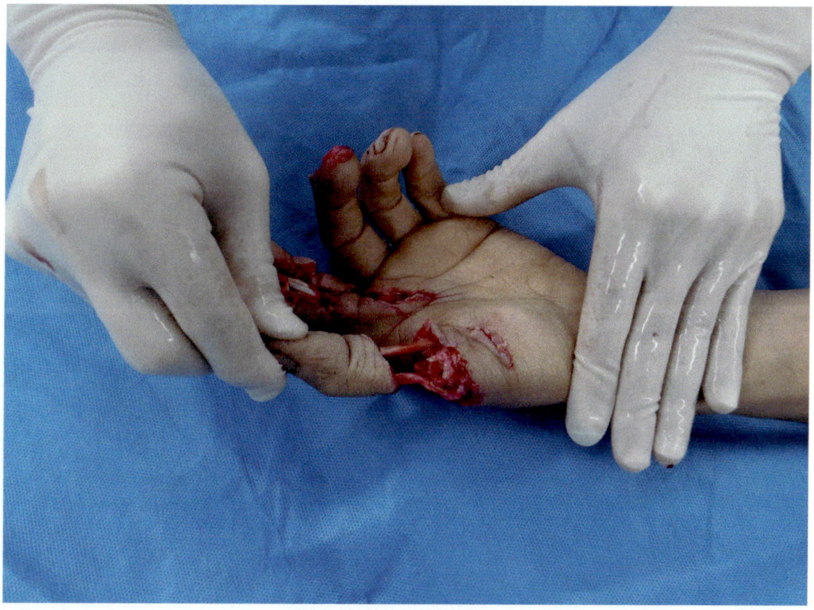

Fig. 18.7 The palm side of the left hand

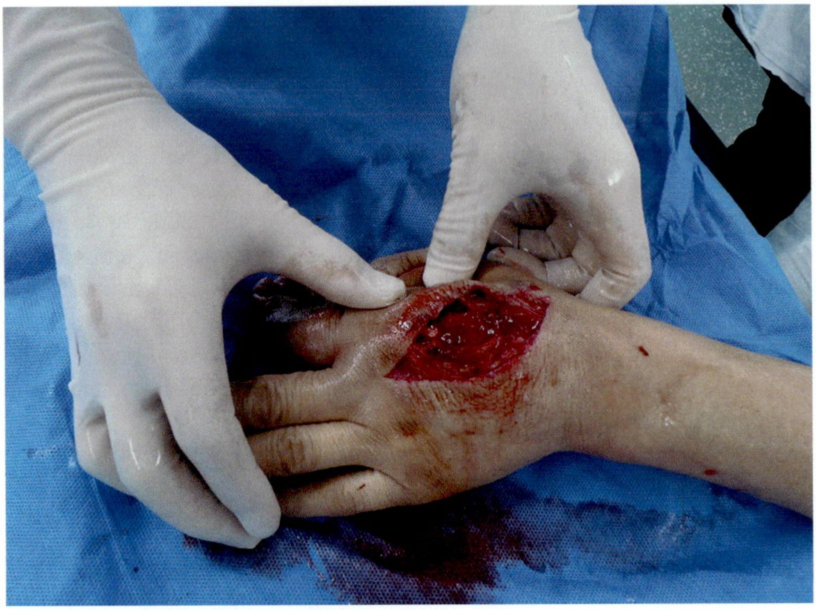

Fig. 18.8 The dorsal side of the left hand

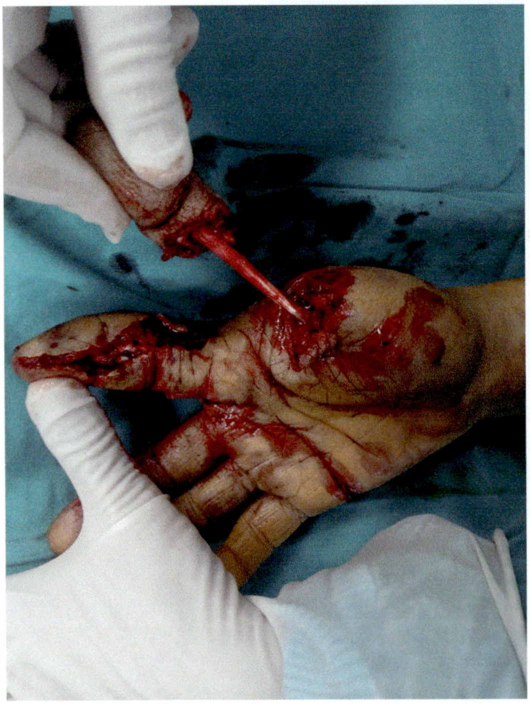

Fig. 18.9 The palm side of the right hand

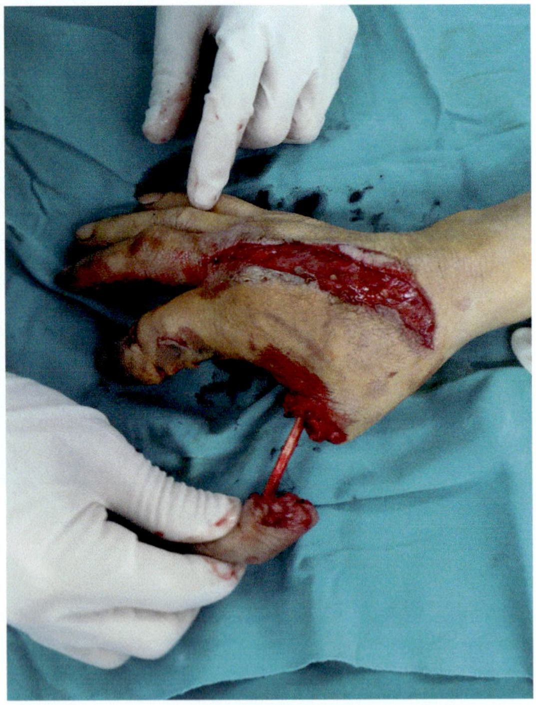

Fig. 18.10 The dorsal side of the right hand

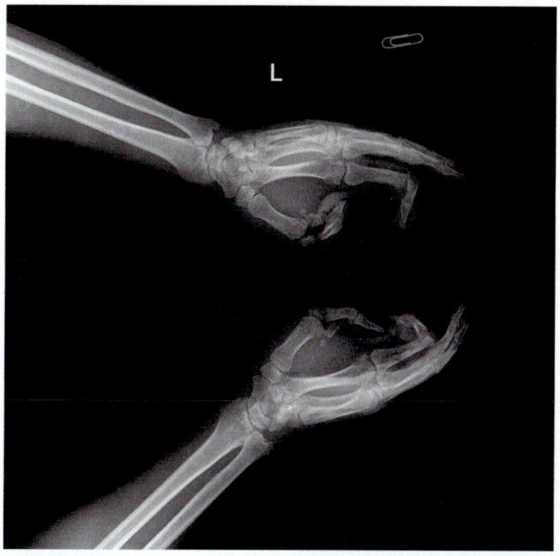

Fig. 18.11 Preoperativer X-rays

Fig. 18.12 The left hand after operation

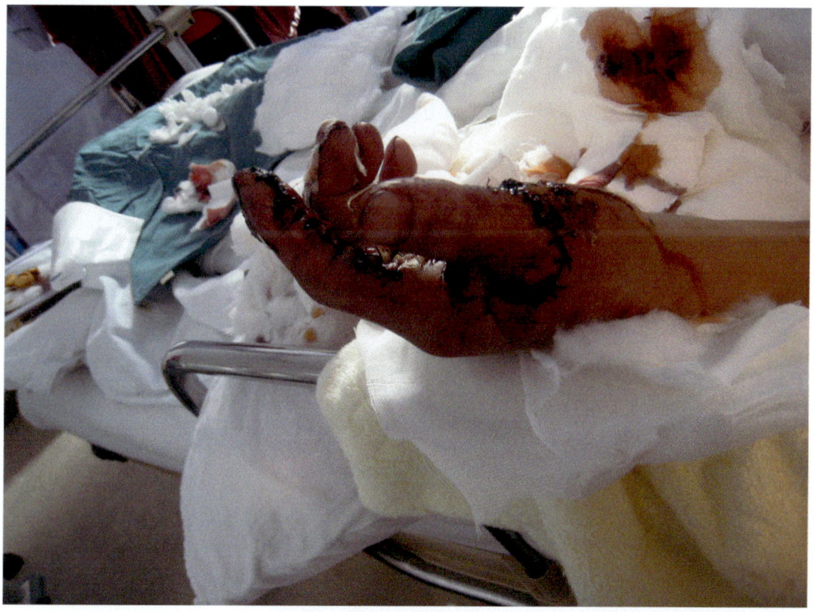

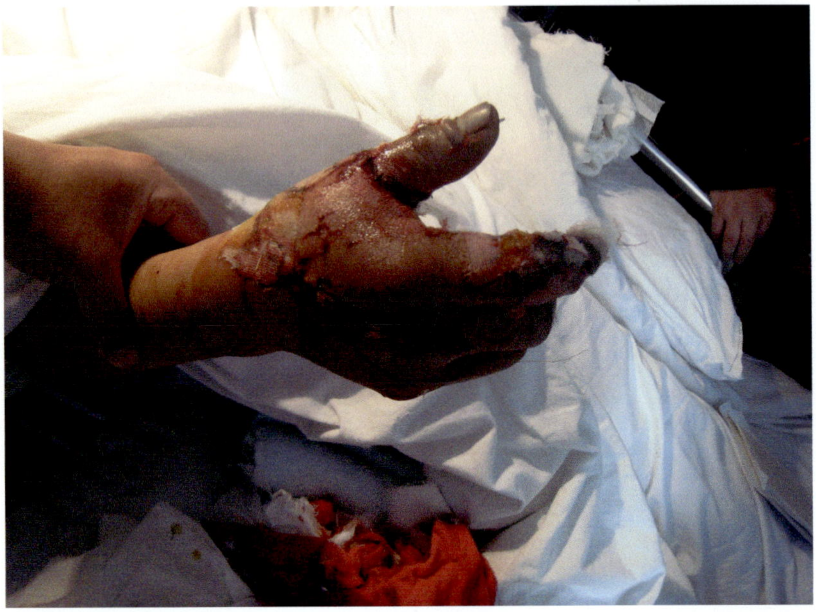

Fig. 18.13 The right hand after surgery

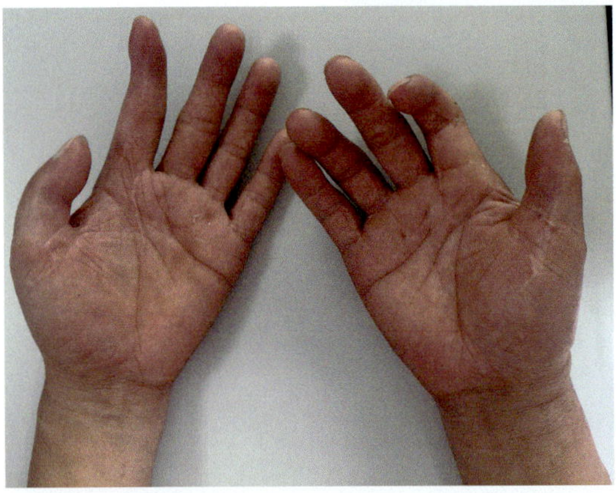

Fig. 18.14 The palm side 34 months after surgery

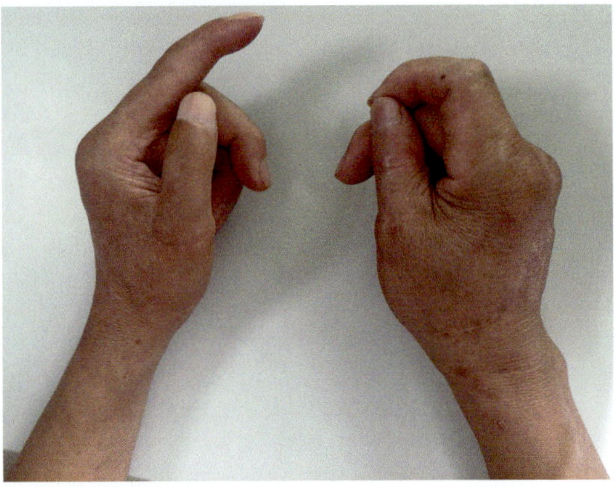

Fig. 18.16 Functionality 34 months after surgery

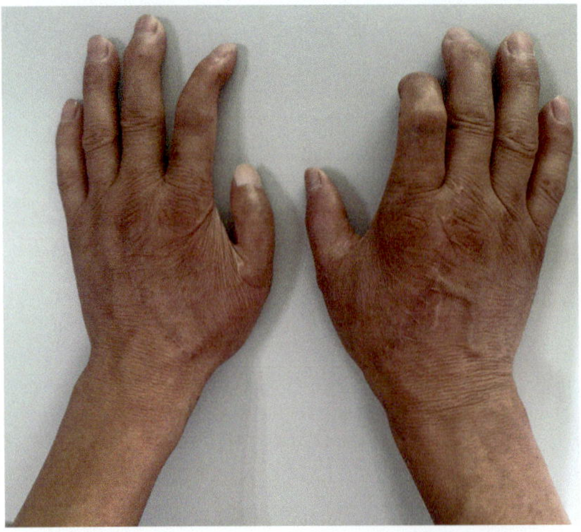

Fig. 18.15 The dorsal side 34 months after surgery

Case 3: Replantation of Final Segments of the Right Thumb of Old Man

The patient, male, 69 years old, admitted to hospital for final segments of the right thumb severed by machine belt and bleeding for 2 hours. Physical examination: the general situation was good and the vital signs were stable. The final segments were completely severed from the interphalangeal joint with joint revealed. The patient described a history of hypertension and diabetes for 4 years, controlled well with blood pressure drugs and insulin. Considering the importance of the thumb and the patient's desire for replantation, successful debridement and replantation were undertaken under anesthesia in the hospital emergency department. The replanted finger was red with moderate tension after relaxing the tourniquet and packed with sterile gauze and padded with broken cotton yarn. The patient was taken back to the ward and given conventional postoperative treatments such as antibiotics, hormone and antispasmodic and treatments for controlling blood glucose and blood pressure. And 2 weeks later, it was evident that the replanted fingers had successfully survived. The appearance and function were good after regular follow-up and functional exercise guidance, and the patient was satisfied (Figs. 18.17, 18.18, 18.19, 18.20, 18.21, 18.22, 18.23, and 18.24).

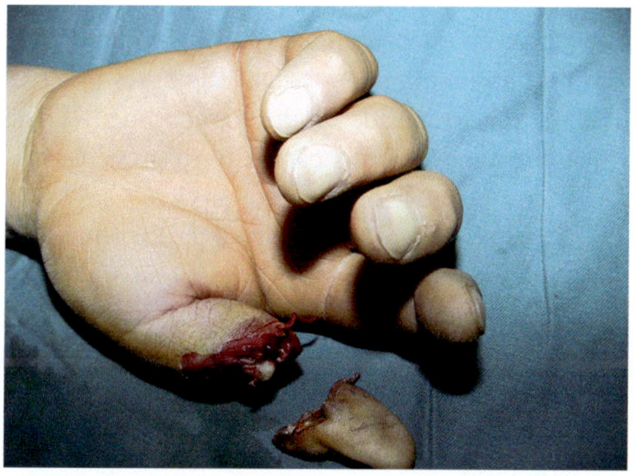

Fig. 18.17 The palm side of the severed finger

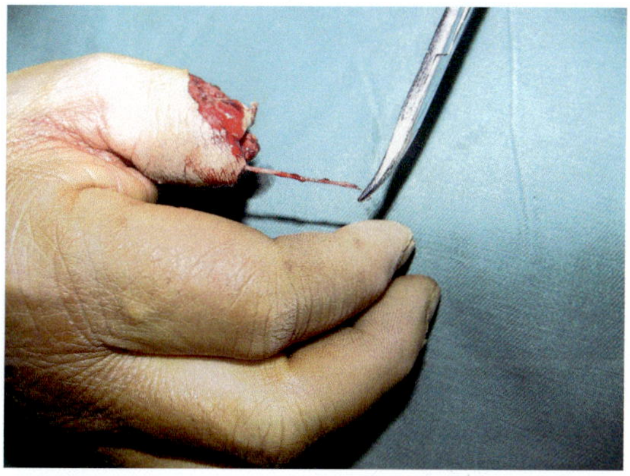

Fig. 18.19 The avulsed finger nerve

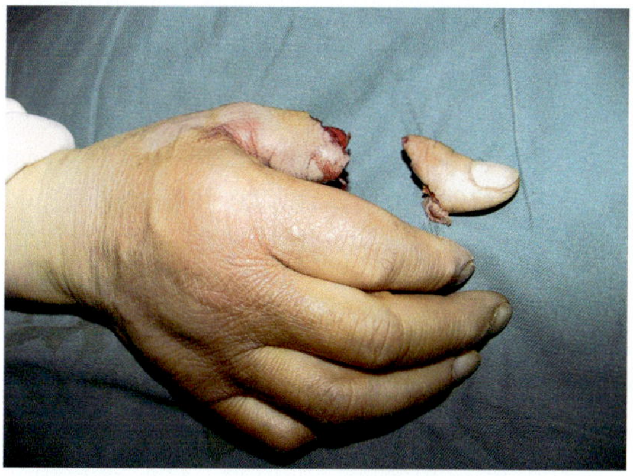

Fig. 18.18 The dorsal side of the severed finger

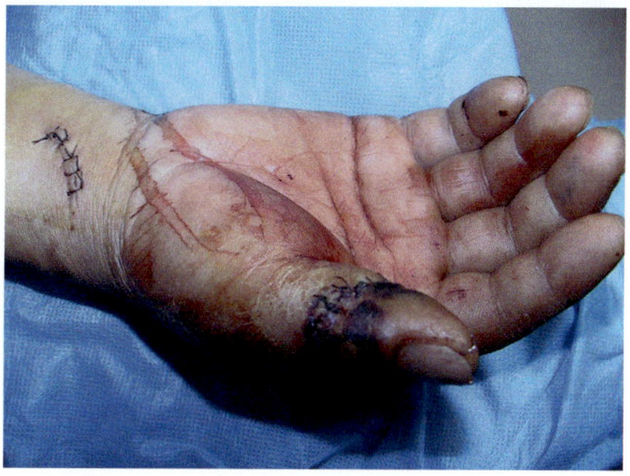

Fig. 18.20 The palm side 2 weeks after surgery

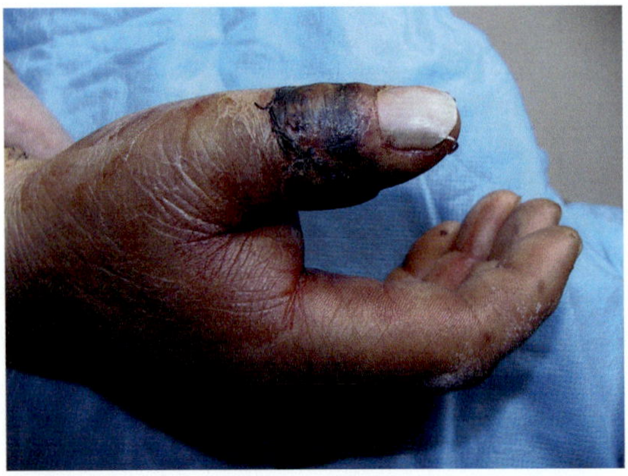

Fig. 18.21 The dorsal side 2 weeks after surgery

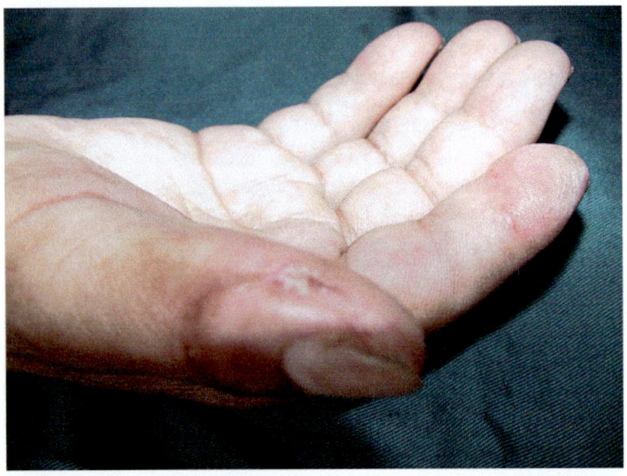

Fig. 18.22 The palm side 13 months after surgery

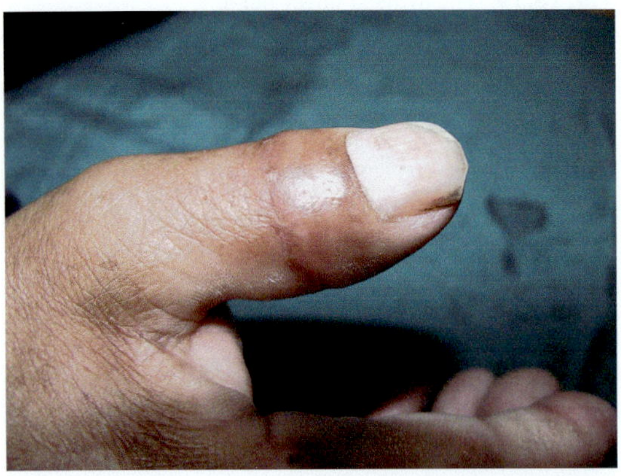

Fig. 18.23 The dorsal side 13 months after surgery

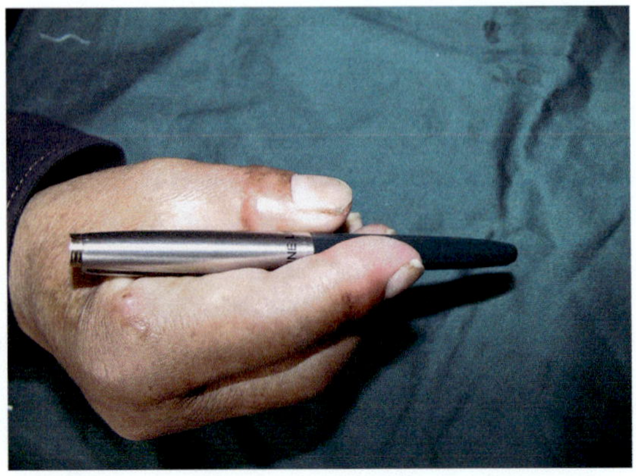

Fig. 18.24 The function 13 months after surgery

18.3 Key Points in Surgery

(a) Through debridement under microscope, find and mark the vessels and nerves that can be anastomosed; at the same time fix the bones and tendons carefully to prevent non-union because of osteoporosis.

(b) Depending on the condition and fractures of the severed finger, the finger can be shortened and the bone fixed with a longitudinal needle of 1.0-1.2 mm, the flexor tendon can be improved by "Kessler" stitching, the extensor tendon can be repaired by "8" stitching.

(c) Anastomosing the arteries before the veins leads to resumption of blood supply, expansion of the capillary network and filling the veins easily to be anastomosed.

(d) Keep more blood vessels or more free parts and less separation of the outer membrane as much as possible since elderly people's vessels are of poor elasticity, low tension and brittleness. Try to minimize the use of vascular clamps to prevent damage to the intima.

(e) The digital artery with thickened wall, loss of elasticity and luminal stenosis and so on easily forms blood clots can be grafted to a relatively normal site and flushed with heparin sodium chloride solution. The operation should be stable, accurate, soft and light, with suitable needle distance and interrupted exstrophy mattress suture.

(f) If vascular tension is high, the carpometacarpal superficial vein can be transplanted.

(g) The stitches should go through the endometrium and outer membrane one time to prevent valve formation which will cause blood clots. Pay attention to skin coverage: if the tension is high, a transfer flap should be used at once.

18.4 Announcements

(a) Understand the patient's tolerance of the operation and eliminate contraindications before surgery. Invite a physician for the appropriate treatment if it is necessary.

(b) Health education is effective to remove negative emotional strains such as fear, anxiety, tension and so on, which will cause complications and affect survival rate.

(c) Old people are not recommended to stay in bed for 5–7 days like other replanted patients, to avoid deep vein thrombosis.

(d) For old people with other systemic diseases, consideration should be given to offering personalized therapy, except for regular postoperative treatments.

(e) Needles should be pulled out after approximately 4-6 weeks but only after X-ray, because of osteoporosis and other possible complications.

(f) Neurological recovery is slower than for other age groups and there is also a loss of feeling, so it is necessary to pay attention to the occurrence of burns, frostbite and so on in the recovery process.

(g) Consider the routine application of small doses of Urokinase for 3 to 4 days except for regular treatment.

(h) If vital signs are stable, proper hydration is useful to prevent high blood coagulation and vasospasm.

Suggested Reading

Barzin A, Hernandez-Boussard T. Adverse events following digital replantation in the elderly. J Hand Surg Am. 2011;36(5):870–4.

Chengqi W, Zhongwei C, Shenxiu Z. Practical microsurgery, vol. 158. Beijing: The People's Army Medical Publishers; 1991.

Komatsu S, Tamai S. Successful replantation of completely cut off thumb. Plast Reconstr Surg. 1968;42:374–7.

Qingmin Y, Chenlin W, Weiwei B, et al. The experience of digital replantation in elderly. Chin J Bone Joint Inj. 2008;23(11):949–50.

Shuqin C. Influencing factors and prevention of vascular crisis after digital replantation. Chin J Nurs. 2009;44(12).

Ximing R, Xiaofeng W, Lifeng M. Report of 6 cases of digital replantation in elder with atherosclerosis in finger arteries. Chin J Pract Hand Surg. 2005;19(2):112.

Xiping L, Zhijian Y, Shengwu L, et al. The characteristic and request of replantation of finger in elderly. J Pract Orthop. 2001;7(5):321–3.

Yudong G, Shuhuan W, De S. Operative hand surgery. Shanghai: Fudan University Press; 2010. p. 726–34.

Yuhong F, Huiqiu G, Min X. The disadvantages and nursing strategies of digital replantation in 45 elderly patients. Chin J Nurs. 2012;47(1):30–2.

Zhengfeng L, Quanrong Z, Kuishui S, et al. Experience in replantation of amputated finger in patients over 60 years old (report of 45 cases) [J]. China J Modern Med. 2010;20(19):2994–6.

Zhongwei C. Traumatic orthopedics and microsurgery. Shanghai: Shanghai Scientific & Technical Publishers; 1995. p. 782–802.

19 Replantation of Amputated Tissue Mass of Fingers

19.1 Summary

With amputated tissue mass of fingers, some parts' continuity with the finger body is broken, including bones, joints, tendons, vessels, and nerves, which cannot survive without vascular anastomosis. It is different from general replantation of severed fingers in these respects:

(a) The tissues are usually separate from each other.
(b) No well-known vessels or nerves to be matched go through.
(c) They are difficult to replant and microsurgical techniques are required because the anatomy of the amputated tissues is not clear, but the appearance and functioning will be good if the surgery succeeds.

There are many types of amputated tissue mass: depending on the vascular conditions, it is divided into the proper digital artery type, small artery type, and total vein type; depending on the amputated position, it is divided into the tissue mass of the final segment, palm tissue mass of the middle and proximal finger phalanx and the dorsal tissue mass of the middle and proximal finger phalanx. Depending on the amputated position, it is divided into type I: different amputated tissue mass of the fingertip; type II: amputated tissue mass of the middle or proximal finger body, with blood supply for the distal part; type III: amputated tissue mass of the middle or proximal finger body, with blood supply for the distal part. These types are all useful for treatment, but in our opinion, it may be more reasonable and useful if it is divided by degree of arterial injury and difficulty of vascular anastomosis, i.e., type I: amputated tissue mass with both artery and vein; type II: amputated tissue mass with only artery; type III: amputated tissue mass with only vein; type IV: amputated tissue mass with neither artery nor vein. With the development of microsurgical techniques, there have been more and more successful reports of small amputated tissue mass, which is great progress.

19.2 Case Description

Case 1: Replantation of Multiple Amputated Tissue Masses of the Right Hand

Male patient, 46 years old, was admitted to hospital for multiple tissue masses amputated from the right hand, caused by a milling machine, and had been bleeding for 1 h. Physical examination: The general situation was good; the vital signs were stable. The amputated tissue masses of the second to fifth fingers, with bone revealed, uneven wounds, and bleeding, were seriously polluted. Successful debridement and replantation were performed under anesthesia under emergency conditions. The replanted tissue masses were red and had moderate tension after

J. Lin et al., *Special Type of Finger Replantation*, https://doi.org/10.1007/978-981-10-6229-2_19

relaxing the tourniquet. They were packed with sterile gauze and padded with broken cotton yarn and the patient was brought back to the ward safely. He was given conventional treatments postoperatively, such as antibiotics, hormones, and antispasmodics. By 2 weeks later, the replanted tissue masses had successfully survived. The appearance and function were good after regular follow-up and functional exercise guidance, and the patient was satisfied (Figs. 19.1, 19.2, 19.3, 19.4, 19.5, 19.6, 19.7, and 19.8).

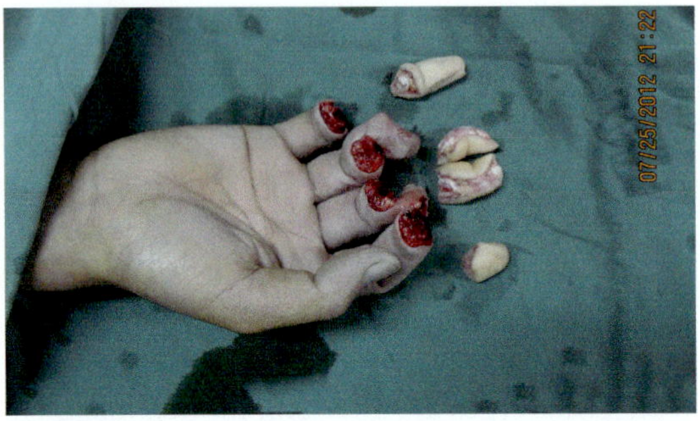

Fig. 19.1 The palm side of multiple amputated tissue masses

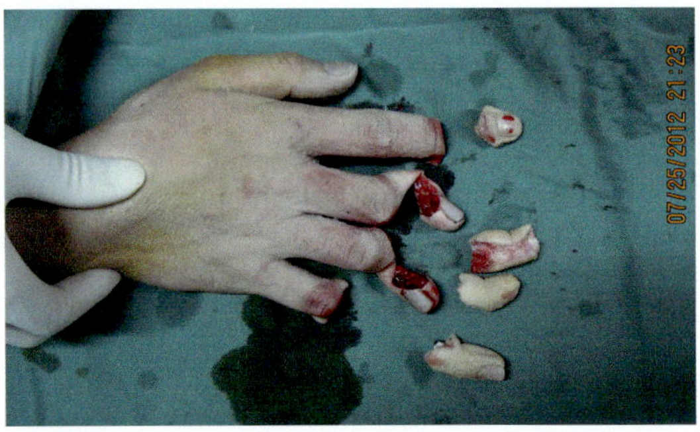

Fig. 19.2 The dorsal side of multiple amputated tissue masses

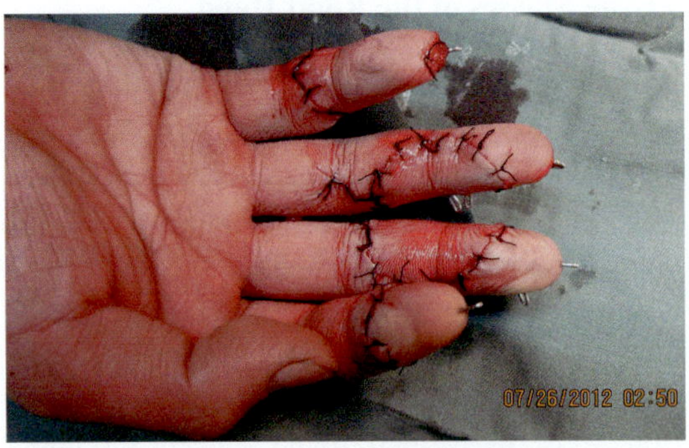

Fig. 19.3 The palm side after replantation

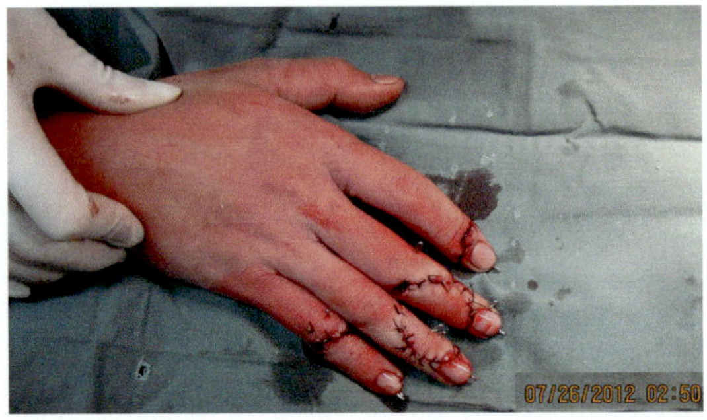

Fig. 19.4 The dorsal side after replantation

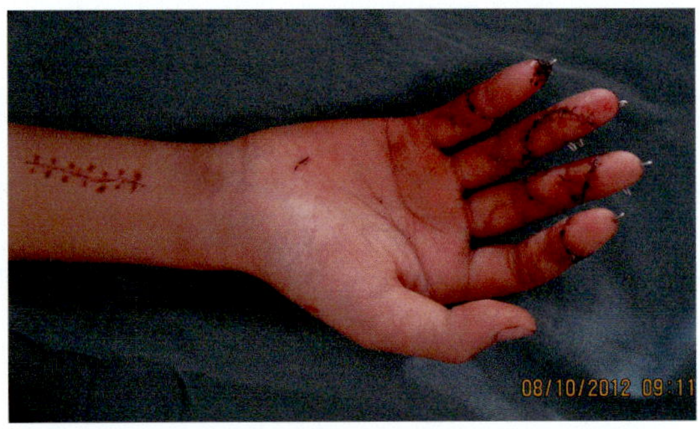

Fig. 19.5 The palm side 2 weeks later

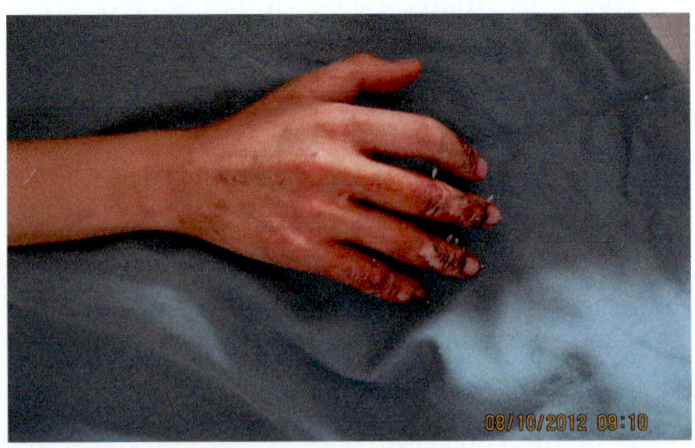

Fig. 19.6 The dorsal side 2 weeks later

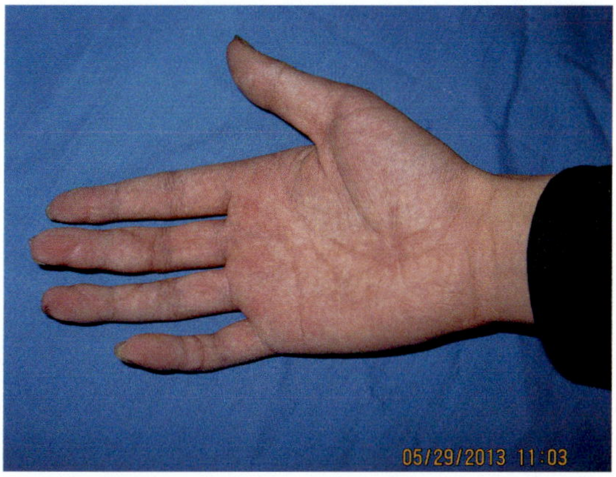

Fig. 19.7 The appearance 3 years later

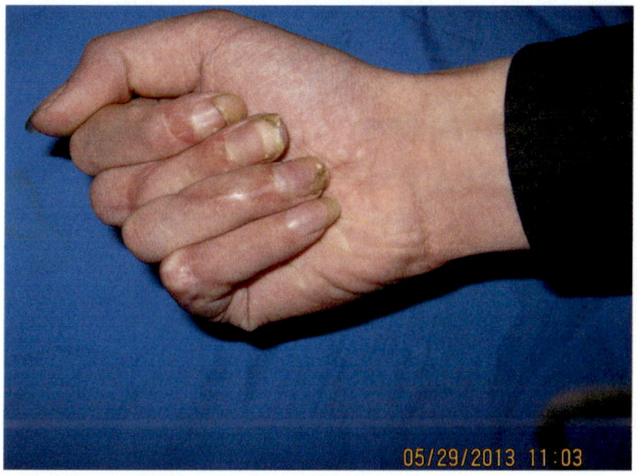

Fig. 19.8 The function 3 years later

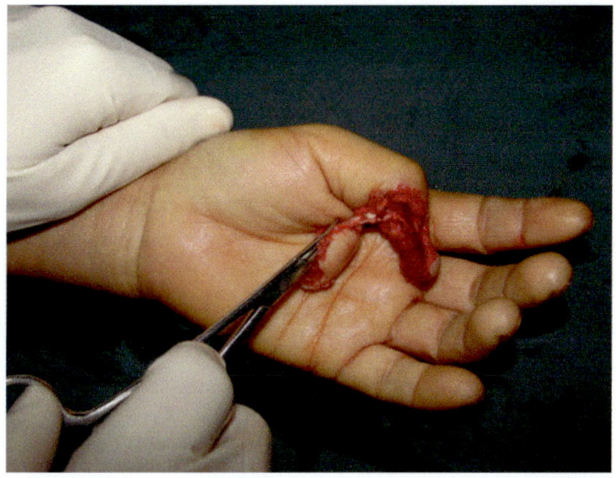

Fig. 19.9 The palm side of the amputated tissue mass

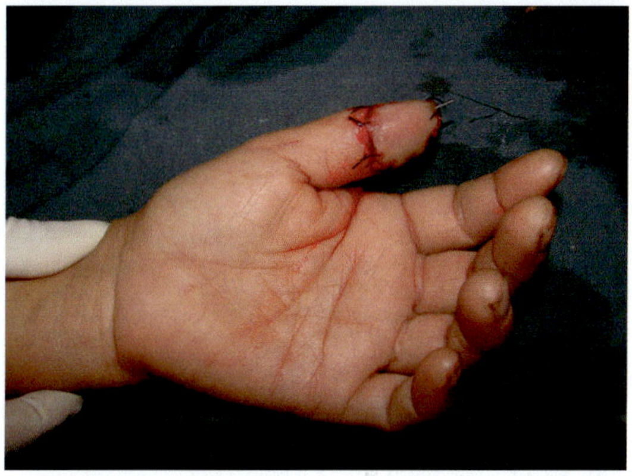

Fig. 19.10 The palm side after replantation

Case 2: Replantation of Amputated Tissue Mass of the Left Thumb

Male patient, 48 years old, was admitted to hospital for an amputated tissue mass from the left thumb pulp caused by a drilling machine, and had been bleeding for 2 h. PE: The general situation was good; the vital signs were stable. The amputated tissue mass of the right thumb, with the bone revealed, and an uneven wound, bleeding, was seriously polluted. Successful debridement and replantation were performed under anesthesia under emergency conditions. The replanted tissue mass was red and had moderate tension after relaxing the tourniquet. It was packed with sterile gauze and padded with broken cotton yarn and the patient was brought back to the ward safely. He was given conventional treatments postoperatively, such as antibiotics, hormones, and antispasmodics. By 2 weeks later, the replanted tissue mass had successfully survived. The appearance and function were good after regular follow-up and functional exercise guidance, and the patient was satisfied (Figs. 19.9, 19.10, 19.11, 19.12, 19.13, 19.14, and 19.15).

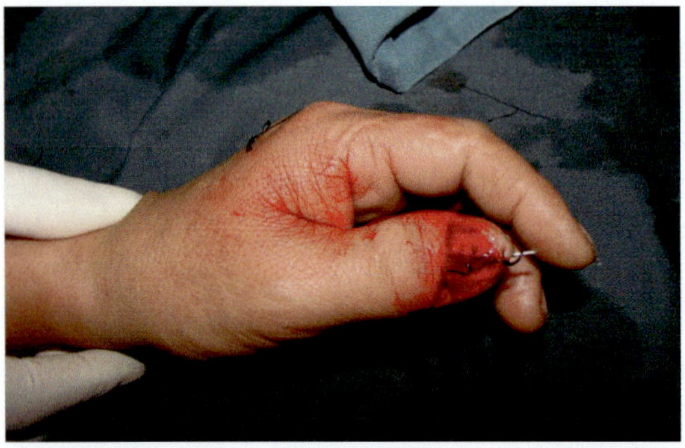

Fig. 19.11 The dorsal side after replantation

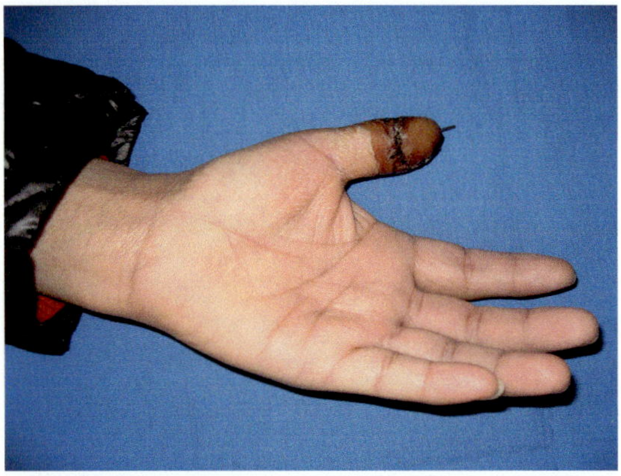

Fig. 19.12 The palm side 3 weeks later

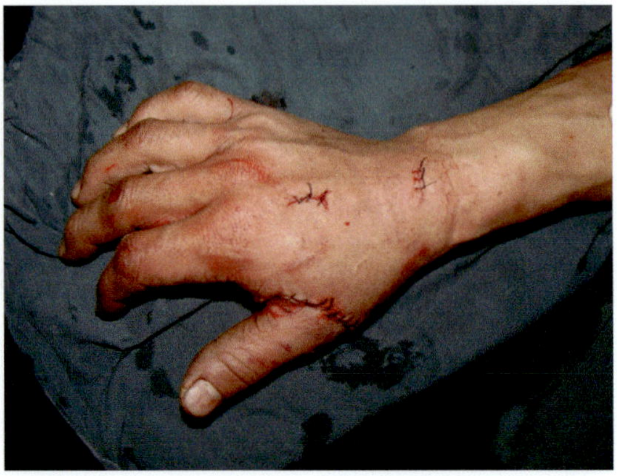

Fig. 19.13 The dorsal side 3 weeks later

Case 3: Replantation of Amputated Tissue Mass of the Palm Side of the Left Thumb

Male patient, 47 years old, was admitted to hospital for an amputated tissue mass of the palmar side of the left thumb caused by a planer, and had been bleeding for 1 h. PE: The general situation was good; the vital signs were stable. The amputated tissue mass of the palm side of the left thumb, with bone revealed, and an uneven wound, bleeding, was seriously polluted. Successful debridement and replantation were performed under anesthesia under emergency conditions. The replanted tissue mass was red

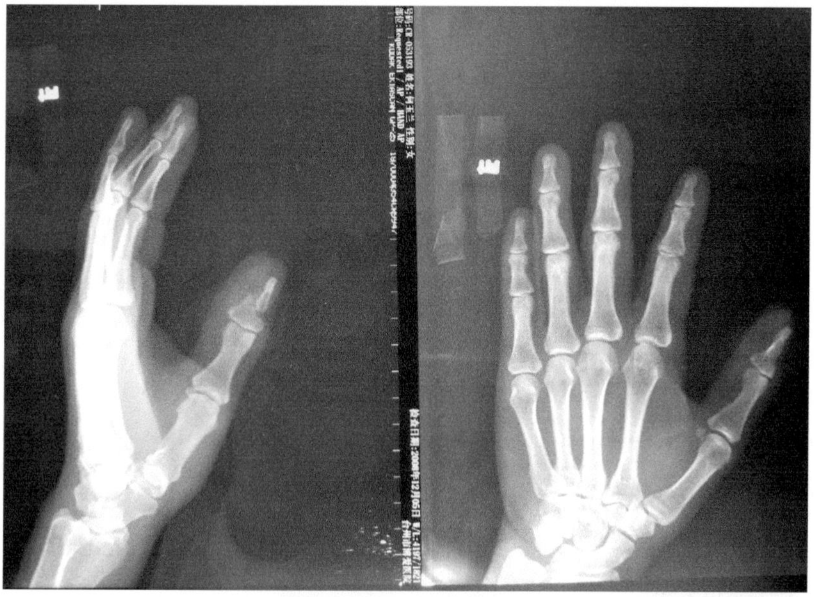

Fig. 19.14 Preoperative X-rays

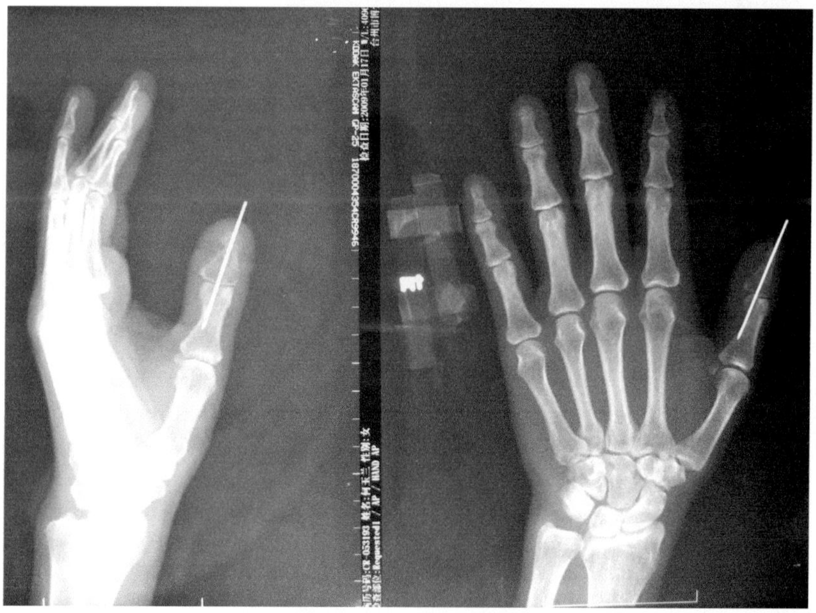

Fig. 19.15 X-rays 3 weeks later

and had moderate tension after relaxing the tourniquet. It was packed with sterile gauze and padded with broken cotton yarn and the patient was brought back to the ward safely. He was given conventional treatments postoperatively, such as antibiotics, hormones, and antispasmodics. By 2 weeks later, the replanted tissue mass had successfully survived. The appearance and function were good after regular follow-up and functional exercise guidance, and the patient was satisfied (Figs. 19.16, 19.7, 19.18, and 19.19).

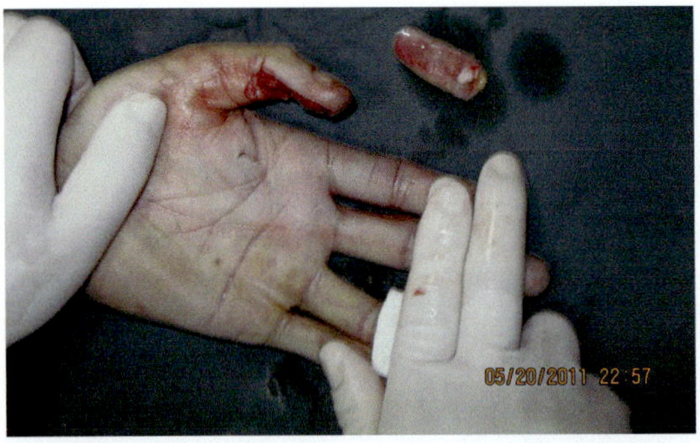

Fig. 19.16 The palm side of the amputated tissue mass

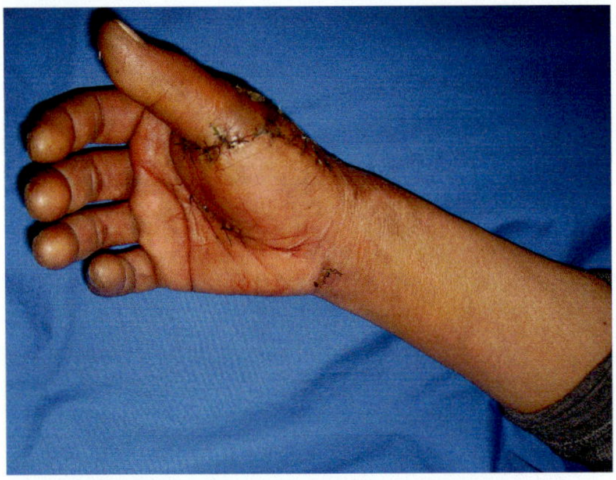

Fig. 19.17 The dorsal side of the amputated tissue mass

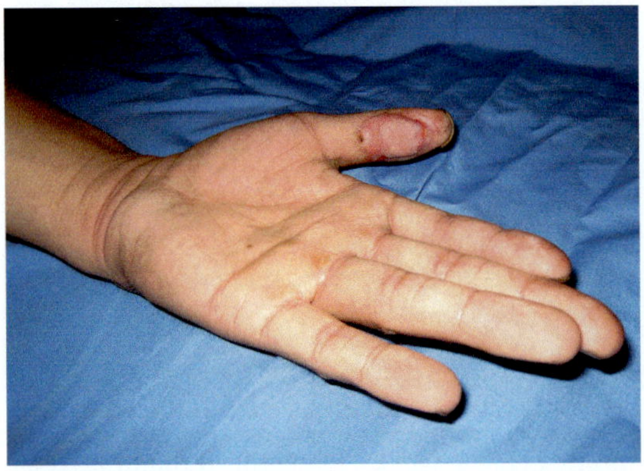

Fig. 19.18 The palm side 15 months later

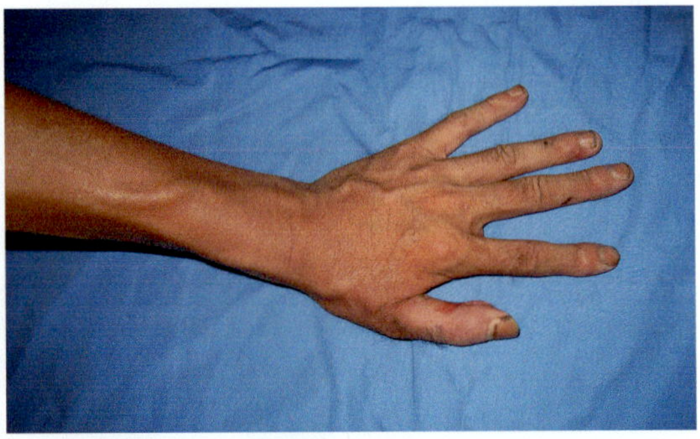

Fig. 19.19 The dorsal side 15 months later

Case 4: Replantation of the Amputated Tissue Mass of the Left Little Finger Palm Body of the Finger

Male patient, 41 years old, was admitted to hospital for an amputated tissue mass from the left little finger abdomen caused by a mold, and had been bleeding for 2 h. PE: The general situation was good; the vital signs were stable. The amputated tissue mass of the left little finger abdomen, with bone revealed, an uneven wound, and bleeding, was seriously polluted. Successful debridement and replantation were performed under anesthesia under emergency conditions. The replanted tissue mass was red and had moderate tension after relaxing the tourniquet. It was packed with sterile gauze and padded with broken cotton yarn and the patient was brought back to the ward safely. He was given conventional treatments postoperatively, such as antibiotics, hormones, and antispasmodics. By 2 weeks later, the replanted tissue mass had successfully survived. The appearance and function were good after regular follow-up and functional exercise guidance, and the patient was satisfied (Figs. 19.20, 19.21, 19.22, 19.23, and 19.24).

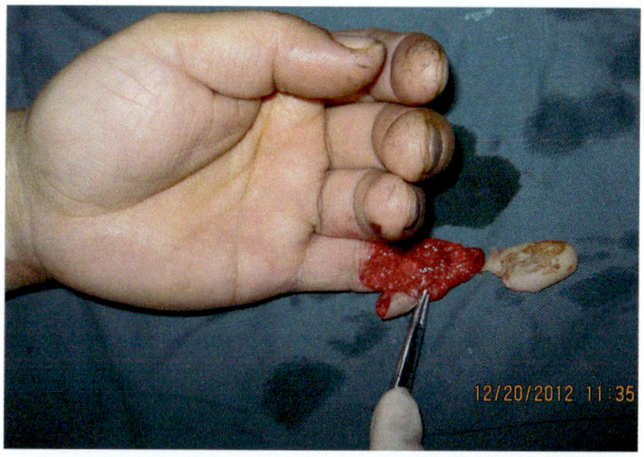

Fig. 19.20 The palm side of the amputated tissue mass

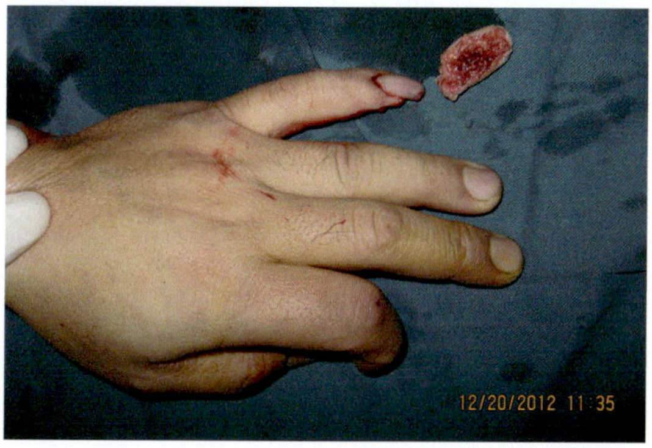

Fig. 19.21 The dorsal side of the amputated tissue mass

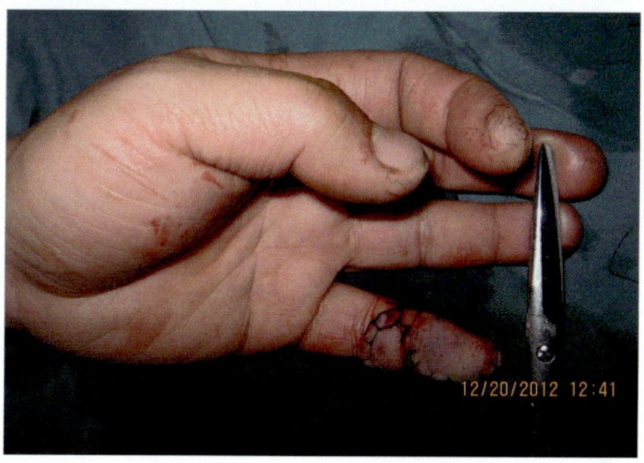

Fig. 19.22 The palm side after replantation

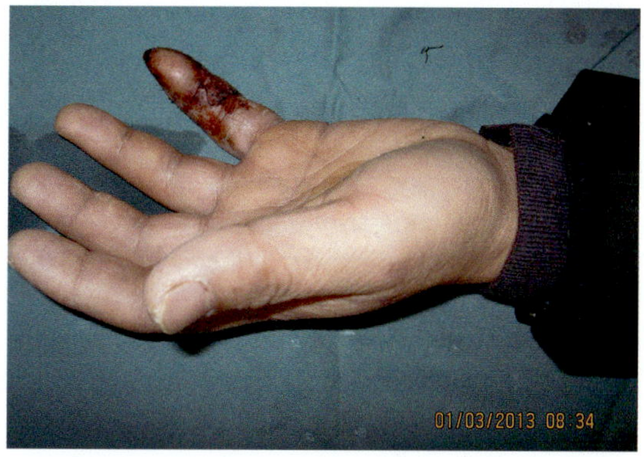

Fig. 19.23 The palm side 4 weeks later

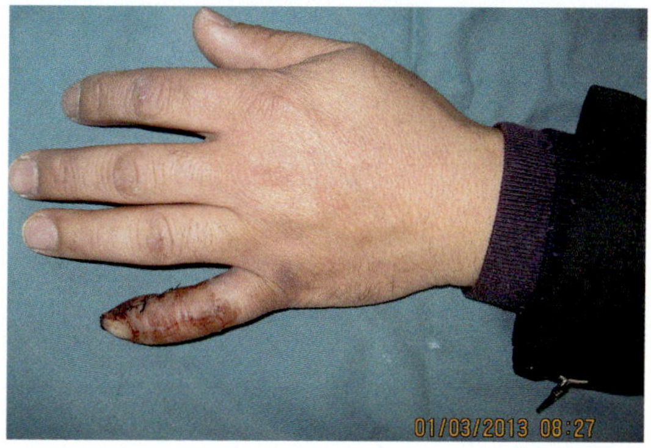

Fig. 19.24 The dorsal side 4 weeks later

Case 5: Replantation of Amputated Tissue Masses of the Right Thumb and Index Finger

Male patient, 53 years old, was admitted to hospital for amputated tissue masses from the right thumb and index finger caused by a lathe, and had been bleeding for 1 h. PE: The general situation was good; the vital signs were stable. The amputated tissue masses of the right thumb and index finger, with bone revealed, uneven wounds, and bleeding, were seriously polluted. Successful debridement and replantation were performed under anesthesia under emergency conditions. The replanted tissue masses were red and had moderate tension after relaxing the tourniquet. They were packed with sterile gauze and padded with broken cotton yarn and the patient was brought back to the ward safely. He was given conventional treatments postoperatively, such as antibiotics, hormones, and antispasmodics. By 2 weeks later, the replanted tissue masses had successfully survived. The appearance and function were good after regular follow-up and functional exercise guidance, and the patient was satisfied (Figs. 19.25, 19.26, 19.27, 19.28, 19.29, 19.30, and 19.31).

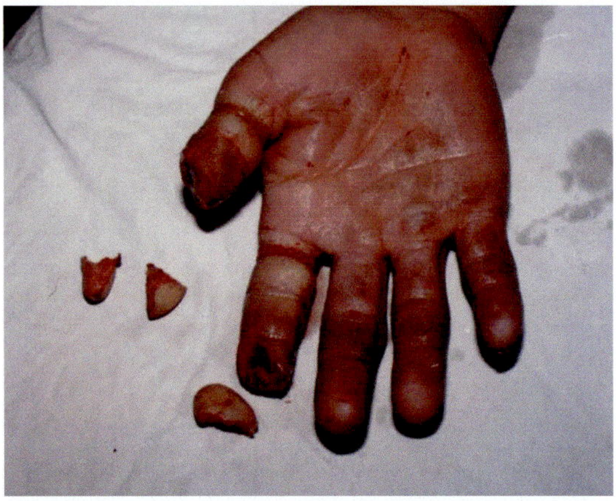

Fig. 19.25 The palm side of the amputated tissue masses

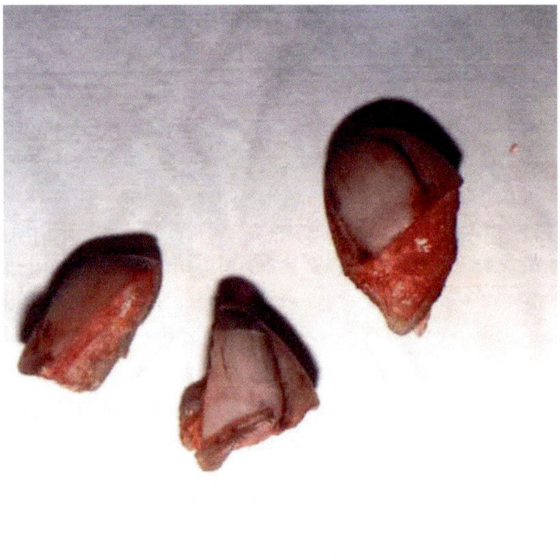

Fig. 19.26 The dorsal side of the amputated tissue masses

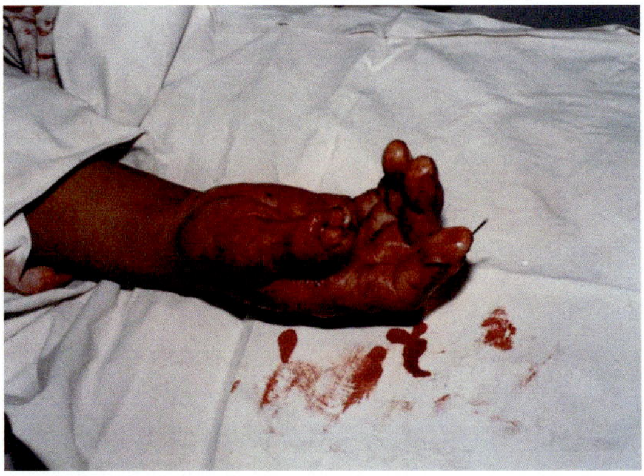

Fig. 19.27 After replantation

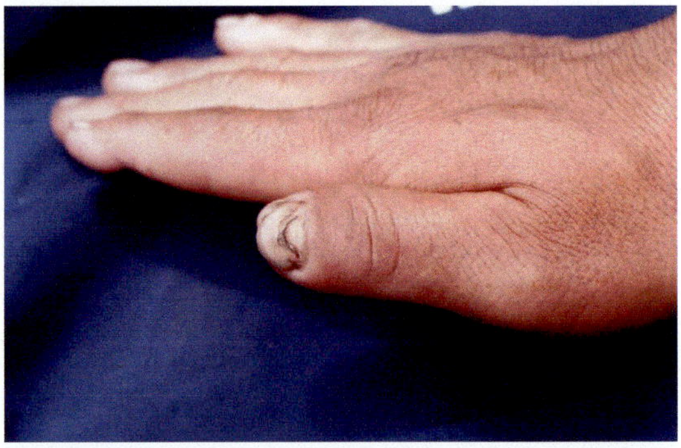

Fig. 19.28 The dorsal side of the thumb 24 months later

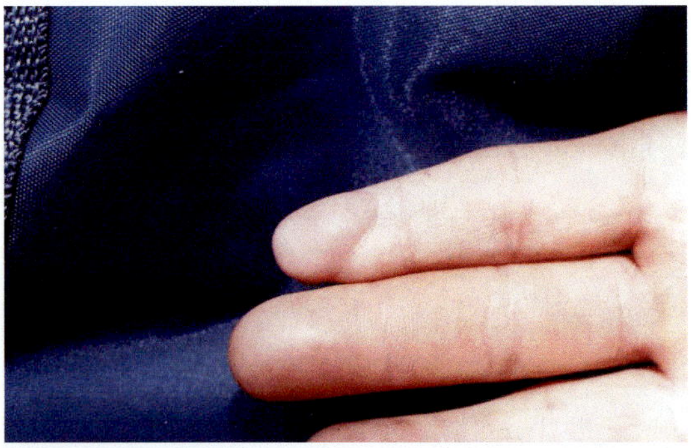

Fig. 19.29 The palm side of the index finger 24 months later

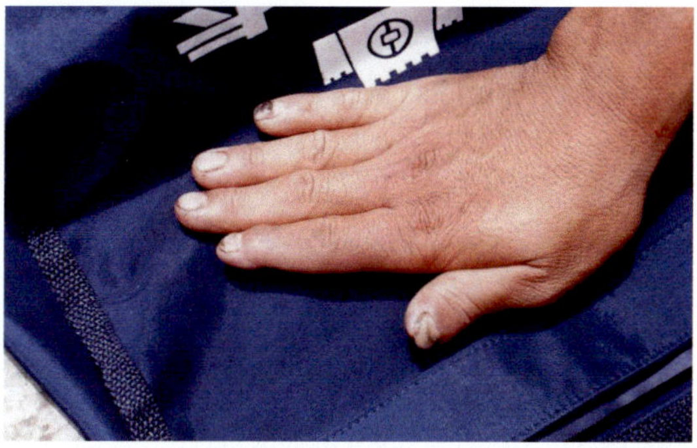

Fig. 19.30 The dorsal side of the index finger 24 months later

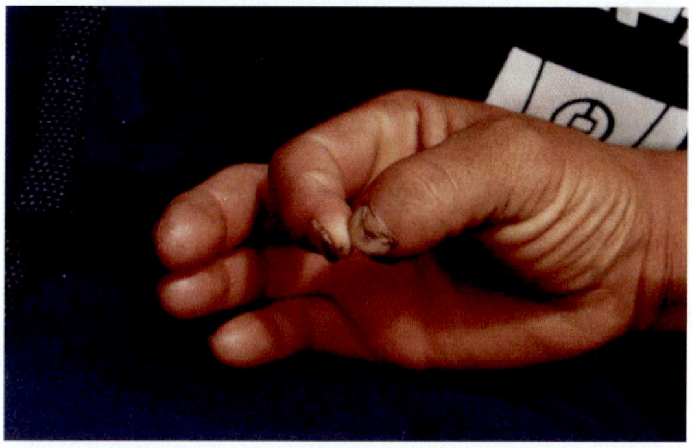

Fig. 19.31 The function 24 months later

Case 6: Replantation of Amputated Tissue Masses of the Right Index and Middle Fingers

Male patient, 26 years old, was admitted to hospital for amputated tissue masses from the right index and middle fingers caused by a lathe, and had been bleeding for 2 h. PE: The general situation was good; the vital signs were stable. The amputated tissue masses of the right thumb tip and radial side of the index finger, with bone revealed, uneven wounds, and bleeding, were seriously polluted. Successful debridement and replantation were performed under anesthesia under emergency conditions. The replanted tissue masses were red and had moderate tension after relaxing the tourniquet. They were packed with sterile gauze and padded with broken cotton yarn and the patient was brought back to the ward safely. He was given conventional treatments postoperatively, such as antibiotics, hormones, and antispasmodics. By 2 weeks later, the replanted tissue masses had successfully survived. The appearance and function were good after regular follow-up and functional exercise guidance, and the patient was satisfied (Figs. 19.32, 19.33, 19.34, 19.35, 19.36, 19.37, and 19.38).

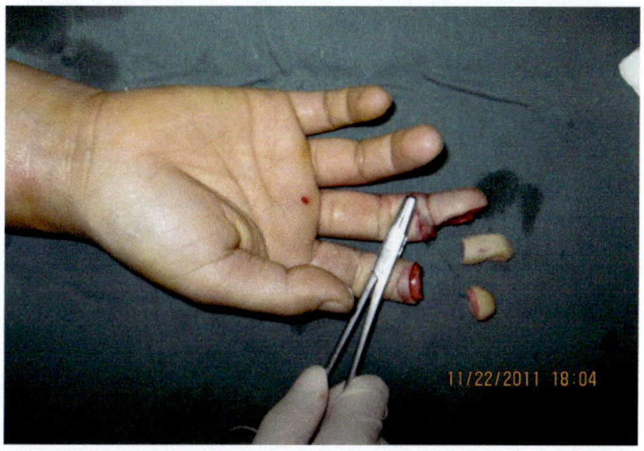

Fig. 19.32 The palm side of the amputated tissue masses

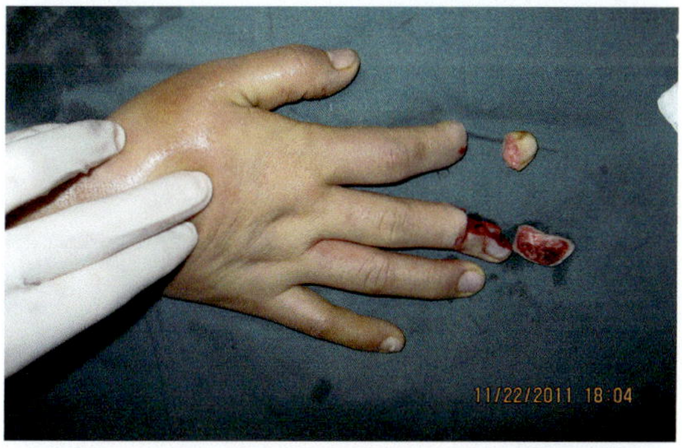

Fig. 19.33 The dorsal side of the amputated tissue masses

Case 7: Replantation of Multiple Tissue Masses of the Right Hand

Male patient, 43 years old, was admitted to hospital for a right-hand injury caused by a lathe, and had been bleeding for 2 h. PE: The general situation was good; the vital signs were

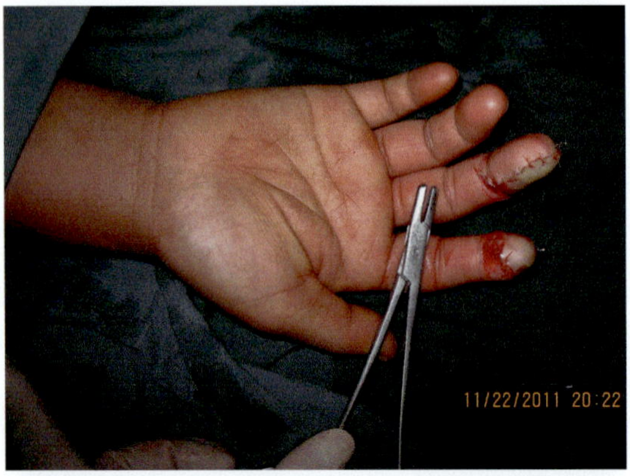

Fig. 19.34 The palm side after replantation

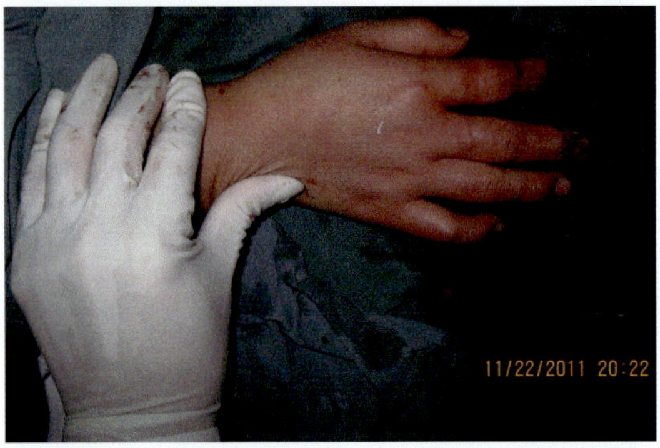

Fig. 19.35 The dorsal side after replantation

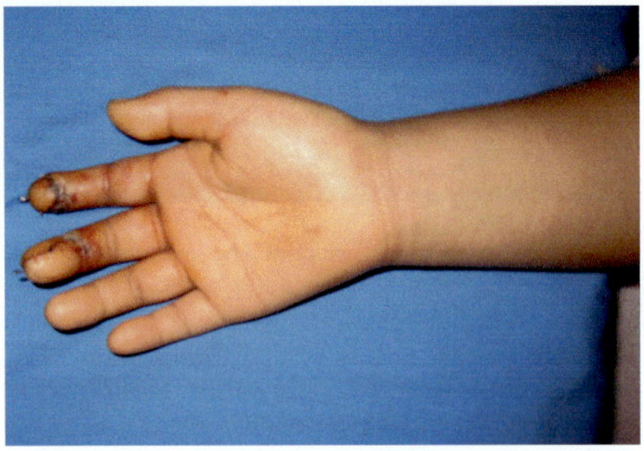

Fig. 19.36 The palm side 8 weeks later

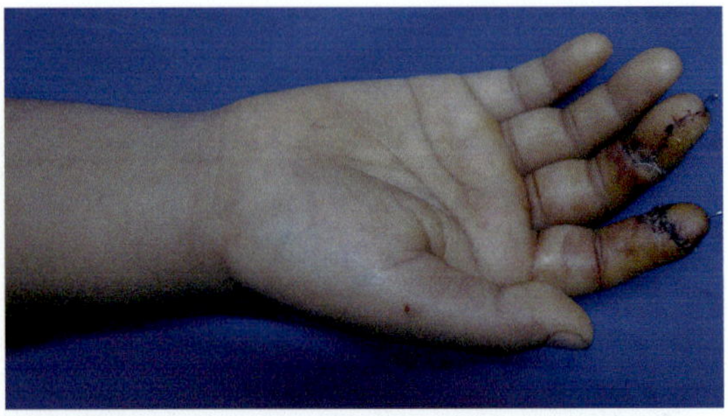

Fig. 19.37 The palm side 6 months later

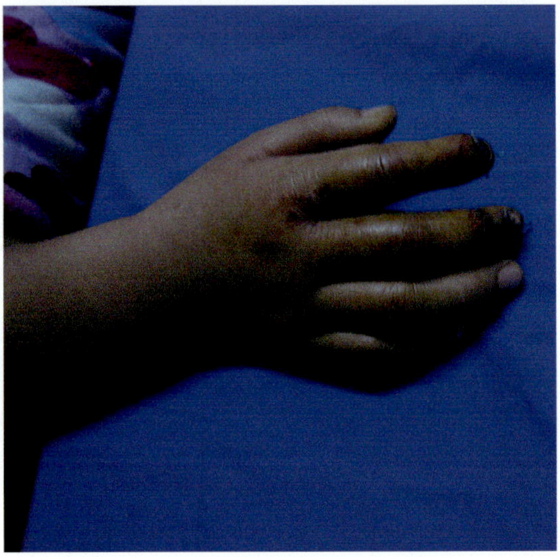

Fig. 19.38 The dorsal side 6 months later

stable. The amputated tissue masses of the right thumb tip, the middle and final segments of the index finger with the flexor tendon attached, the proximal segment of the ring finger with the flexor tendon attached, a soft-tissue defect of the little finger tip, with bone revealed, uneven wounds, bleeding, were seriously polluted. Successful debridement and replantation were performed under anesthesia under emergency conditions. The replanted tissue masses were red and had moderate tension after relaxing the tourniquet. They were packed with sterile gauze and padded with broken cotton yarn and the patient was brought back to the ward safely. He was given conventional treatments postoperatively, such as antibiotics, hormones, and antispasmodics. By 2 weeks later, the replanted tissue masses had successfully survived. The appearance and function were good after regular follow-up and functional exercise guidance and the patient was satisfied (Figs. 19.39, 19.40, 19.41, 19.42, 19.43, 19.44, 19.45, and 19.46).

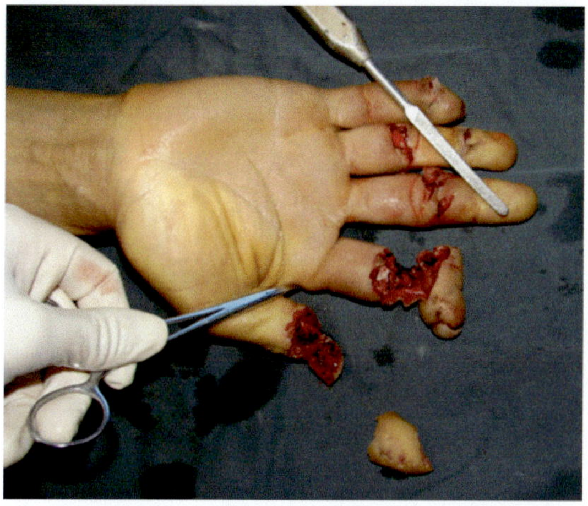

Fig. 19.39 The palm side of the amputated tissue masses

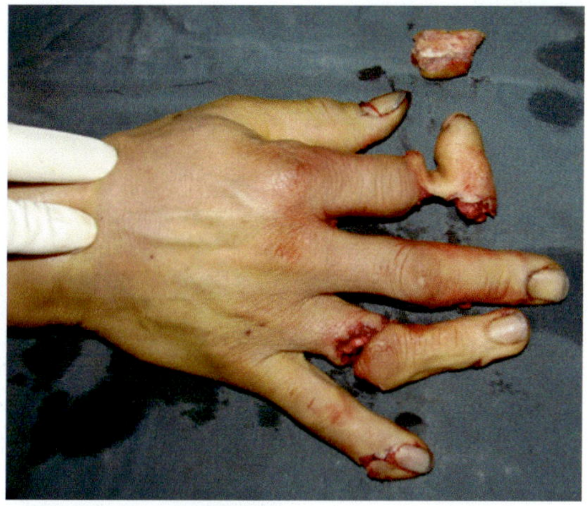

Fig. 19.40 The dorsal side of the amputated tissue masses

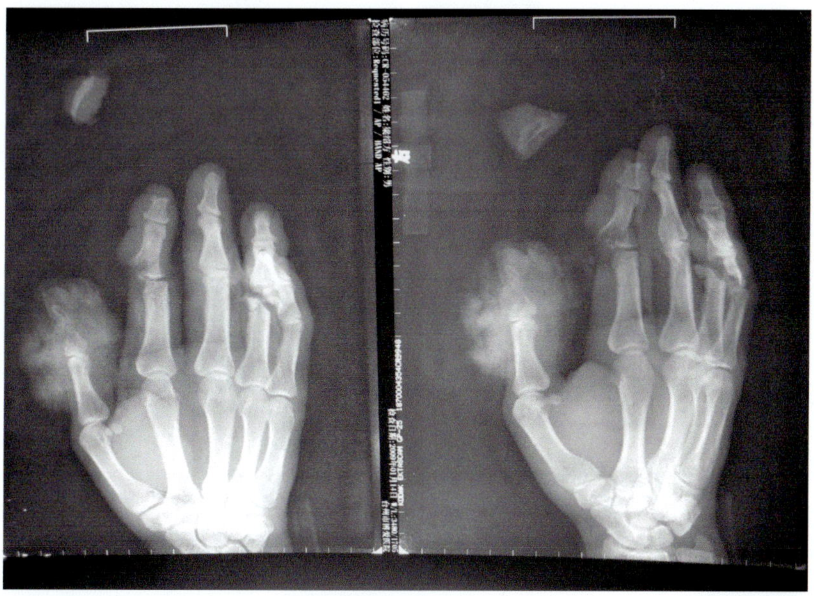

Fig. 19.41 Preoperative X-rays

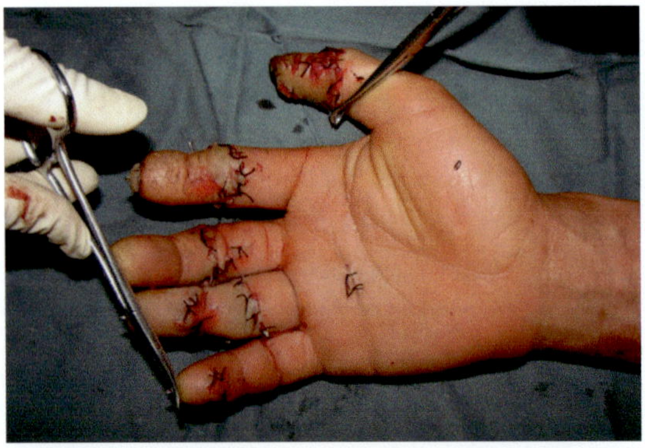

Fig. 19.42 The palm side postoperatively

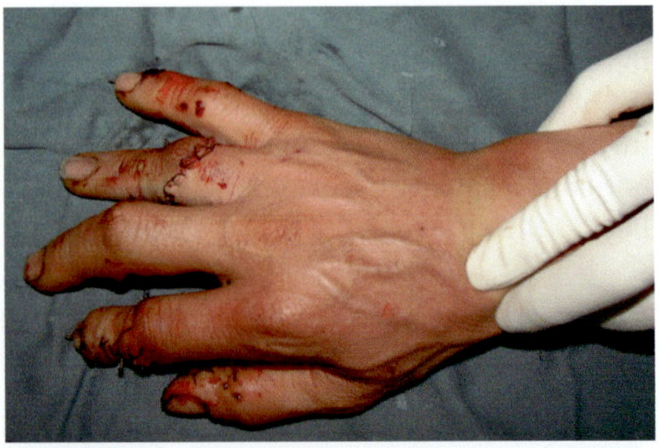

Fig. 19.43 The dorsal side postoperatively

Fig. 19.44 X-rays 3 weeks later

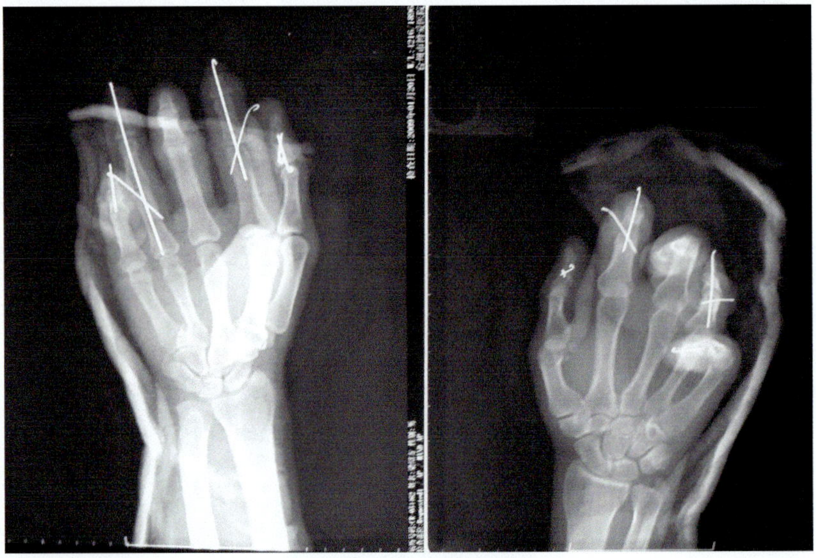

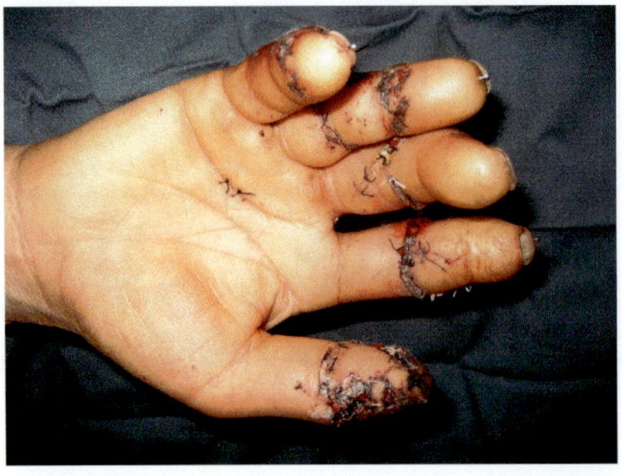

Fig. 19.45 The palm side 6 weeks later

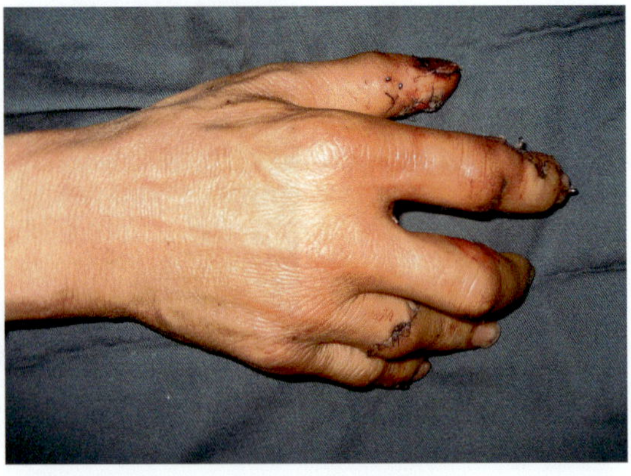

Fig. 19.46 The dorsal side 6 weeks later

Case 8: Replantation of Amputated Tissue Mass of the Right Palm

Male patient, 29 years old, was admitted to hospital for a right-hand injury caused by a punch, and had been bleeding for 1 h. PE: The general situation was good; the vital signs were stable. The amputated tissue mass was of the right palm, the diameter was about 2.5 cm, with an uneven wound, bleeding, and a poor blood supply. Successful debridement and replantation were performed under anesthesia under emergency conditions. The replanted tissue mass was red and had moderate tension after relaxing the tourniquet. It was packed with sterile gauze and padded with broken cotton yarn, and the patient was brought back to the ward safely. He was given conventional treatments postoperatively, such as antibiotics, hormones, and antispasmodics. By 2 weeks later, the replanted tissue mass had successfully survived. The appearance and function were good after regular follow-up and functional exercise guidance, and the patient was satisfied (Figs. 19.47, 19.48, 19.49, 19.50, 19.51, 19.52, and 19.53).

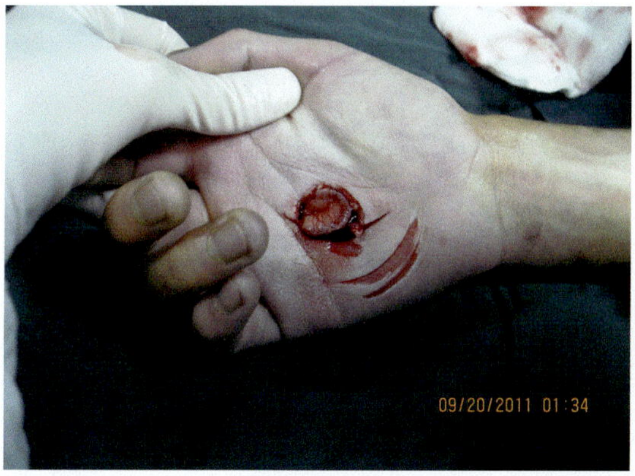

Fig. 19.47 The palm side of amputated tissue masses

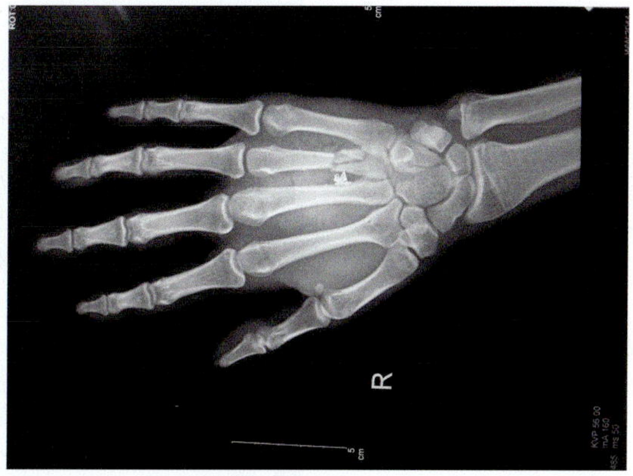

Fig. 19.49 Preoperative X-ray

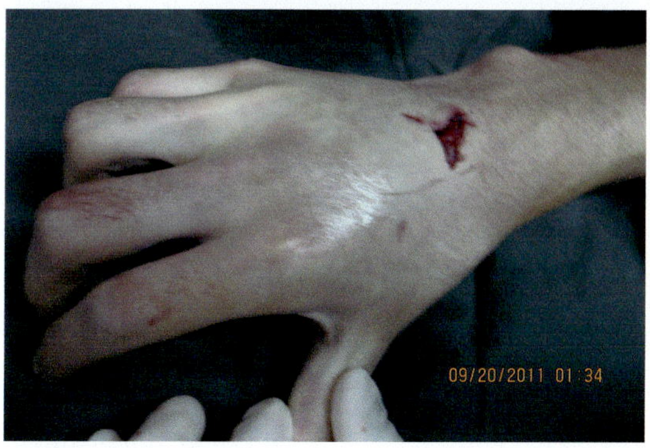

Fig. 19.48 The dorsal side

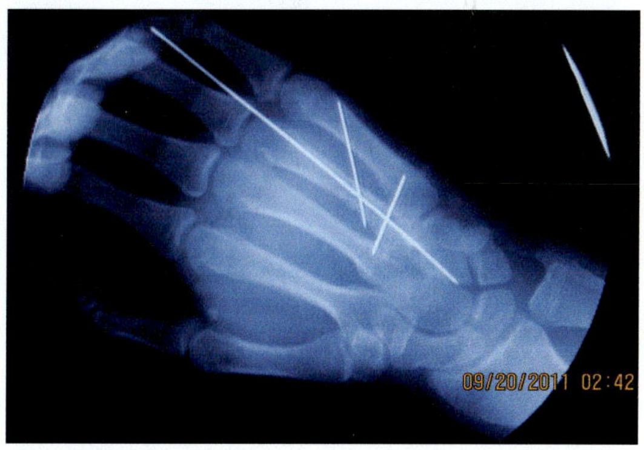

Fig. 19.50 Postoperative X-ray

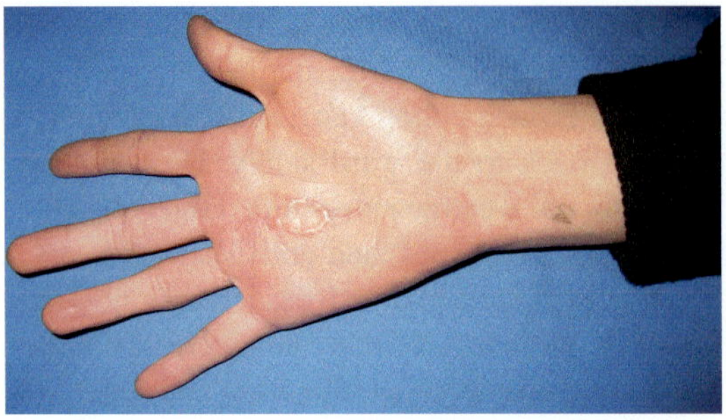

Fig. 19.51 The palm side 2 years later

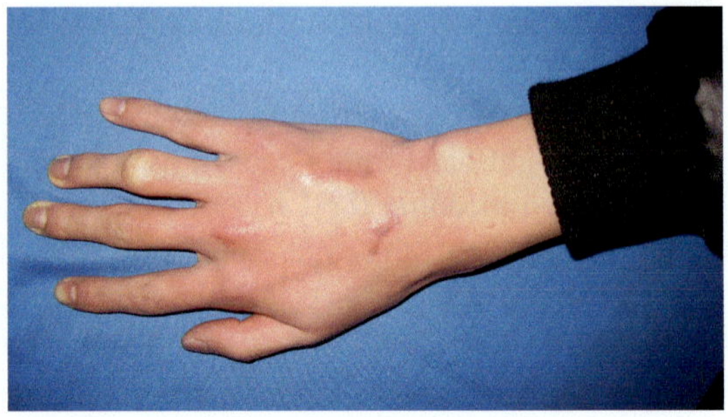

Fig. 19.52 The dorsal side 2 years later

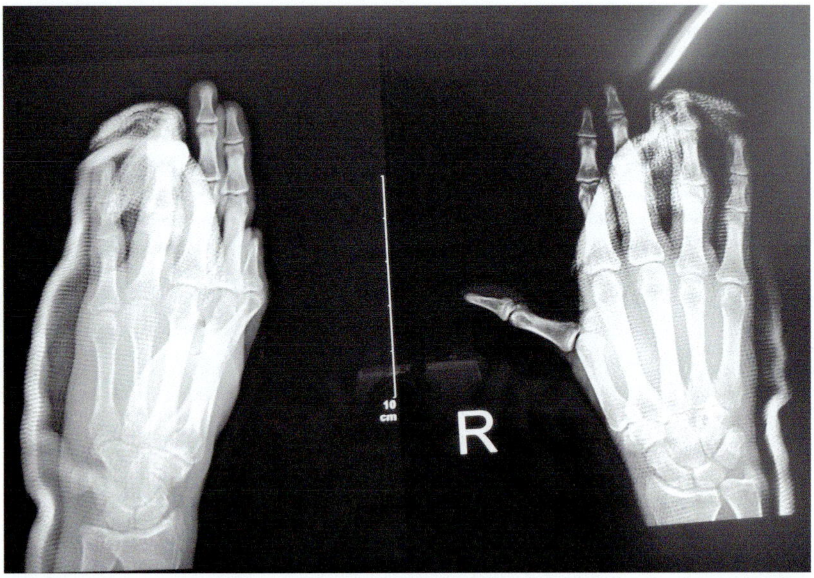

Fig. 19.53 X-rays 2 months later

19.3 Key Points in Surgery

(a) Fine debridement under microscope to find any line material and mark it, which may be vessels.
(b) Finger pulp tissue mass usually combined with fractures of the phalanx tuberosity and injury of the tendons, which should be fixed with 0.8- to 1.0-mm needles.
(c) To expose the digital arteries and digital palm body of the finger veins by suturing the pulp tissue mass to the distal in reverse.
(d) Find the veins according to the bleeding points after relaxing the tourniquet and anastomose them with 12-0 noninvasive stitches; 3–4 needles are sufficient.

19.4 Announcements

(a) Assess whether the amputated tissue mass could be replanted before surgery.
(b) Fine debridement under ×10 microscope to avoid injury to the vessels.
(c) Wash with sterile normal saline, not disinfectant, after debridement, to avoid injury to the vessels.
(d) Transplant veins to resume the blood supply when there are no arteries to be anastomosed.
(e) Pay attention to the exact fit of the nerve to restore finger sensation.
(f) Loosen stitches and leave the flap of the drainage and local saline drip to keep wet when there are no veins to be anastomosed.

(g) The disease of amputated tissue mass is complicated; debridement should not only be thorough, but also keep as much of the active tissue as possible to repair the soft-tissue defect.

Suggested Reading

Barbary S, Dap F, Dautel G. Finger replantation: surgical technique and indications. Chirurgie de la main. 2013;32:363–72.

Fanyu P, Xue M, Kuishui S, et al. The clinical experience of replantation of avulsed finger pulp. Chin J Hand Surg. 2014;30(6):209–11.

Huang H-F, Yeong E-K. Surgical treatment of distal digit amputation: success in distal digit replantation is not dependent on venous anastomosis. Plast Reconstr Surg. 2015;135:174–8.

Jian H, Hong C, Peng W. The experience of 38 cases of replantation of amputated complex tissue mass of finger. Mod Pract Med. 2004;16(10):591–2.

Jianmin L, Wu J. The clinical research of the use of papaverine after replantation of amputated tissue mass of finger. Zhejiang J Trauma Surg. 2014;4:588–9.

Jianwen Z, Zihu B, Dajiang H, et al. Replantation of amputated complex mass of fingers. Chin J Hand Surg. 2003;19(1):29–30.

Lee C, Wei C-Y. Fingertip replantation without venous anastomosis. Ann Plast Surg. 2014;73(4):473–4.

Mingwu Z, Kunde L, Dongsheng Z, et al. Application of veno-arterialization in digit replantation and reconstruction. Chin J Hand Surg. 2006;22(2):101–2.

Shen X, Xu Y, Yongjun R, et al. Replantation of degloved fingertips. Chin J Hand Surg. 2010;26(2):104–6.

Wei F, Danmo X, Dong R, et al. Replantation of severed complex tissue mass of the hand. Chin J Hand Surg. 2012;28(4):227–9.

Weiwen Z, Hong C, Wang X, et al. Replantation of special types of amputated fingers. Chin J Hand Surg. 2003;19(3):135–8.

Xue J, Huabo F. 11 cases of replantation of amputated tissue mass of fingertip[J]. Chin J Microsurg. 2004;27(3):192.

Yanchun F, Jian Z, Zhongtian F, et al. The experience of replantation of amputated tissue mass of finger. China Med Herald. 2010;7(9):166–7.

Yujie L, Xiaoheng D, Hongsheng J, et al. Replantation methods of mini tissue mass of amputated finger. Chin J Hand Surg. 2011;34(2):109–12.

20 Ectopic Implantation of Severed Fingers

20.1 Summary

If the severed part is complete, but the proximal part is seriously damaged or the general condition of the patient does not permit surgery, the severed part could be implanted to another position before being implanted to the in-situ position to recover the appearance and function. This therapy method is called ectopic implantation.

In 1986, Godina et al. (1986) proposed that the chest wall could be the accepting site for severed limbs when the proximal limbs were not in a good condition, which made microsurgery feasible for ectopic implantation. Chernofsky and Sauer (1990) ectopically transplanted a severed limb forearm to the abdomen and successfully replanted it to the in-situ position after 11 weeks in 1990. Hallock (1992) suggested that the upper abdominal blood vessels could be used to keep a single severed finger alive. Miao Kaixi successfully ectopically implanted the second to fifth fingers with fingerwebs to the foot back in 1992. Gao Weiyang carried out successful ectopically implantation of a severed finger to the groin in 1996. This method, of course, expands the indications for replantation of severed fingers, which can save the functions of the hand as far as possible.

20.2 Case Description

Case 1: Ectopic Implantation of the Severed Left Thumb

Female patient, 34 years old, was admitted to hospital for a completely severed left thumb caused by a high-speed machine, and had been bleeding for 8 h. Physical Examination. The general situation was good; the vital signs were stable. The left thumb was completely severed, with the bone revealed, an uneven wound, a soft-tissue defect of about 3*4 cm, bleeding, and was seriously polluted. The severed thumb was packed with gauze whose finger pulf and nail were black. The interphalangeal joints had an intercondylar fracture. The flexor pollicis longus muscle tendon and the extensor pollicis longus muscle tendons were avulsed about 25 cm. Both sides of the digital nerves were avulsed about 8 cm and both sides of the proper digital arteries were avulsed about 4 cm. Successful debridement and ectopic implantation were performed under anesthesia under emergency conditions. The severed thumb was implanted to the anterolateral thigh flap and successfully survived after second-stage surgery. The patient was given conventional treatments postoperatively, such as antibiotics, hormones, and antispasmodics. By 1 year later, the replanted severed thumb

J. Lin et al., *Special Type of Finger Replantation*, https://doi.org/10.1007/978-981-10-6229-2_20

achieved sensory recovery. The appearance and function were good after regular follow-up and functional exercise guidance, and the patient and her family were satisfied (Figs. 20.1, 20.2, 20.3, 20.4, 20.5, 20.6, 20.7, 20.8, 20.9, 20.10, 20.11, and 20.12).

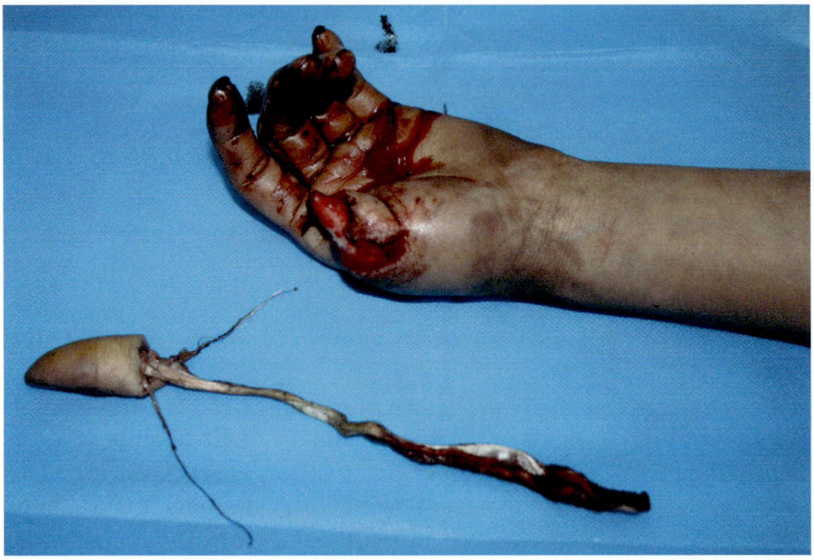

Fig. 20.1 The condition of the severed left thumb

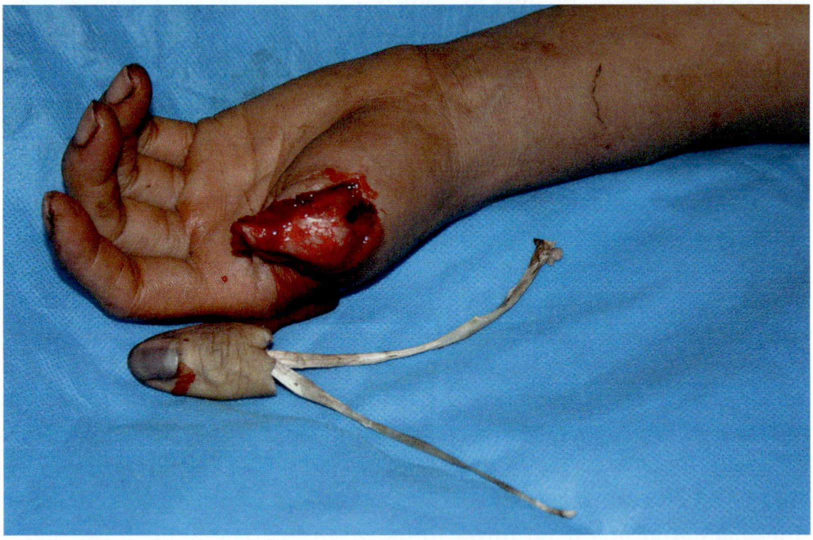

Fig. 20.2 The condition after debridement

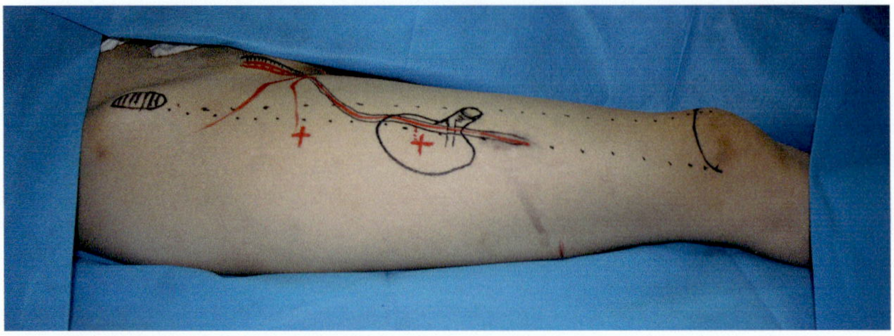

Fig. 20.3 The design of the ectopic implantation

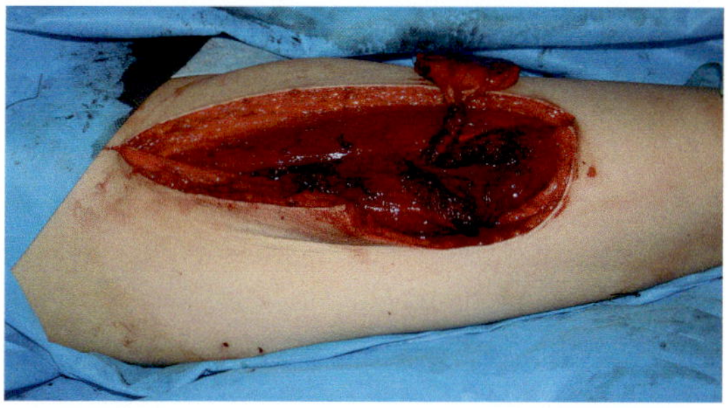

Fig. 20.4 Flap is cut out

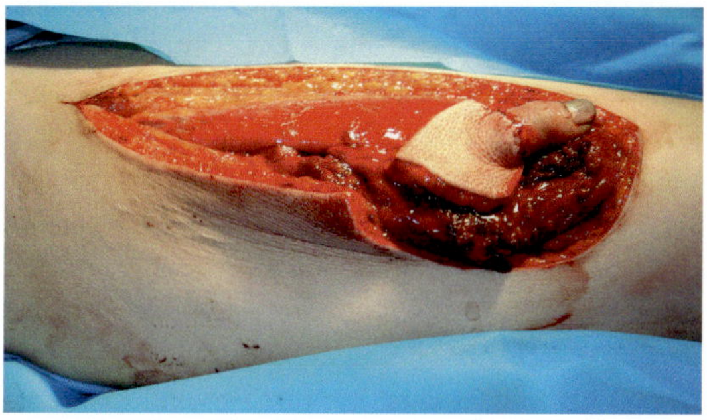

Fig. 20.5 Repairing the defect of the severed left thumb

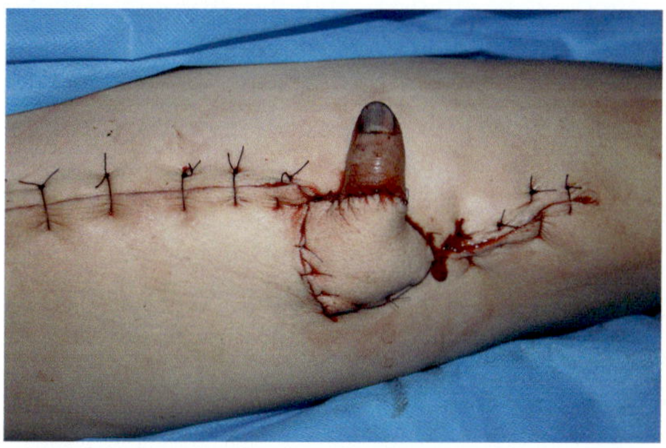

Fig. 20.6 The blood supply after ectopic implantation

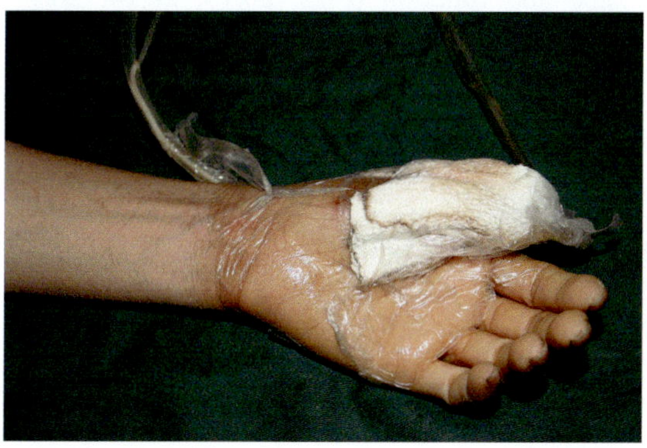

Fig. 20.7 The treatment administered to the amputation ending

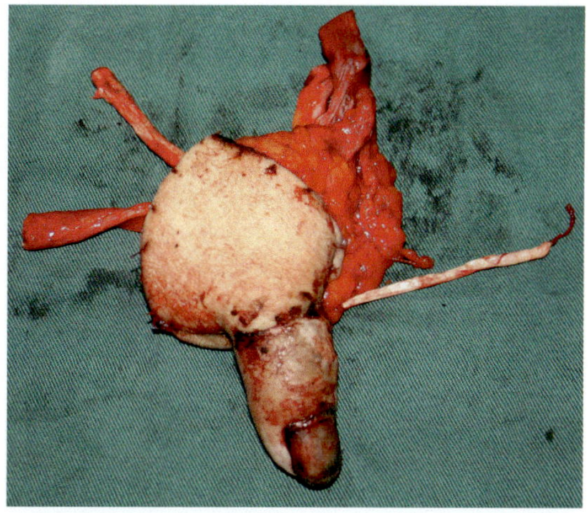

Fig. 20.8 Fifteen days later

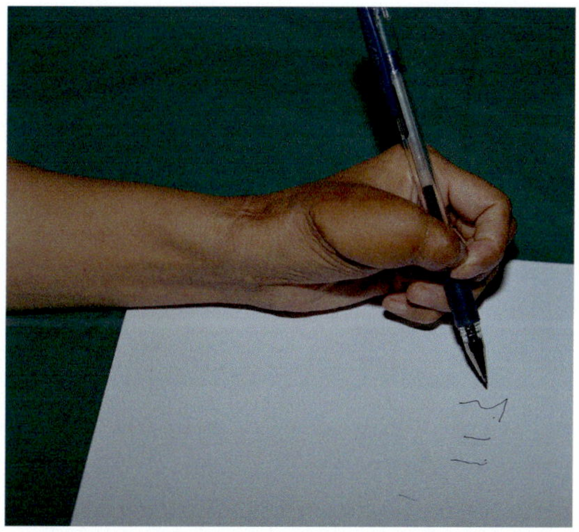

Fig. 20.9 Ectopic implanted finger is cut out

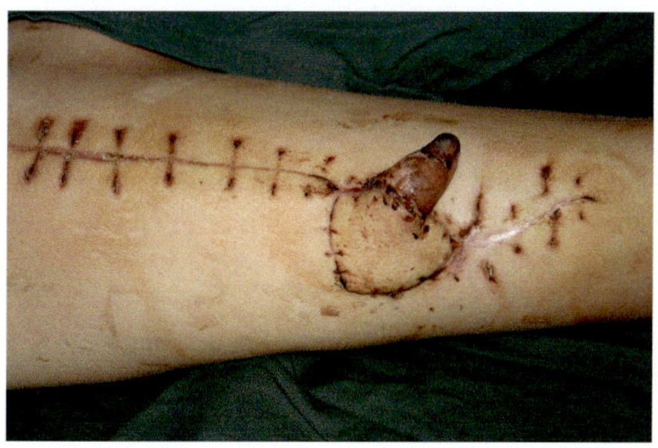

Fig. 20.10 The appearance and function 12 months later

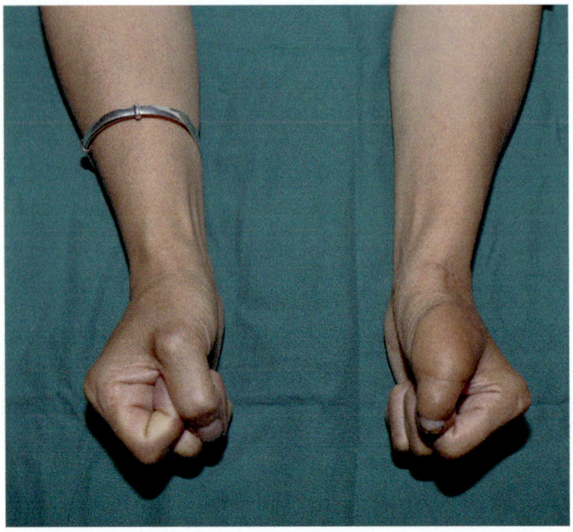

Fig. 20.11 The appearance and function 12 months later

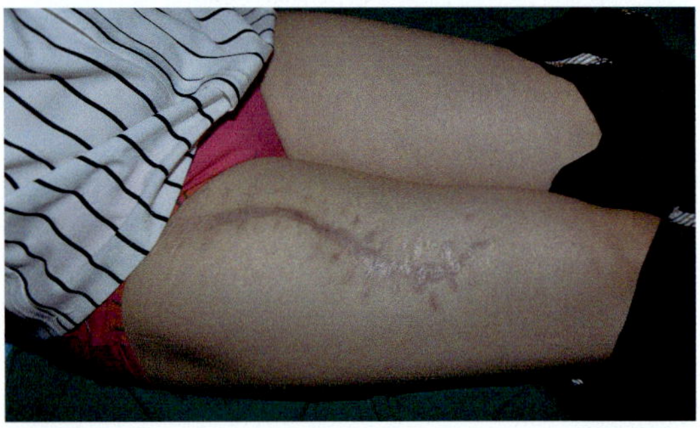

Fig. 20.12 The condition of the accepting site 12 months later

Case 2: Foster Replantation of Amputated Right Fingers

The patient, male, 39 years old, machine twist led to the injury of the right hand and wrist for 3 hours. Physical examination: soft tissue defects from the ulnar and distal site of the right forearm to the area between the thumb and the index fingers, comminuted fracture at the distal part of the ulna; open fracture of the right thumb with a relatively intact dorsal skin; metacarpophalangeal joints of the right index and middle fingers were avulsion off, the distal part of the finger bodies were relatively intact and connected with the fingerwebs. The metacarpophalangeal joints were damaged, the distal site to the fourth and fifth palm bases were badly damaged, with a seriously wounded area. In the hospital emergency department, we undertook debridement and foster replantation of index and the middle fingers at the dorsum of right foot. According to stump skins of the finger bodies, we fixed the index and middle fingers with Kirschner wire on the first and second metatarsal of the dorsal foot, anastomosed the finger vein and dorsal venous, common artery the of the second finger and the plantar dorsal artery, and finally we sutured the skins. After the blood transfusion, the fingers showed a ruddy colour. After the debridement of right forearm and the hand, the Vacuum sealing drainage (VSD) was put to cover the wound. The anteroposterior lateral anterolateral flap was used to repair the wound of the forearm and the hand. After the wound healed, we grafted the fingers back. During the surgery, the index and the middle fingers were grafted, and the first and second metacarpal were fixed. Using a modified Kessler method, we sutured the flexor tendon while the extensor tendon was with sutured by an "8" suture method. We anastomosed radial artery and plantar dorsal artery of fostered finger, great saphenous vein and radial artery accompanying vein, finger inherent nerve and common finger nerves, respectively. After a successful blood pass, we sutured the wound, made a dressing and used gypsum external fixation, performed a conventional treatment postoperative replantation. The fingers survived well. The patient was satisfied with both the shape and function (Figs. 20.13, 20.14, 20.15, 20.16, 20.17, 20.18, 20.19, 20.20, 20.21, 20.22, 20.23, and 20.24).

The cases are generally provided by Dr. Ming wu Zhou.

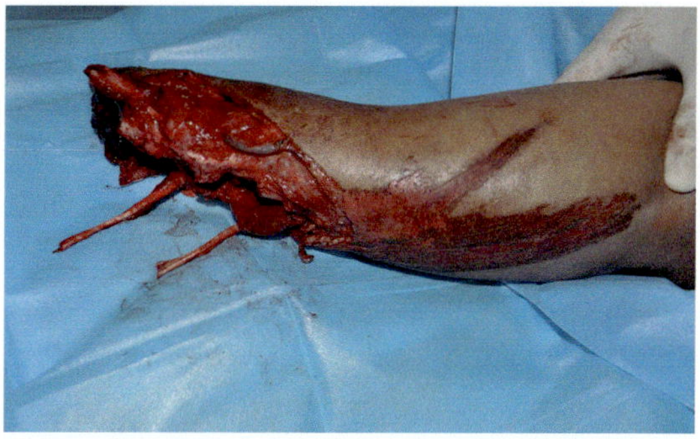

Fig. 20.13 Injury situation of right hand

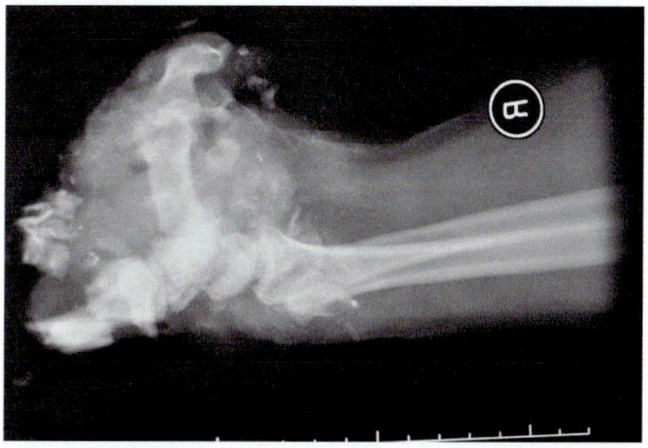

Fig. 20.14 X-ray before the operation

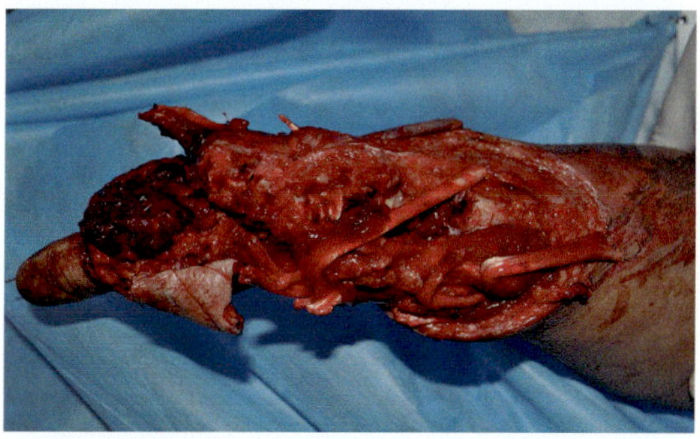

Fig. 20.15 Volar view of the right hand after debridement

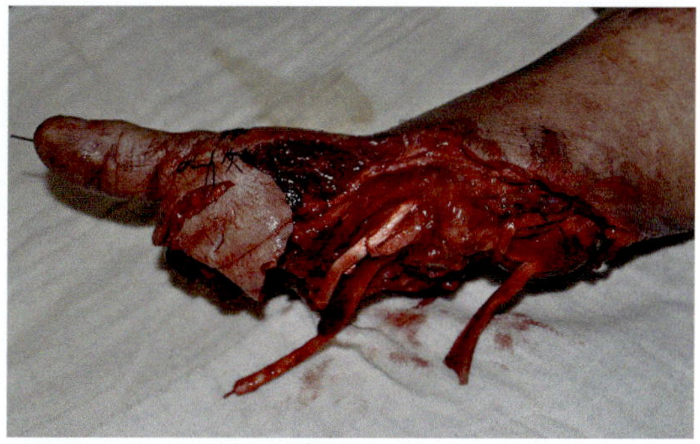

Fig. 20.16 Dorsal view of the right hand after debridement

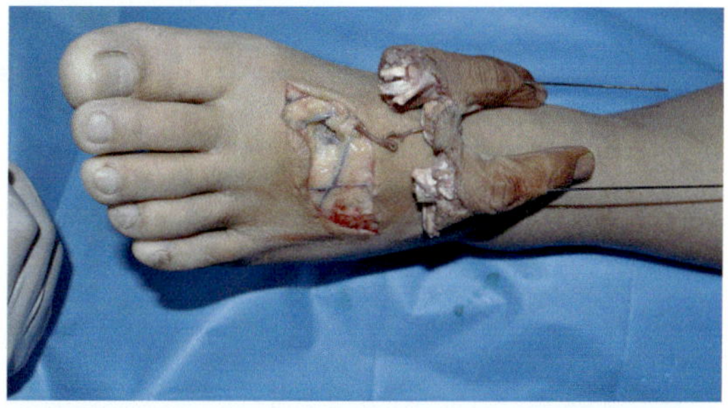

Fig. 20.17 Foster replantation of index and the middle fingers at the dorsum of right foot.

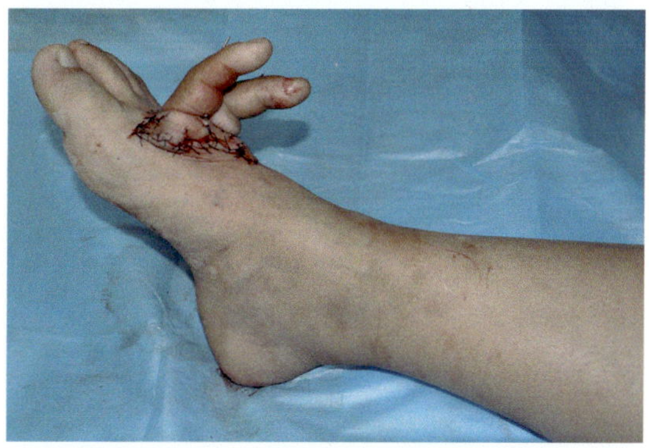

Fig. 20.18 Successful foster replantation of right index and middle fingers

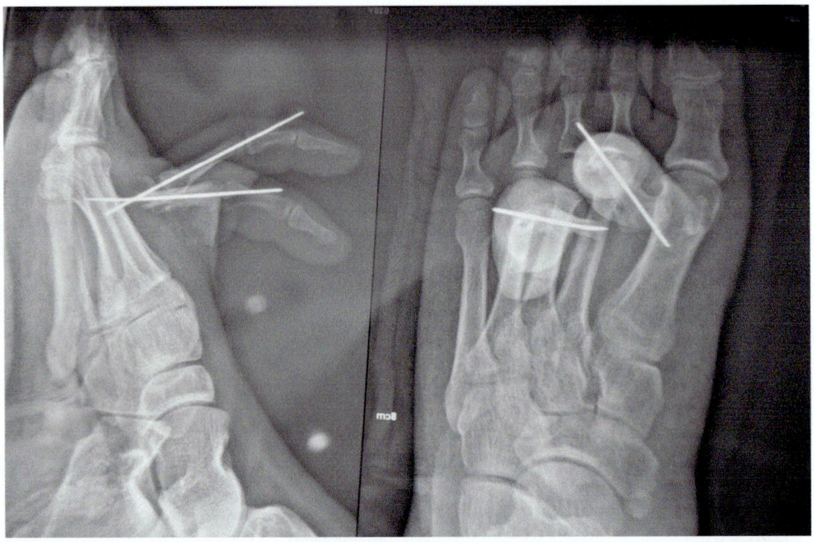

Fig. 20.19 X ray after the foster replantation

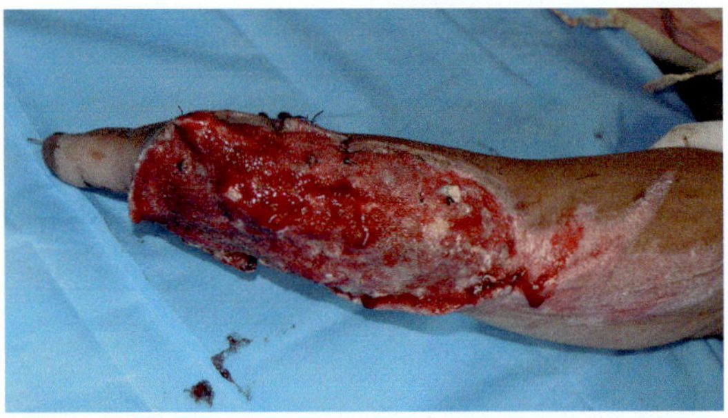

Fig. 20.20 The wound after VSD treatment to the right hand

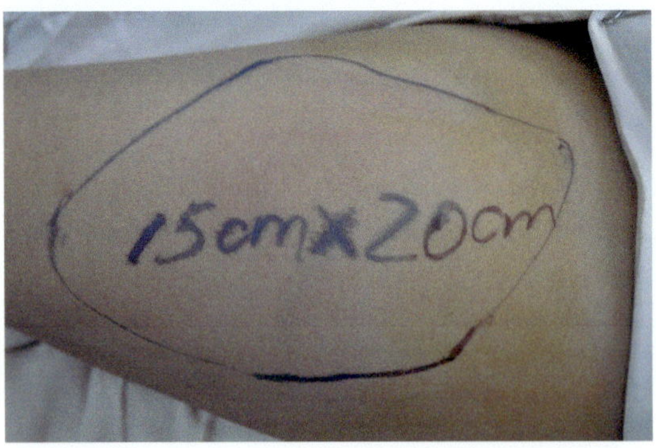

Fig. 20.21 Design of left anteroposterior lateral anterolateral flap

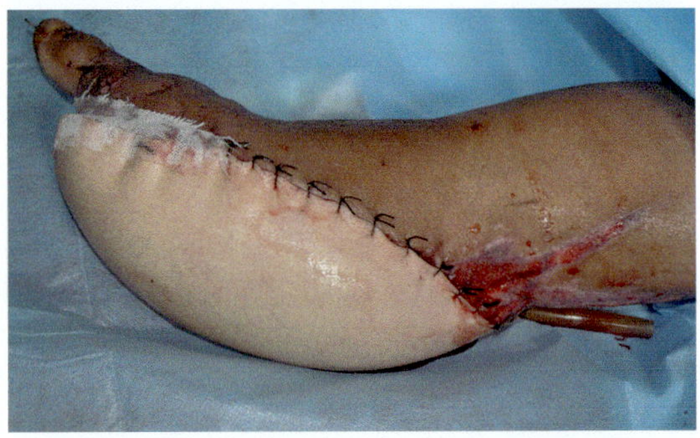

Fig. 20.22 Wound repair by a anteroposterior lateral anterolateral flap

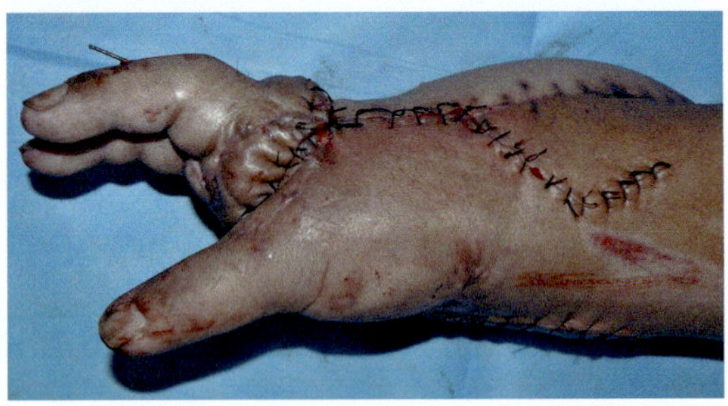

Fig. 20.23 Right index and middle fingers were grafted back

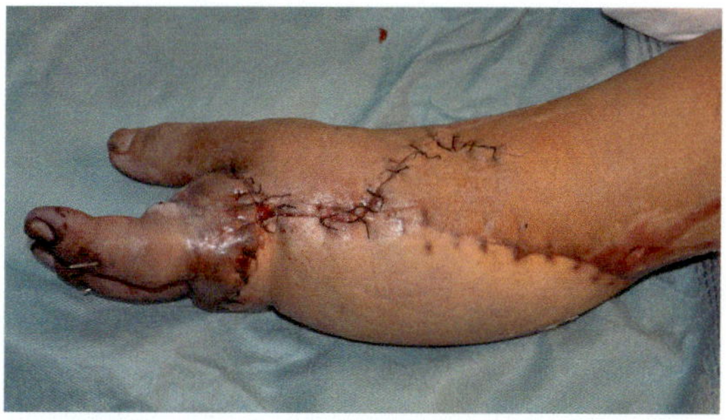

Fig. 20.24 15 days after the right index and middle fingers grafted back

Case 3: Foster Replantation of Left Thumb

The patient, male, 33 years old, left hand suffered machine crushing injury leading to skin and soft tissue avulsion, severed thumb of left hand for 7 hours. Physical examination: there was sneak stripping of the soft tissues from the distal part of the lower part of the left forearm to the metacarpophalangeal joints of the palm, and the wound was seriously contaminated. There little skin on the ulnar side of the palm connected with deep tissues. The thumb was avulsion off at the metacarpophalangeal joint. The severed thumb was intact. Due to the injury, serious pollution, high risk of both infection and skin necrosis, no intravenous anastomosis could be performed in situ replantation. Under anesthesia, we did the left forearm and hand debridement and grafted the skin back, taking the ipsilateral inguinal pedicle flap to repair the dorsal side of the left hand and the wound between the thumb and the index fingers. The thumb was fostered in the contralateral. We sutured the skin and closed the wound. After the blood transfusion, the thumb showed a ruddy colour. One week later, the fostered finger had survived well. Four weeks later, we replanted the fostered finger. Conventional treatment was made following postoperative replantation. After follow-up, the shape and function recovery of the left hand was ideal (Figs. 20.25, 20.26, 20.27, 20.28, 20.29, 20.30, 20.31, 20.32, and 20.33).

The cases are generally provided by Dr. Ming wu Zhou.

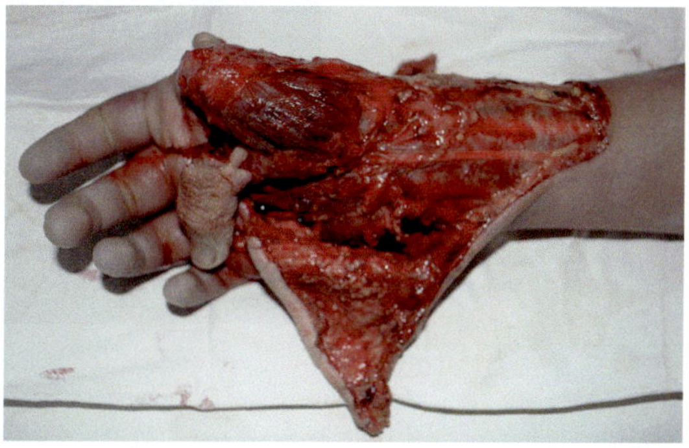

Fig. 20.25 Volar side view of the left hand

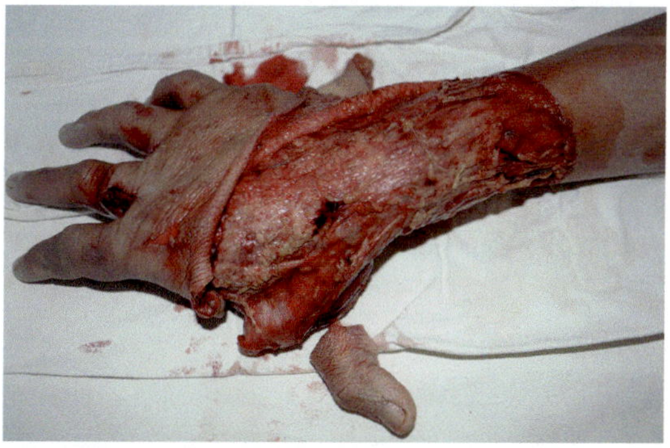

Fig. 20.26 Dorsal side view of the left hand

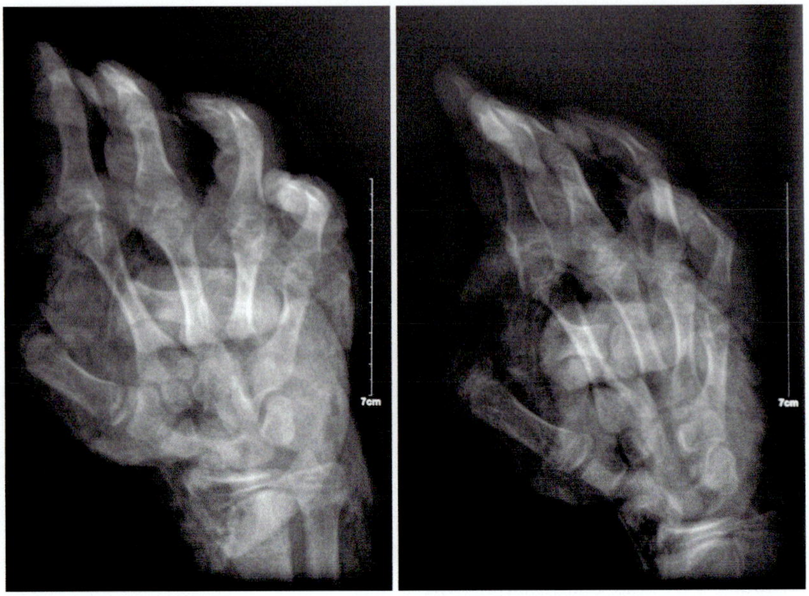

Fig. 20.27 X-ray of the left hand before the surgery

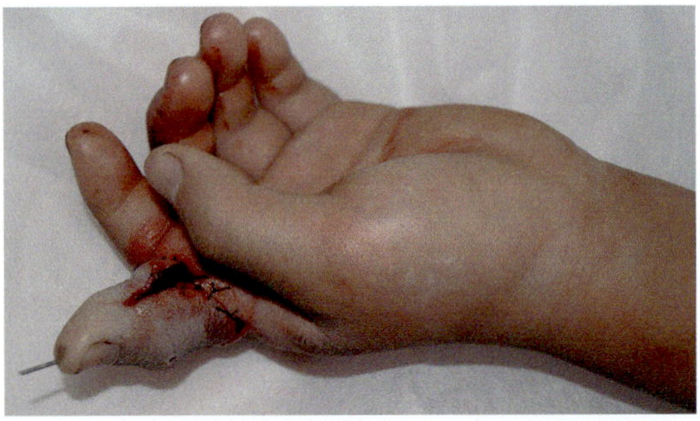

Fig. 20.28 Right index finger foster replantation

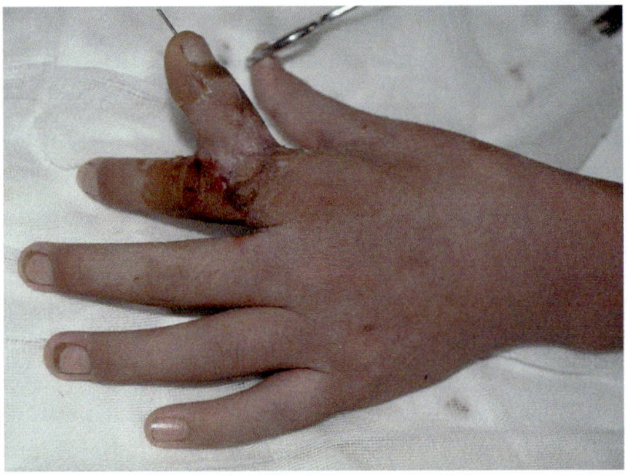

Fig. 20.30 Dorsal side view of left thumb 2 weeks after the foster replantation

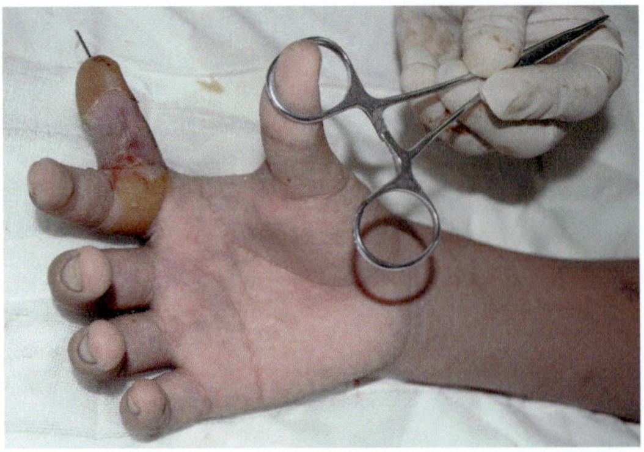

Fig. 20.29 Volar side view of left thumb 2 weeks after the foster replantation

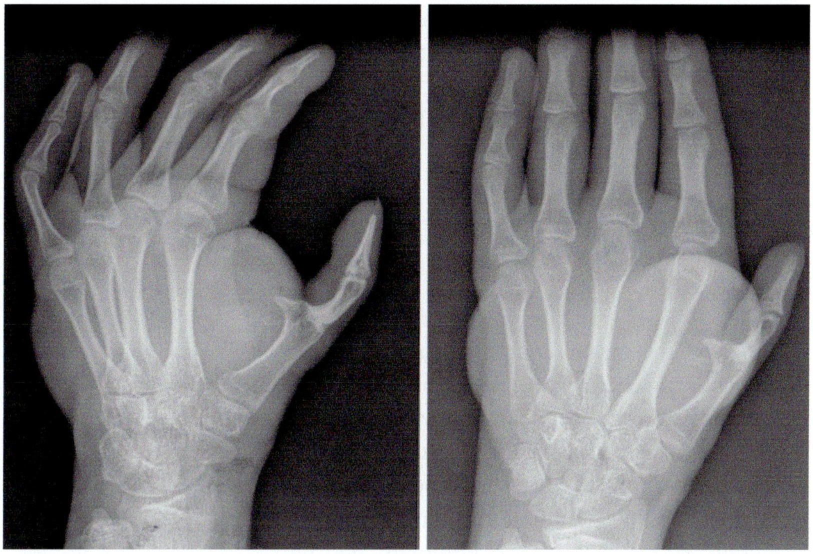

Fig. 20.31 X ray after foster replantation

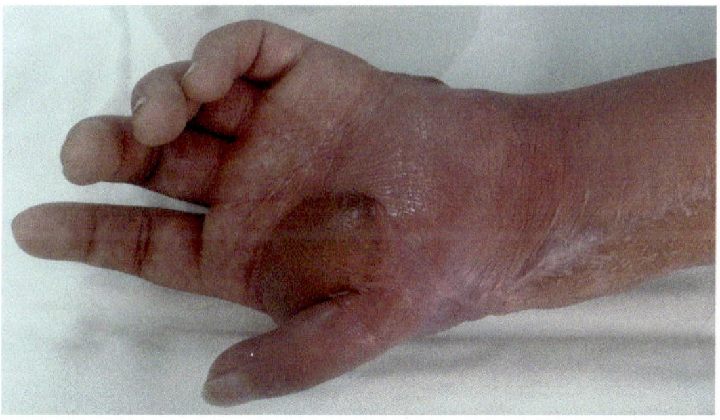

Fig. 20.32 Volar side view 3 months after foster replantation

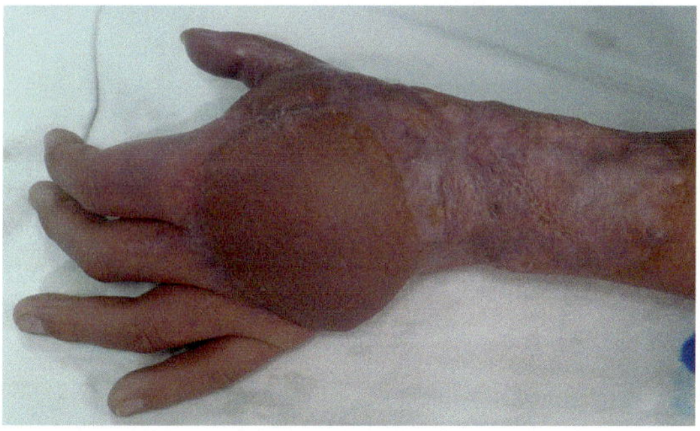

Fig. 20.33 Dorsal side view 3 months after foster replantation

20.3 Key Points in Surgery

(a) The operation should be carried out with groups, one group to take the debridement for the proximal and distal parts of the severed finger, the other group to design the accepting site, flap, repair the ectopic finger, etc.
(b) The diameter of the accepting vessel and the ectopic finger vessel should be the same and the anastomosis should be performed under a ×8 microscope.
(c) The nerves can be matched in the second phase.
(d) Depending on the soft-tissue defect, the finger could be ectopically replanted with some soft tissue. If the soft-tissue defect is to be repaired with an adjacent tissue flap, pedicle amputation should be carried out.
(e) Design the incision at the accepting site and separate the vessels that should be anastomosed under a microscope according to the principle of an arteriovenous ratio of 1:2. The vascular defect can be solved by vessel transplantation.

(f) Find the nerve end in the severed finger and anastomose it with the nerve at the accepting site.
(g) Repair the soft-tissue defect with the flap of the ectopic implantation site.

20.4 Announcements

(a) In the case of completely severed fingers combined with a serious compound injury that cannot tolerate long-term replantation surgery, the fingers can be ectopically implanted after debridement and replanted in a second phase.
(b) Ectopic implantation should be considered when the important finger is completely severed, whose distal part is complete, and the proximal is seriously damaged. Replantation in situ or transposition is not permitted; otherwise, the function will not be good.
(c) The principle for the choice of accepting site is:
    - The location is concealed and the effect is small.
    - It is easy to fix the severed finger. The diameter of the accepting vessel and the ectopic finger vessel should be the same, constant, easily separated, and obtained. There should be a nerve for anastomosis that does not affect body function.
    - There should be a flap to repair the soft-tissue defect.
    - The most commonly used sites are the abdomen, the thigh, the calf, etc.

References

Chernofsky MA, Sauer PF. Temporary ectopic implantation. J Hand Surg [Am]. 1990;15:910–4.

Godina M, Bajec J, Baraga A. Salvage of the mutilated upper extremity with temporary ectopic implantation of the undamaged part. Plast Reconstr Surg. 1986;78:295–9.

Hallock GG. Transient single-digit ectopic implantation. J Reconstr Microsurg. 1992;8:309–11.

Replantation of Fingers with Rotational Avulsion

21

21.1 Summary

Rotation avulsion of fingers is usually caused by a fast rotating machine with a roller and occurs in the left thumb. In most patients, it is characterized by the following:

(a) The skin is stripped with the subcutaneous tissue, which is like a flap or avulsion injury.
(b) The extensor and flexor tendons are usually pulled out.
(c) The digital veins are usually broken near the edge of the skin.
(d) The digital nerves are usually pulled out with uneven ends because they are relatively strong.
(e) The toughness of the arteries is stronger than that of the veins, but they are weaker than the nerves; thus, they are broken earlier than nerves and later than veins, which is easily understood.

Fingers with rotational avulsion is most complicated in all types of severed fingers. Opinions differ with the changes in the times and in microsurgical techniques as to whether they should be replanted. So many scholars have tried different methods of repair to achieve better appearance and function of the avulsed thumb. That it was difficult to replant an avulsed finger and only very few cases could succeed. Only avulsed thumbs could be attempted and if the vessels were avulsed too much, the procedure should be terminated. The extensor and flexor tendons that are usually broken on the border and the vessels and nerves that were usually not broken in the plane in which the fingers were severed were not suitable for replantation. There are many ways to replant a finger with rotational avulsion, but the effect is not ideal. However, with the development of microsurgical techniques, the anastomosis of small-diameter vessels and the transplantation of vessels and nerves are possible, which have been reported by Pho et al. (1979) and Cheng Guoliang (since 1978) (Cheng et al., 1982).

21.2 Case Description

Case 1: Replantation of a Left Thumb with Rotational Avulsion

Male patient, 48 years old, was admitted to hospital for a rotational avulsion of the left thumb caused by a bench drill, and had been bleeding for 1 h. Physical Examination. The general situation was good; the vital signs were stable. The left thumb was completely avulsed with about 20 cm of avulsed tendon attached and with the bone revealed, an uneven wound, a soft-tissue defect, bleeding, and no blood supply. Successful debridement and replantation were performed under anesthesia under emergency conditions. The replanted thumb was red and had moderate

J. Lin et al., *Special Type of Finger Replantation*, https://doi.org/10.1007/978-981-10-6229-2_21

tension after relaxing the tourniquet. It was packed with sterile gauze and padded with broken cotton yarn and the patient was brought back to the ward safely. He was given conventional treatments postoperatively, such as antibiotics, hormones, and antispasmodics. By 2 weeks later, the replanted severed thumb had successfully survived. The appearance and function were good after regular follow-up and functional exercise guidance, and the patient was satisfied (Figs. 21.1, 21.2, 21.3, 21.4, 21.5, 21.6, 21.7, 21.8, and 21.9).

Case 2: Replantation of a Left Thumb with Rotational Avulsion

Male patient, 48 years old, was admitted to hospital for rotational avulsion of the right thumb caused by a bench drill, and had been bleeding for 1 h. PE: The general situation was good; the vital signs were stable. The left thumb was com-

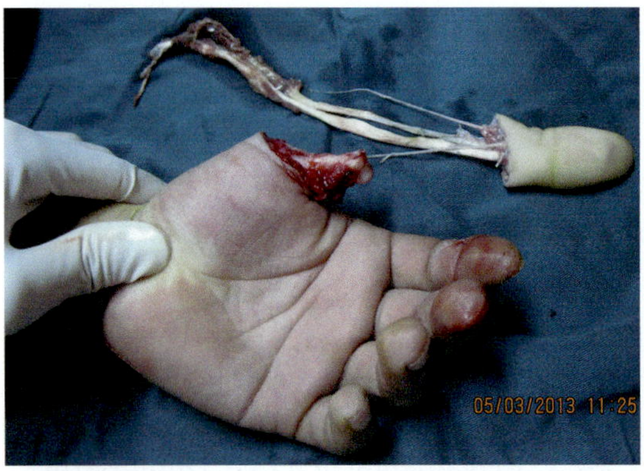

Fig. 21.1 The palm side of the avulsed finger

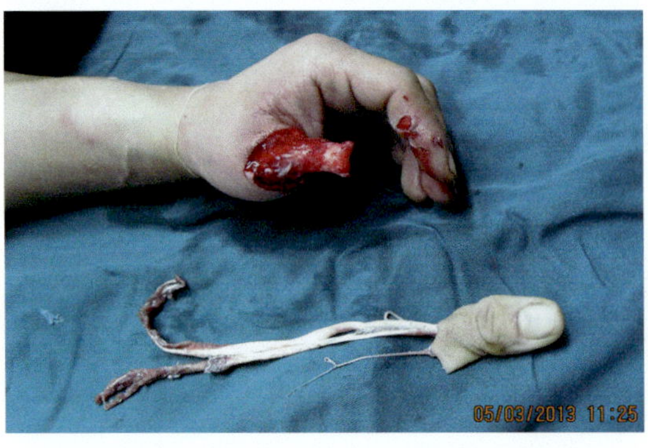

Fig. 21.2 The dorsal side of the avulsed finger

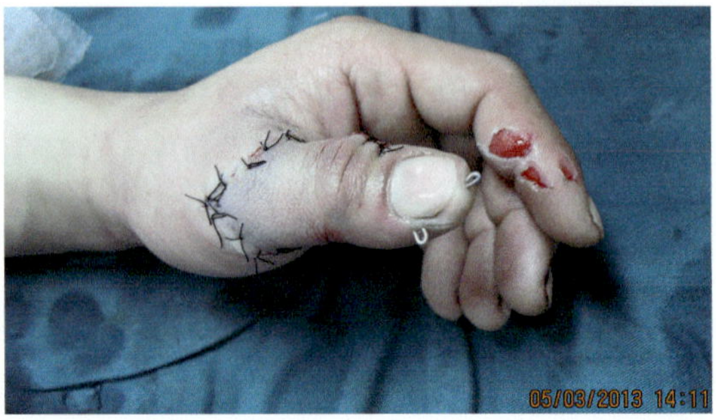

Fig. 21.3 The dorsal side after replantation

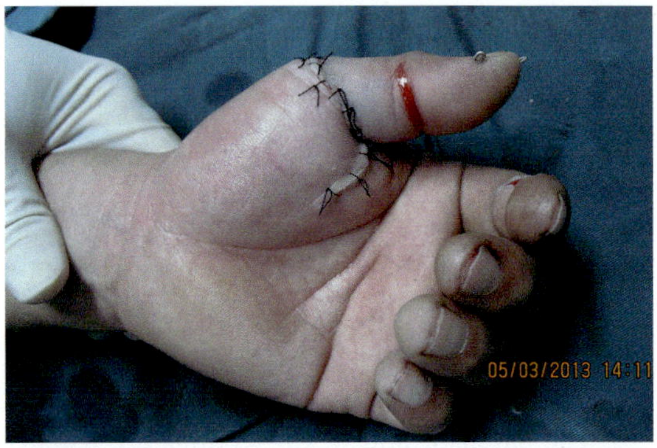

Fig. 21.4 The palm side after replantation

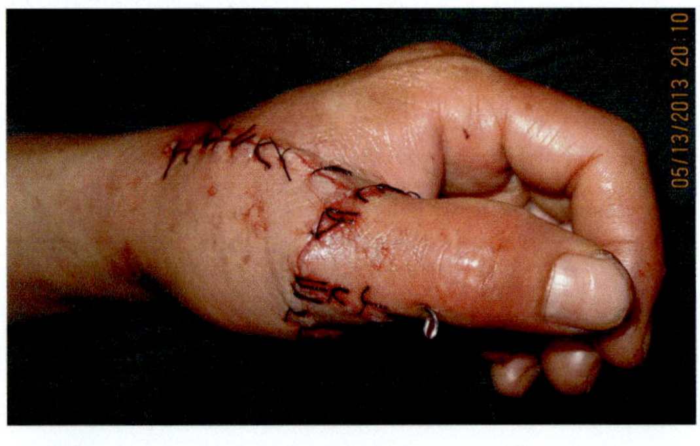

Fig. 21.5 Survival 2 weeks later

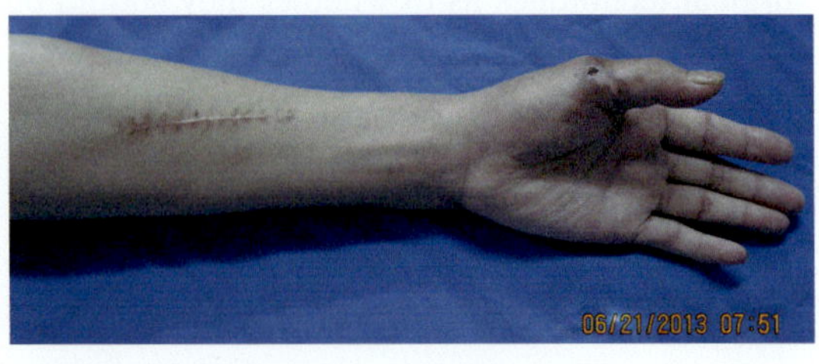

Fig. 21.6 The palm side 15 months later

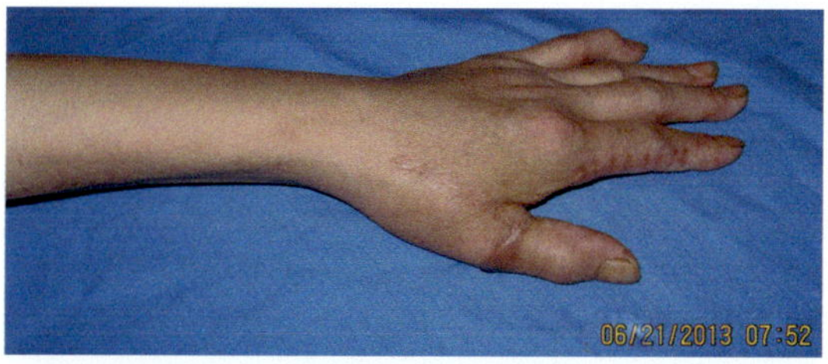

Fig. 21.7 The dorsal side 15 months later

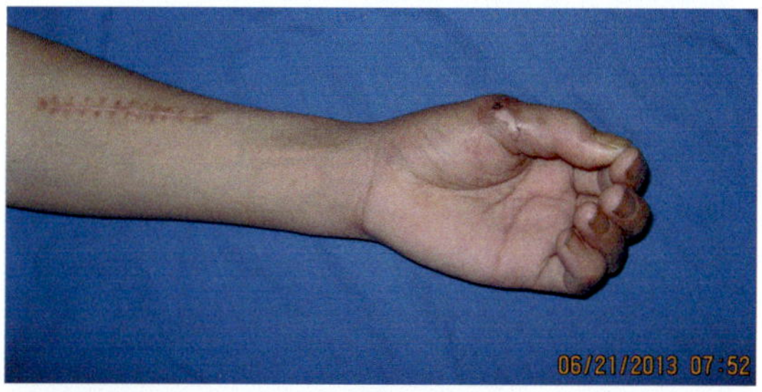

Fig. 21.8 Function 15 months later

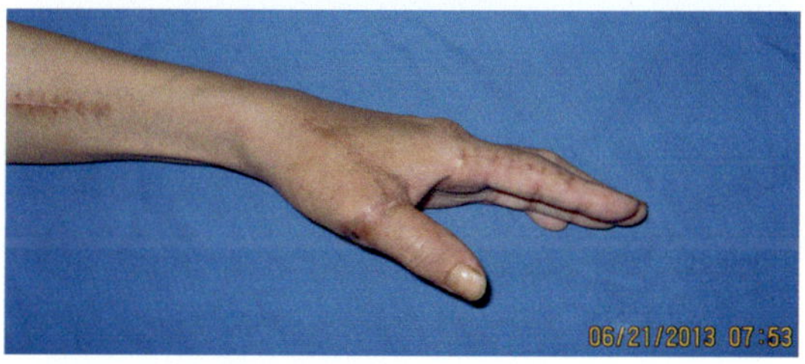

Fig. 21.9 Function 15 months later

pletely avulsed with about 20 cm of avulsed tendon attached and with the bone revealed, an uneven wound, a soft-tissue defect, bleeding, and no blood supply. Successful debridement and replantation were performed under anesthesia under emergency conditions. The replanted thumb was red and had moderate tension after relaxing the tourniquet. It was packed with sterile gauze and padded with broken cotton yarn and the patient was brought back to the ward safely. He was given conventional treatments postoperatively, such as antibiotics, hormones, and antispasmodics. By 2 weeks later, the replanted severed thumb had successfully survived. The appearance and function were good after regular follow-up and functional exercise guidance and the patient was satisfied (Figs. 21.10, 21.11, 21.12, 21.13, 21.14, 21.15, 21.16, and 21.17).

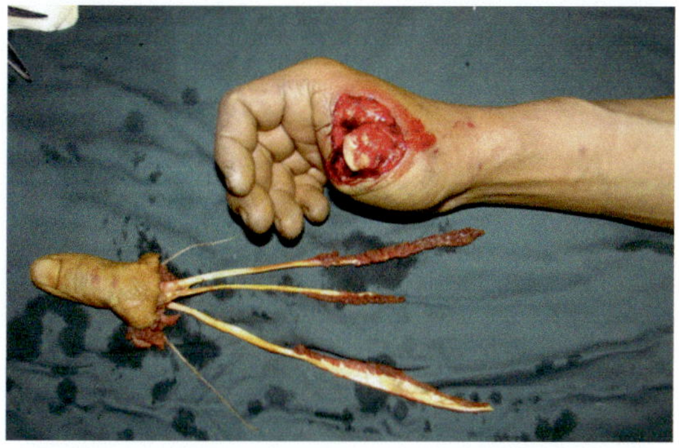

Fig. 21.10 The dorsal side of the avulsed finger

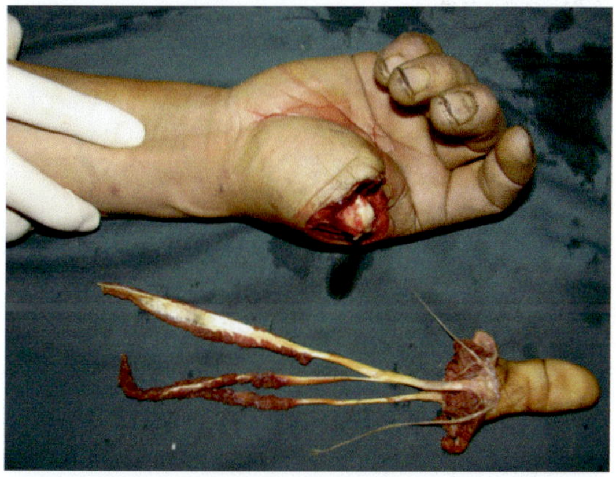

Fig. 21.11 The palm side of the avulsed finger

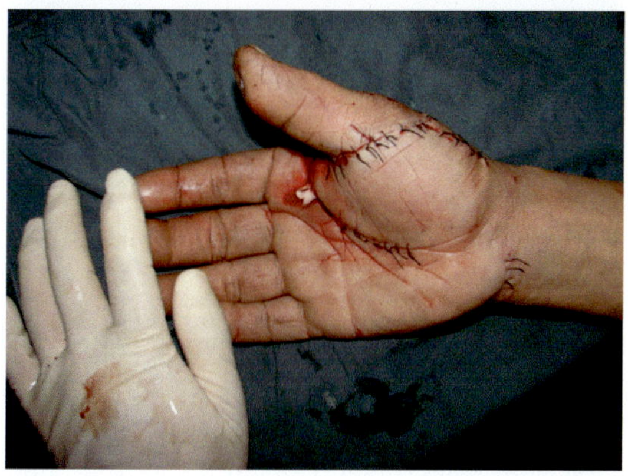

Fig. 21.12 The palm side after replantation

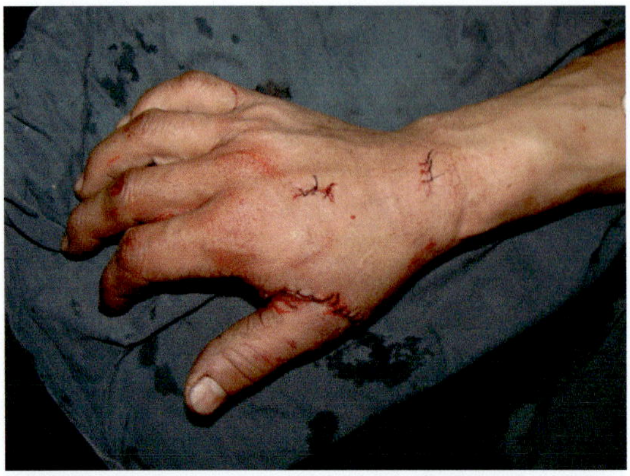

Fig. 21.13 The dorsal side after replantation

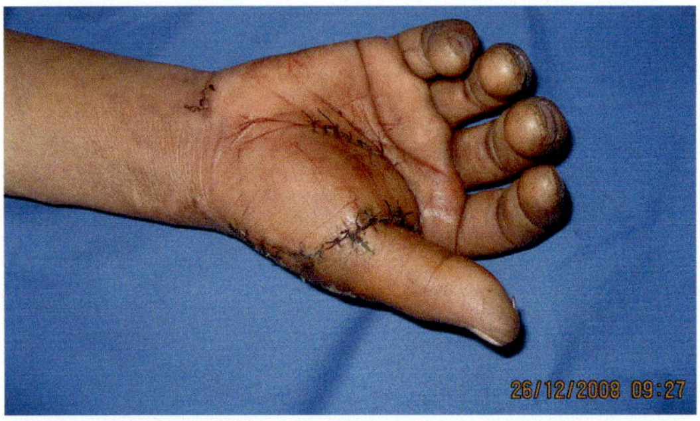

Fig. 21.14 The palm side 2 weeks later

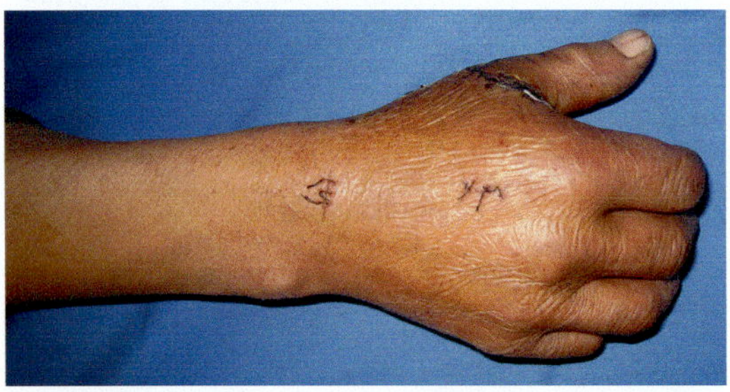

Fig. 21.15 The dorsal side 2 weeks later

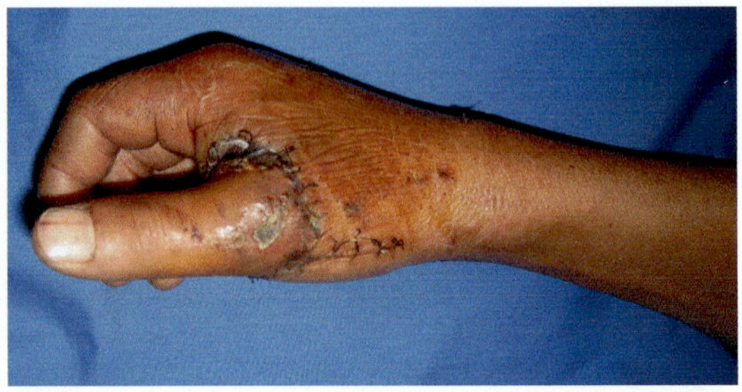

Fig. 21.16 The thumb dorsal side 2 weeks later

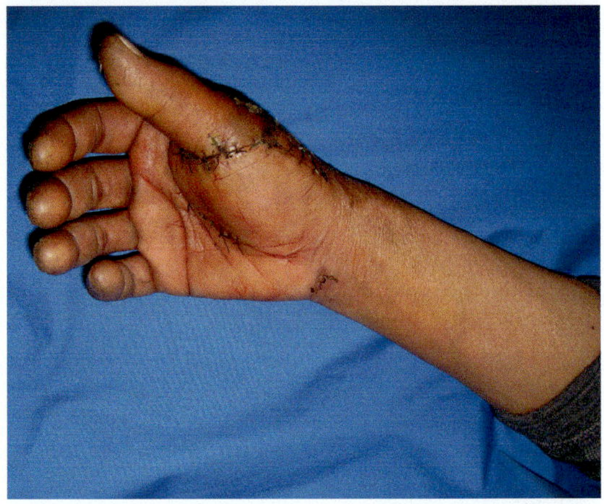

Fig. 21.17 The thumb palm side 2 weeks later

Case 3: Replantation of a Left Thumb with Rotational Avulsion

Male patient, 35 years old, was admitted to hospital for the rotational avulsion of the right thumb caused by a lathe, and had been bleeding for 1.5 h. PE: The general situation was good; the vital signs were stable. The left thumb was completely avulsed with about 20 cm of avulsed tendon and about 5 cm of avulsed nerve attached and with the bone revealed, an uneven wound, a soft-tissue defect, bleeding and without blood supply. Successful debridement and replantation were performed under anesthesia under emergency conditions. The replanted thumb was red and had moderate tension after relaxing the tourniquet. It was packed with sterile gauze and padded with broken cotton yarn and the patient was brought back to the ward safely. He was given conventional treatments postoperatively, such as antibiotics, hormones, and antispasmodics. By 2 weeks later, the replanted severed thumb had successfully survived. We transplanted the sural nerve to reconstruct the sensory function 9 months later. The appearance and function were good after regular follow-up and functional exercise guidance, and the patient was satisfied (Figs. 21.18, 21.19, 21.20, 21.21, 21.22, 21.23, 21.24, 21.25, 21.26, 21.27, and 21.28).

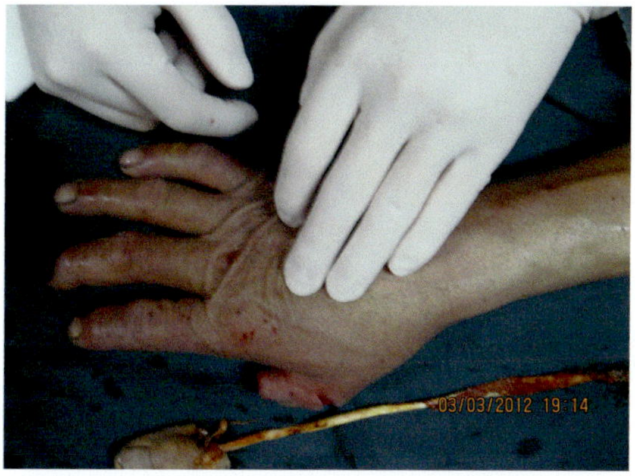

Fig. 21.18 The dorsal side of the avulsed finger

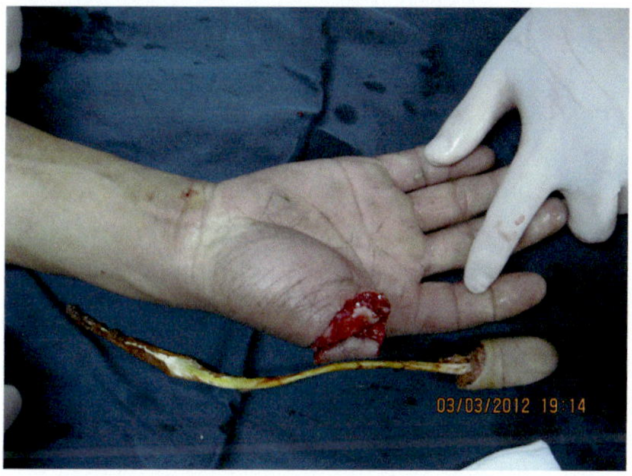

Fig. 21.19 The palm side of the avulsed finger

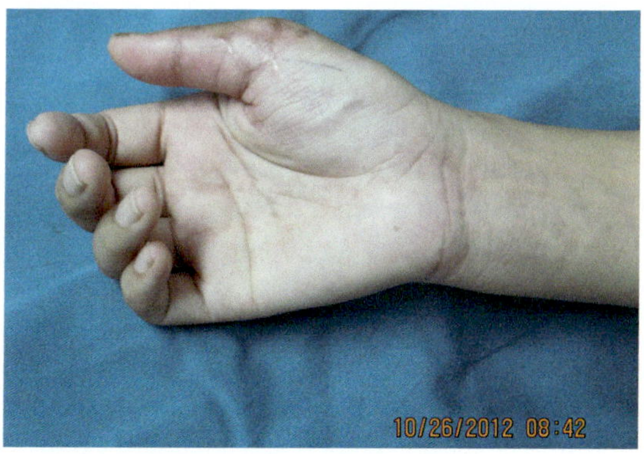

Fig. 21.20 The palm side 3 months later

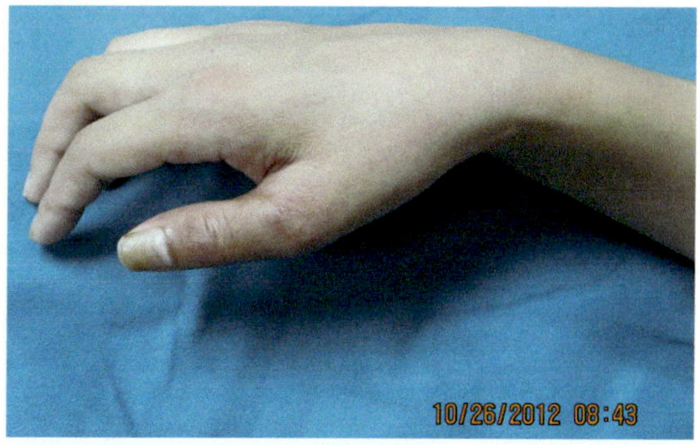

Fig. 21.21 The dorsal side 3 months later

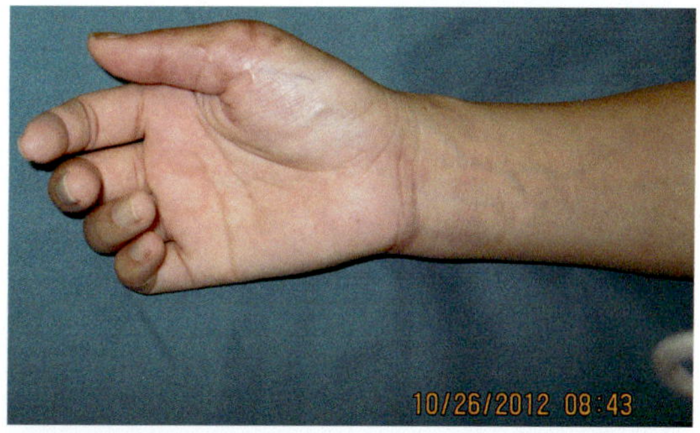

Fig. 21.22 The palm side 9 months later

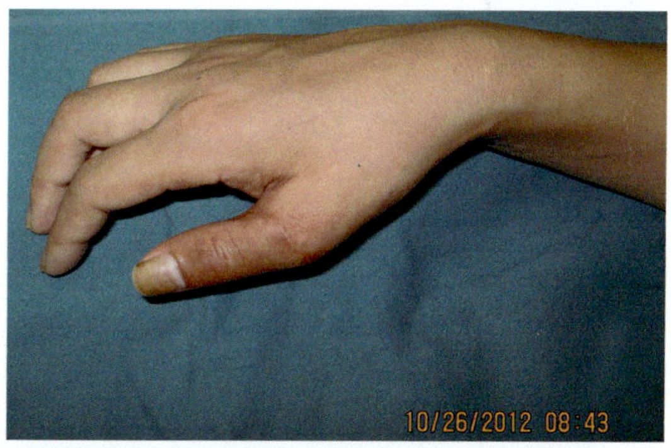

Fig. 21.23 The dorsal side 9 months later

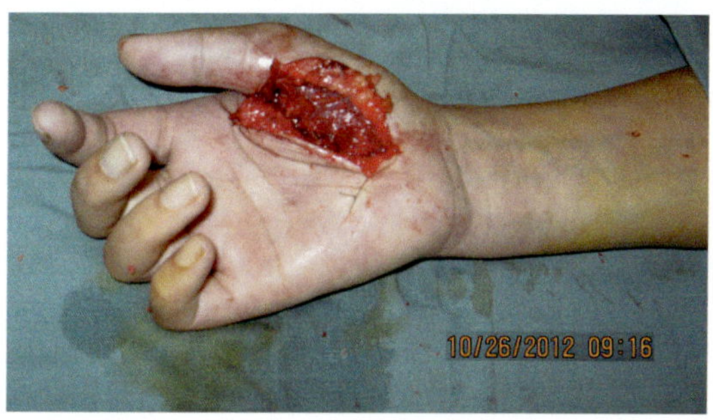

Fig. 21.24 Nerve defect 9 months later

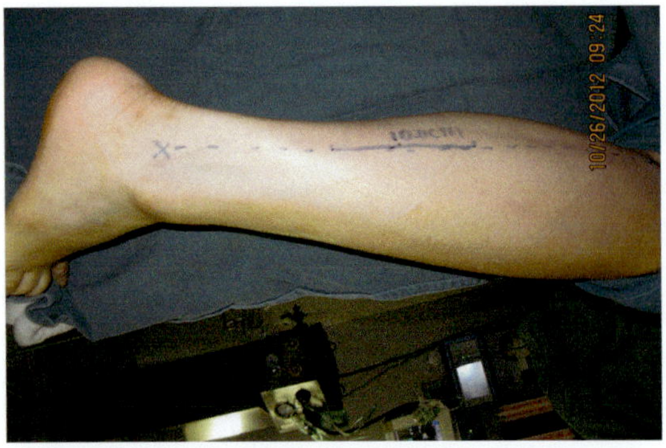

Fig. 21.25 The design of the cutting of the sural nerve

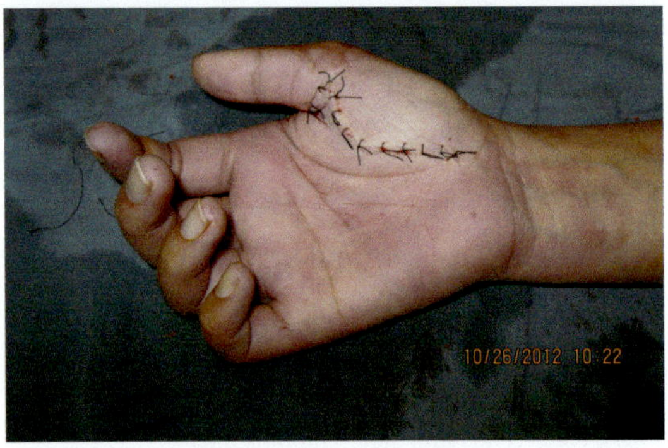

Fig. 21.26 The cutting of the sural nerve

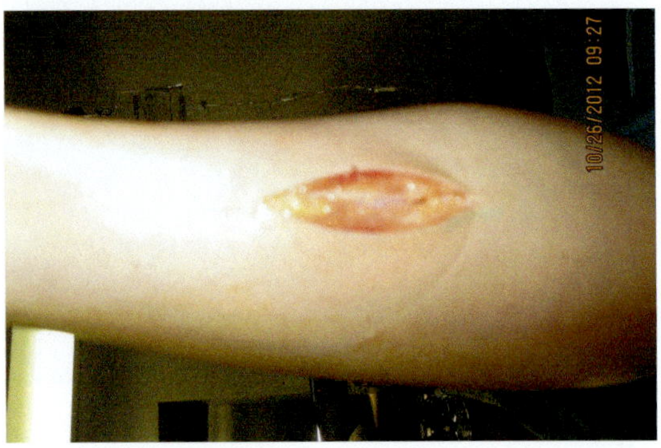

Fig. 21.27 The accepting- site of the nerve

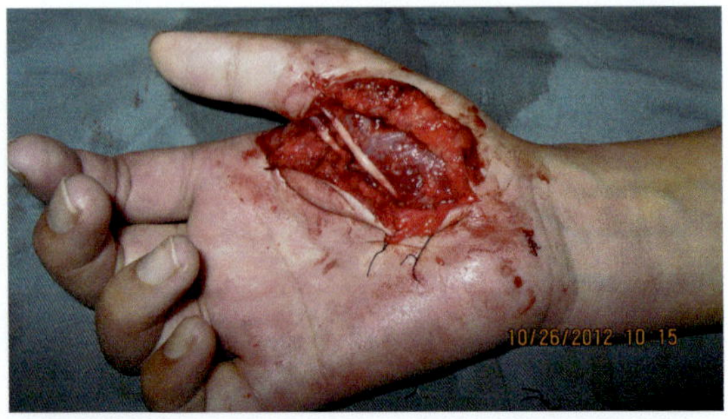

Fig. 21.28 Wound closure

Case 4: Replantation of a Rotationally Avulsed Right Little Finger

Female patient, 26 years old, was admitted to hospital for the right little finger rotational avulsed caused by bench drill and bleeding for 2 h. PE: The general situation was good; the vital signs were stable. The right little finger was completely avulsed with about 20 cm of avulsed tendon attached and with the bone revealed, an uneven wound, a soft-tissue defect, bleeding, and no blood supply. Successful debridement and replantation were performed under anesthesia under emergency conditions. The replanted finger was red and had moderate tension after relaxing the tourniquet It was packed with sterile gauze and padded with broken cotton yarn and the patient was brought back to the ward safely. She was given conventional treatments postoperatively, such as antibiotics, hormones, and antispasmodics. By 2 weeks later, the replanted severed finger had successfully survived. The appearance and function were good after regular follow-up and functional exercise guidance, and the patient was satisfied (Figs. 21.29, 21.30, 21.31, 21.32, and 21.33).

Case 5: Finger Replantation After the Avulsion Injury; The Lateral Skin Flap to Repair the Skin Defect Area Between the Thumb and Index

Patient, male, 46 years old, machine twist led to severed left thumb, with great pain and bleeding. He came to the hospital 4 hours after the injury. Physical examination: the general situation was good, the left thumb was rotatably avulsed from the metacarpophalangeal joint, both the flexor pollicis longus muscle tendon and tendon of extensor pollicis longus were proximally withdrawn. From the area between the thumb and index to the first metacarpal dorsal, the skin tissues were seriously defected. In emergency, during brachial plexus anesthesia, we undertook thumb debridement replantation: we used the upper arm lateral flap which was on the same side to cover the wound

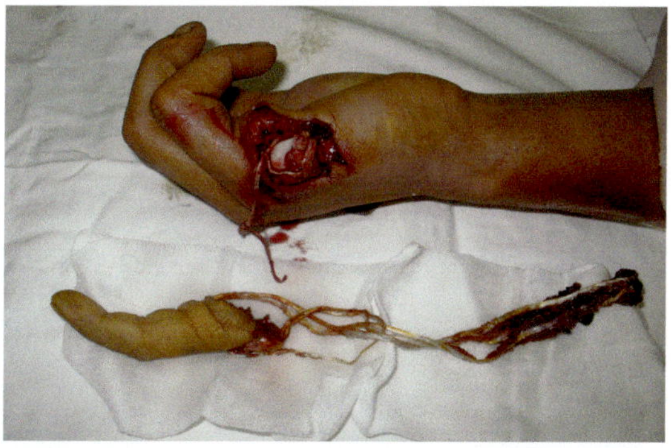

Fig. 21.29 The palm side of the avulsed finger

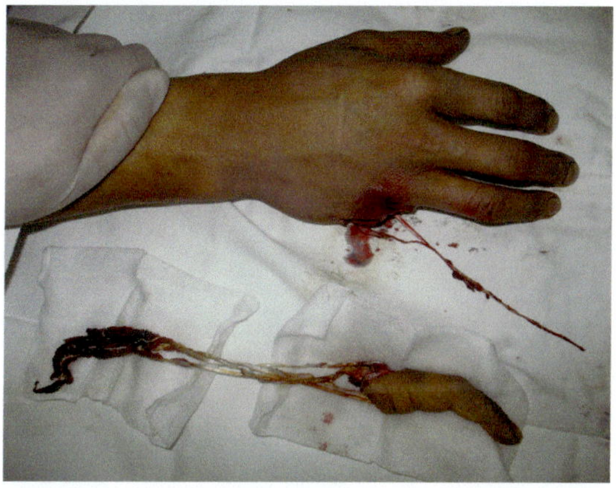

Fig. 21.30 The dorsal side of the avulsed finger

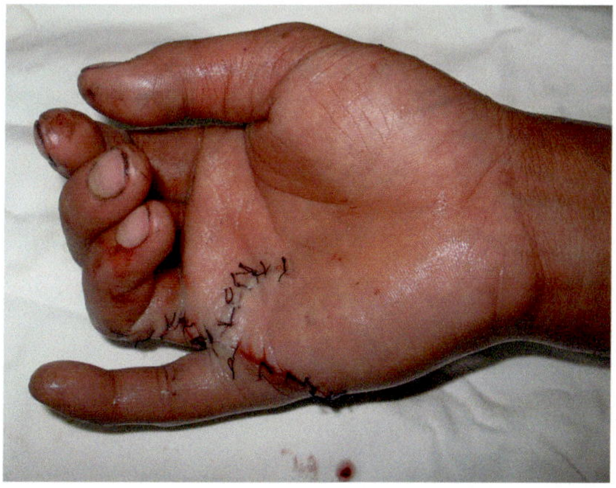

Fig. 21.31 The palm side after replantation

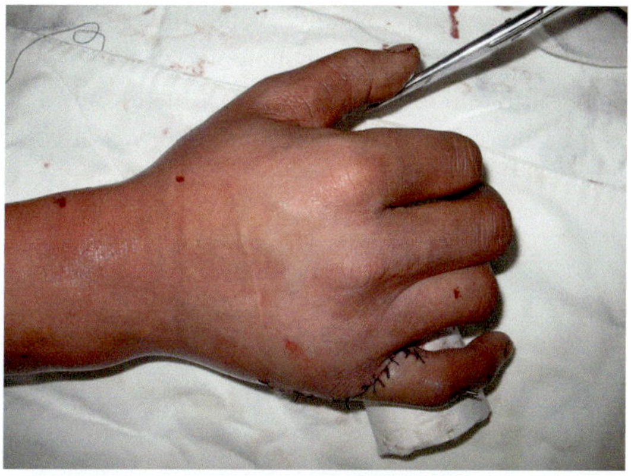

Fig. 21.32 The dorsal side after replantation

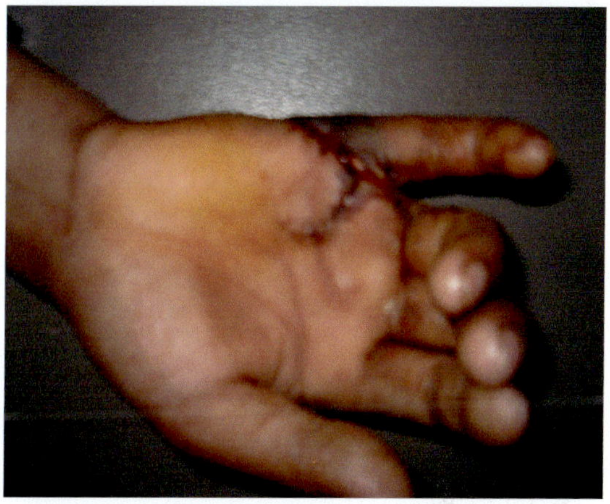

Fig. 21.33 Survival 2 weeks later

and bridge the finger blood vessels. During the operation, we replaced the flexor pollicis longus muscle tendon and tendon of extensor pollicis longus with the superficial flexor tendon of ring finger and indicis proprius tendon respectively. Under the microscope, we separated and debrided the lateral ulnar artery, the dorsal vein and the radial artery, we graft the lateral flap of the upper arm to cover the wound and bridged the broken vascular. From the ending point of the deltoideus triangularis to the lateral epicondyle of humerus, which was the axis, we grafted the free skin flap including the radial artery and its accompanying veins, the posterior medial cutaneous nerve of the upper arm, to cover the skin defect, we anastomosed the radial artery, radial collateral artery, thumb ulnar artery, the thumb dorsal vein, the accompanying veins of radial side vein, cephalic vein, the superficial radial nerve, posterior cutaneous nerve of the upper arm and radial side nerve of the thumb. The same side of the upper arm donor site was directly sutured. The replanted fingers and flap survived the operation and both the function and shape were very good (Figs. 21.34, 21.35, 21.36, 21.37, 21.38, 21.39, 21.40, 21.41, and 21.42).

The cases are generally provided by Dr. Guang jun Liu.

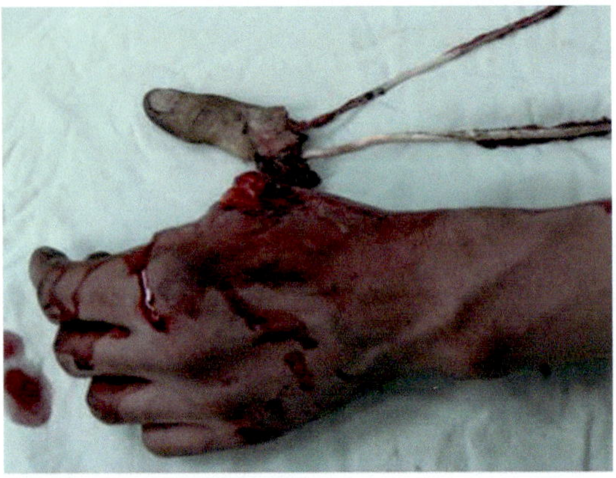

Fig. 21.34 The injury situation

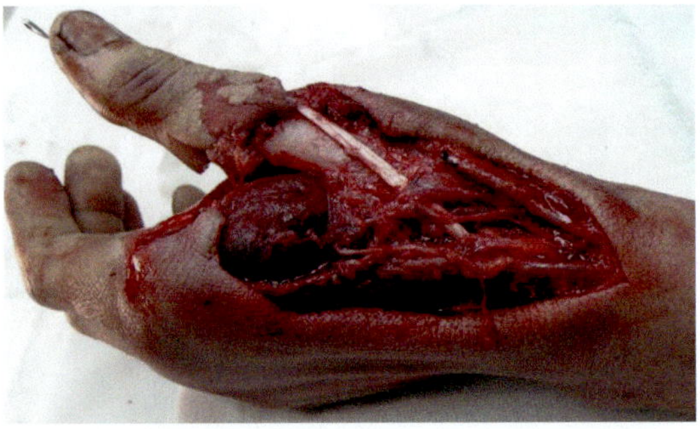

Fig. 21.35 Skin defect after the thumb replantation

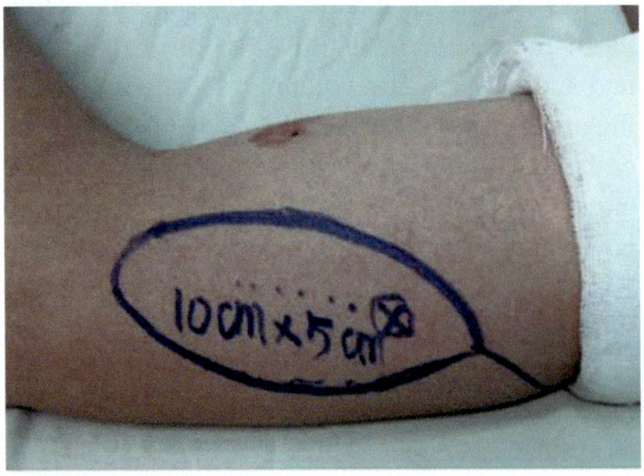

Fig. 21.36 Flap design

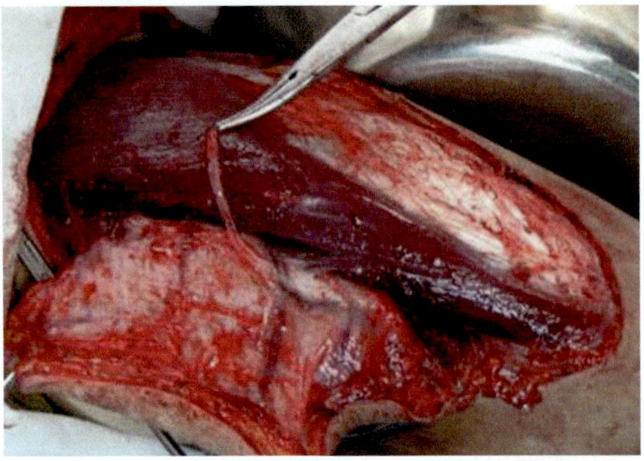

Fig. 21.37 Flap graft

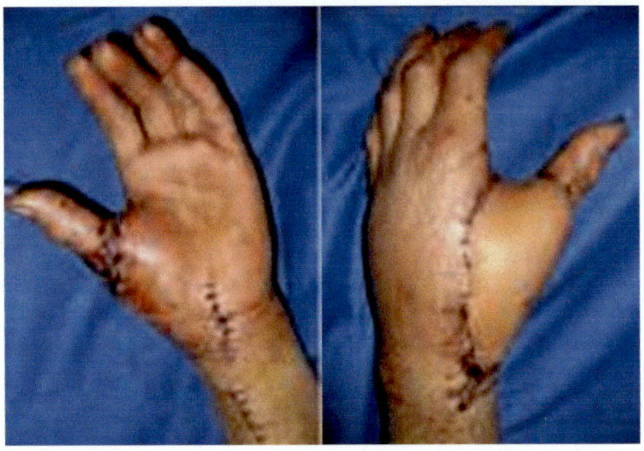

Fig. 21.38 Hand view 2 weeks after surgery

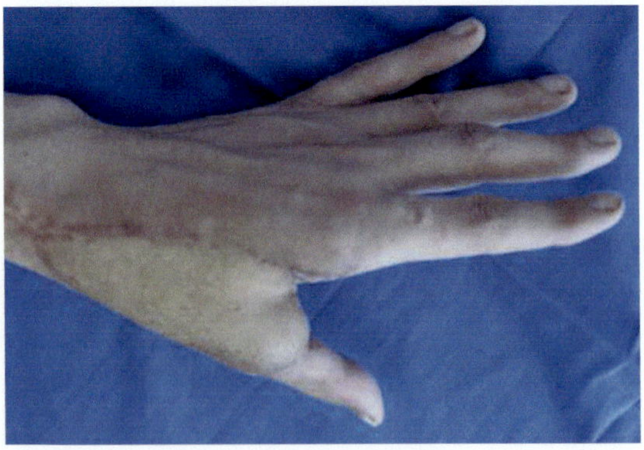

Fig. 21.39 Hand view after surgery

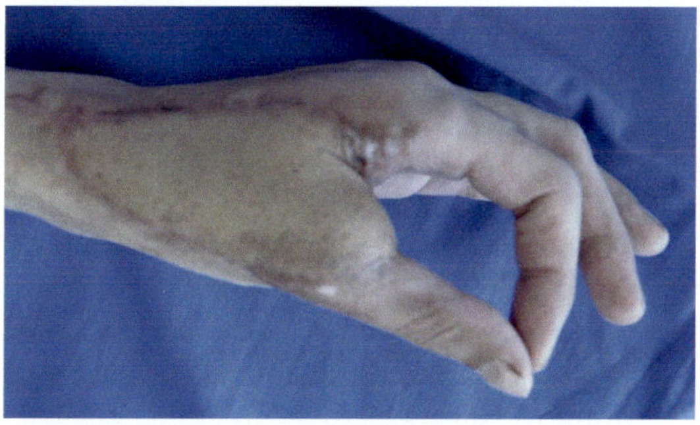

Fig. 21.40 The function of the hand after surgery

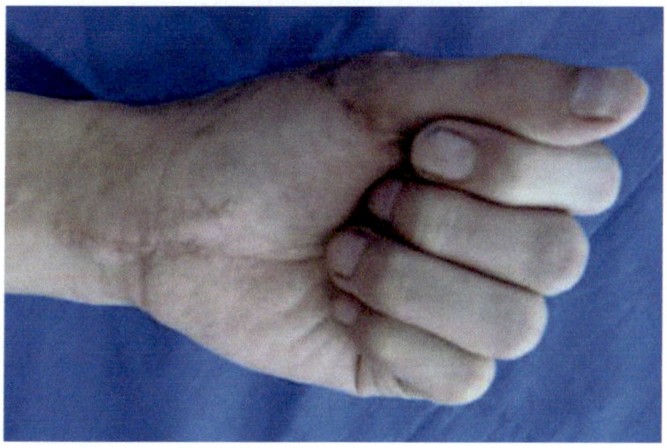

Fig. 21.41 Finger function after surgery

21.3 Key Points in Surgery

(a) There are many ways to fix the phalanx, of which longitudinal fixation with a single needle is simple and reduces the operation time. Functional exercise should be started just after the needle has been withdrawn 4 weeks later.

(b) b) Avoid fixing the needle across the joints as far as possible. In those fingers severed through the joints, the distal ones could be fused and the proximal ones may save the joint function if the soft tissue is good.

(c) It does not make sense to retain the joint if skin bruising and pollution are serious, as the replanted finger will not function. In fingers severed through the metacarpophalangeal joints, the thumb could be fused, the second to fifth fingers should retain the joints and attention should be paid to the repair of the joint capsules and collateral ligaments.

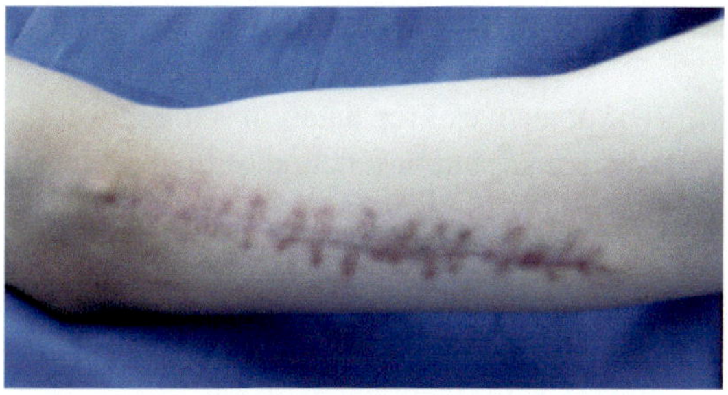

Fig. 21.42 The donor site view after surgery

(d) There are three basic ways to repair the vessels and nerves:
- Transplant of veins and cutaneous nerves to bridge the digital vessels and nerves.
- Transplant of the nearby digital vessels and nerves.
- Shorten the phalanx to anastomose the vessels and nerves.

(e) The common method of repairing the avulsed tendons is as follows:
- Repair the flexor digitorum profundus tendon first if the profundus tendon and the superficialis tendon can be cross-repaired.
- Tendon avulsed from the muscle belly of a single finger could be repaired by the nearby flexor digitorum superficialis tendon and the tendons of multiple fingers should be matched to the in-situ site through an additional proximal incision.
- The extensor tendons should be repaired in situ.
- Tendon defects that are too large could be left to be repaired by transplanting tendons in the second phase. The insertion of the tendon should be reconstructed.
- The tendons of fingers severed from the metacarpophalangeal joint of the thumb and from the distal interphalangeal joint of the other fingers do not need to be handled.

(f) After the veins have been repaired, the dorsal skin should be sutured right away to protect the repaired veins. If the skin defect is too large, a local flap or free transplanted skin could be used to cover it.

(g) The use of the nearby digital nerves for repair is a simple but effective method.

21.4 Announcements

(a) The objective of replantation is to recover the appearance and/or function of finger. Thus, it should be strictly assessed before surgery.
(b) Debridement under the microscope could clear the injury planes and extents of the vessels and nerves, but it is not always useful for fingers with rotational avulsion.
(c) The defects of the digital arteries could be repaired by transposition of the wrist vein or nearby digital vessels. Ensure that the veins are reversed when anastomosed. Defects of the dorsal digital veins could be repaired directly by the wrist vein.
(d) If the avulsed vessel is longer than 4 cm, or the finger needs to be shortened too much, or if the soft tissue bruises badly, replantation should not be undertaken.
(e) Postoperative rehydration with normal saline (500 mL) and heparin (100 mg) maintained for 24 h is useful for increasing the survival rate.
(f) The vascular crisis rate of multiple avulsed fingers is much higher than for a single finger, which should be closely observed.
(g) The transposition of the patient's own small veins makes it possible to clear the injured vessels and nerves and reduce the rate of blood clots. The transposition of the nearby digital arteries, veins, and nerves could achieve better functional recovery and repair of the vessels because of the same diameter and physiological functions.
(h) It is necessary to take early, reasonable, and long-term functional exercise.

References

Cheng G, Pan D, Zhiyong Q, et al. Report of 12 cases of replantation of the rotational avulsed thumb. Chin J Surg. 1982;20:712–3.

Pho RW, Chacha PB, Yeo KQ. Rerouting vessels and nerves from other digits in replanting an avulsed and degloved thumb. Plast Reconstr Surg. 1979;64(3):330–5.

22 Replantation of Severed Fingers with Avulsion

22.1 Summary

Severed finger with avulsion is also called a ring avulsed finger that is combined with avulsed arteries and nerves, which are difficult to repair. It usually occurs in workers wearing gloves to operate a high-speed spinning machine or a finger with a ring whose entire soft tissue was avulsed like taking off the gloves, including skin, subcutaneous tissue, vessels, and nerves, just leaving the bones, joints, and tendons. It is characterized by:

(a) The destroyed finger has a blunt injury, which is much heavier than the distal part.
(b) The avulsed tissues are not in the same plane or even the same tissue.
(c) The avulsed vessels and nerves are usually long and may not be able to be used.
(d) The finger body of the destroyed finger is usually contused to different degrees.

In the literature, replantation in this type of injury is not suggested, or even repair by flaps, which cannot take the place of hand-specific tissue. With the development of microsurgical techniques, destroyed finger will also be indications for replantation, which may be the best way to recover the appearance and function lost to this type of injury.

22.2 Case Description

Case 1: Replantation of an Avulsed Right Thumb

Male patient, 41 years old, was admitted to hospital for a right-hand injury caused by a mold, and had been bleeding for 1 h. Physical examination: The general situation was good; the vital signs were stable. The soft tissues of the thumb were completely destroyed, with no blood supply and with the bone revealed, an uneven wound, and bleeding. The middle and final segments of the ring finger were damaged and could not be replanted. The vessels and nerves of the index, middle, and little fingers were contused, with a poor blood supply. Successful debridement and replantation were performed under anesthesia under emergency conditions. The replanted fingers were red and had moderate tension after relaxing the tourniquet. They were packed with sterile gauze and padded with broken cotton yarn and the patient was brought back to the ward safely. He was given conventional treatments postoperatively, such as antibiotics, hormones, and antispasmodics. By 2 weeks later, the replanted fingers had successfully survived. The appearance and function were good after regular follow-up and functional exercise guidance, and the patient was satisfied (Figs. 22.1, 22.2, 22.3, 22.4, 22.5, 22.6, 22.7, 22.8, 22.9, and 22.10).

J. Lin et al., *Special Type of Finger Replantation*, https://doi.org/10.1007/978-981-10-6229-2_22

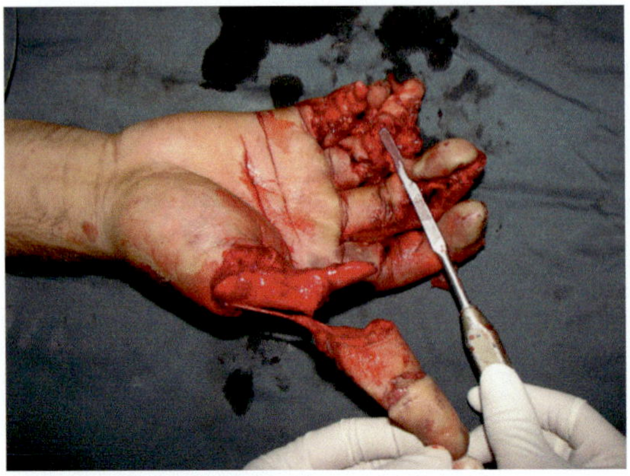

Fig. 22.1 The palm side of the right hand

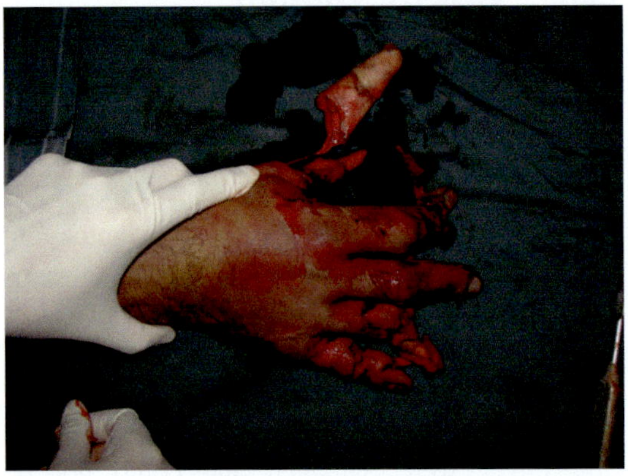

Fig. 22.2 The dorsal side of the right hand

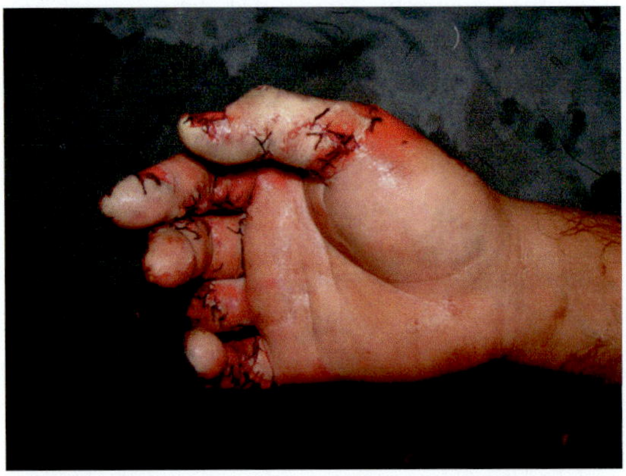

Fig. 22.3 The palm side after replantation

Case 2: Replantation of an Avulsed Index Finger

Female patient, 35 years old, was admitted to hospital for a right-hand injury caused by a mold, and had been bleeding for 2 h. PE: The general situation was good; the vital signs were stable. The soft tissues of the index finger were completely

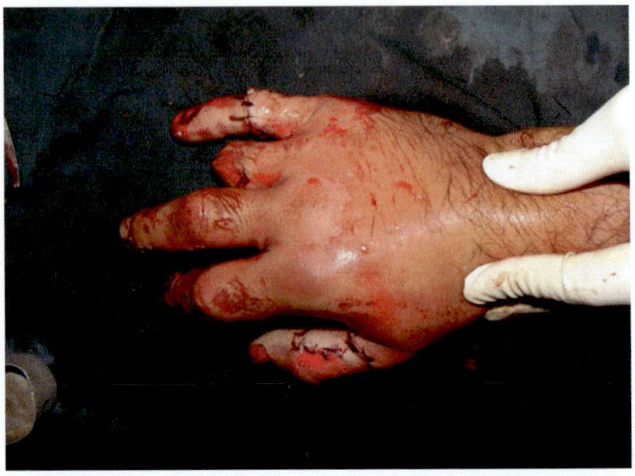

Fig. 22.4 The dorsal side after replantation

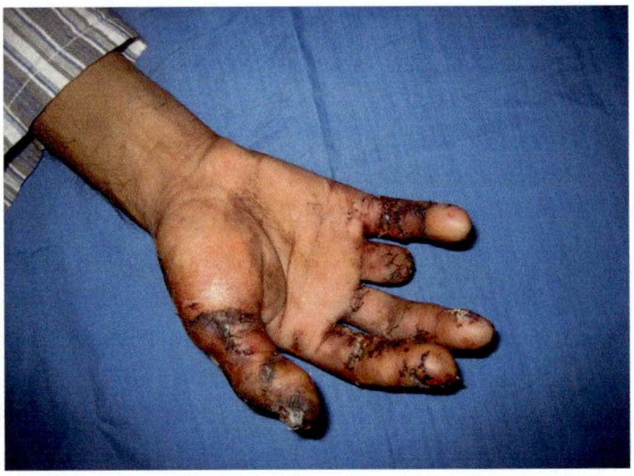

Fig. 22.5 The palm side 2 weeks later

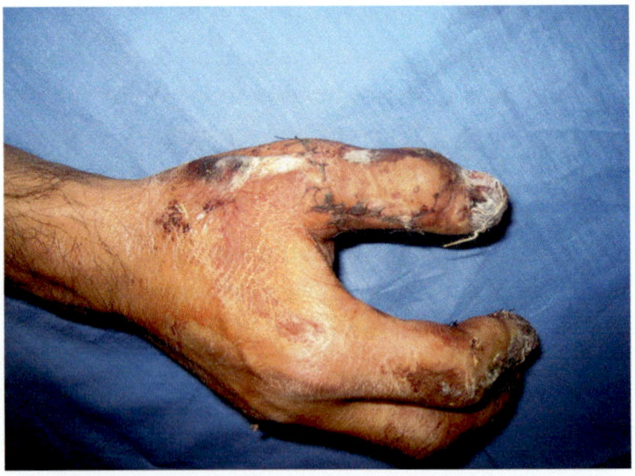

Fig. 22.6 The dorsal side 2 weeks later

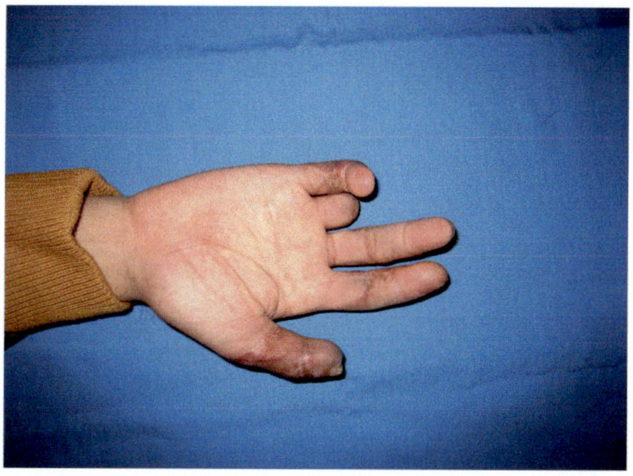

Fig. 22.7 The palm side 11 months later

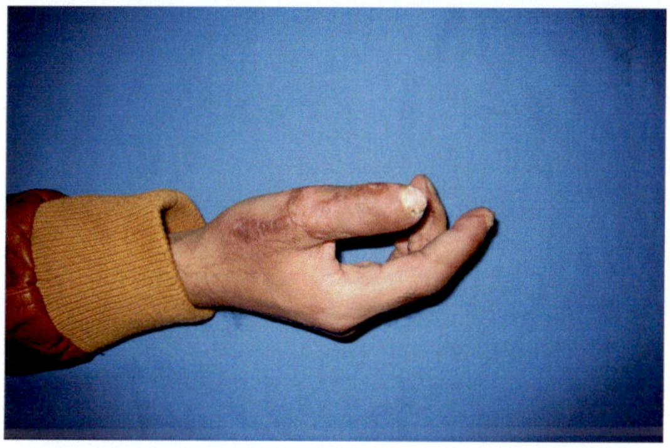

Fig. 22.8 The dorsal side 11 months later

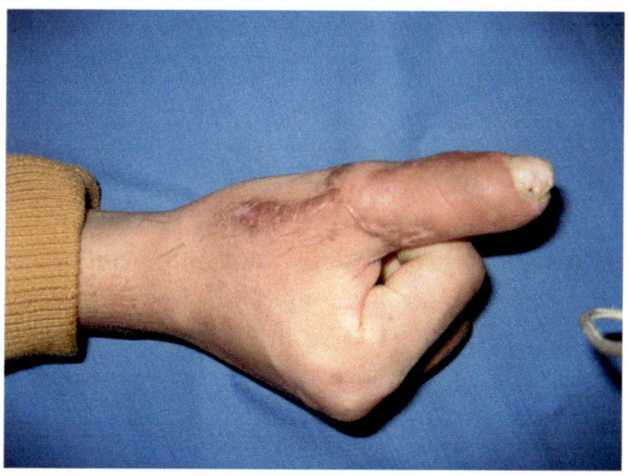

Fig. 22.9 Function 11 months later

destroyed, with no blood supply and with the bone revealed, uneven wounds, and bleeding. Successful debridement and replantation were performed

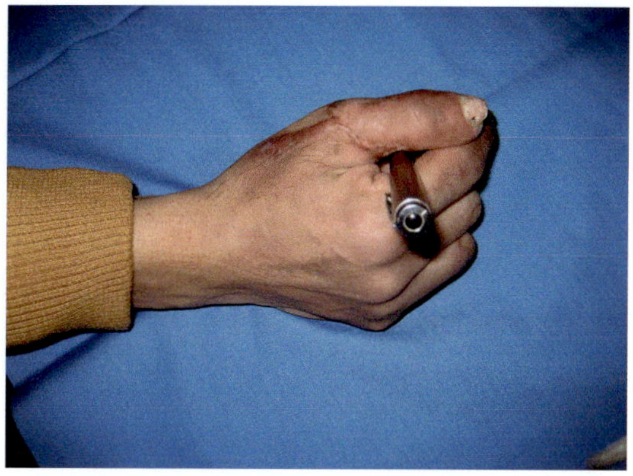

Fig. 22.10 The function 11 months later

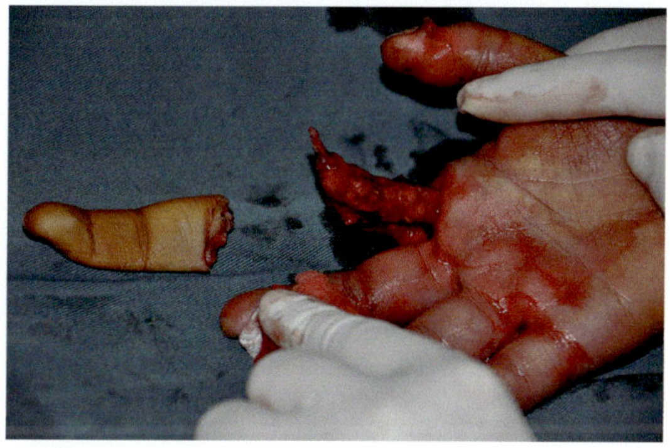

Fig. 22.11 The palm side of the right hand

under anesthesia under emergency conditions. The replanted finger was red and had moderate tension after relaxing the tourniquet. It was packed with sterile gauze and padded with broken cotton yarn, and the patient was brought back to the ward safely. The patient was given conventional treatments postoperatively, such as antibiotics, hormones, and antispasmodics. By 2 weeks later, the replanted finger had successfully survived. The appearance and function were good after regular follow-up and functional exercise guidance, and the patient was satisfied (Figs. 22.11, 22.12, 22.13, 22.14, 22.15, and 22.16).

Case 3

Male patient, 24 years old, was admitted to hospital for a left-hand injury caused by a machine tool, and had been bleeding for 1.5 h. PE: The general situation was good; the vital

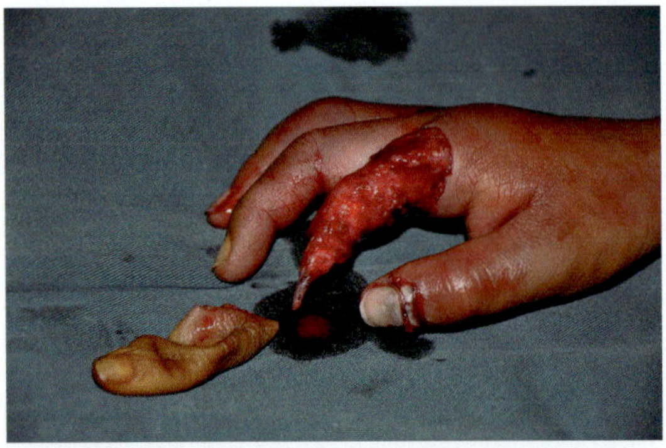

Fig. 22.12 The dorsal side of the right hand

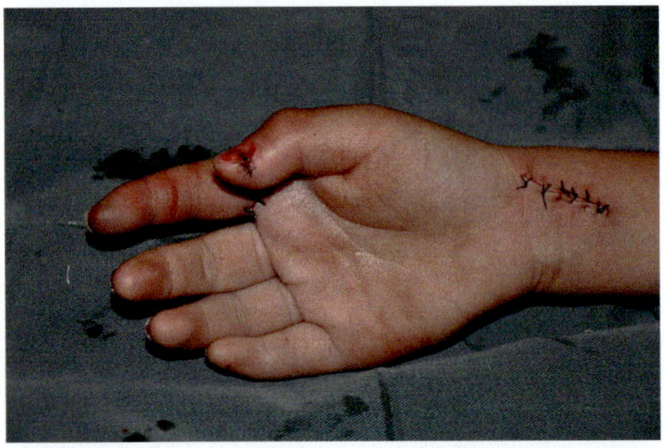

Fig. 22.13 The palm side after replantation

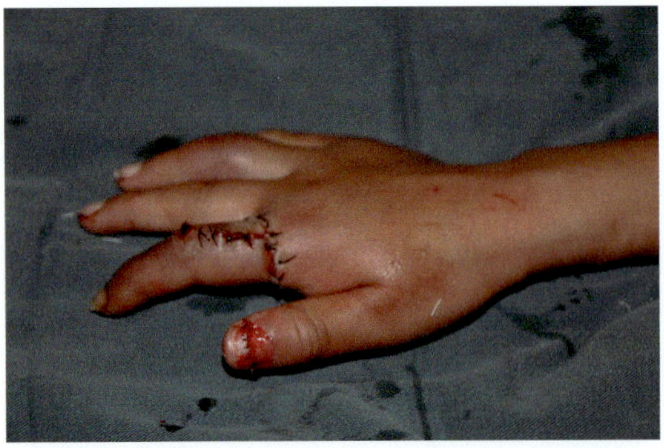

Fig. 22.14 The dorsal side after replantation

signs were stable. The soft tissues of multiple fingers were completely destroyed, with no blood supply and with the bone revealed,

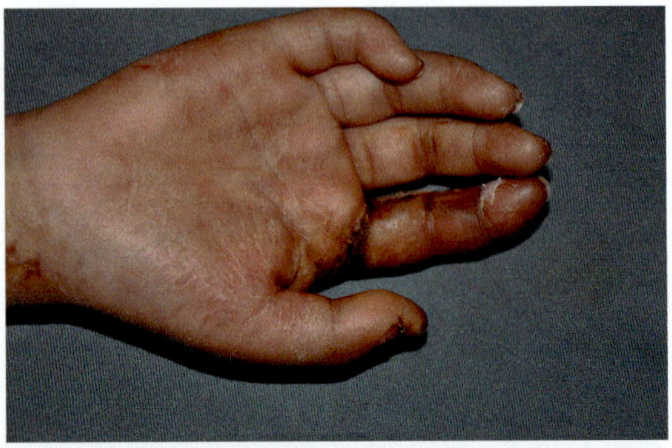

Fig. 22.15 The palm side 2 weeks later

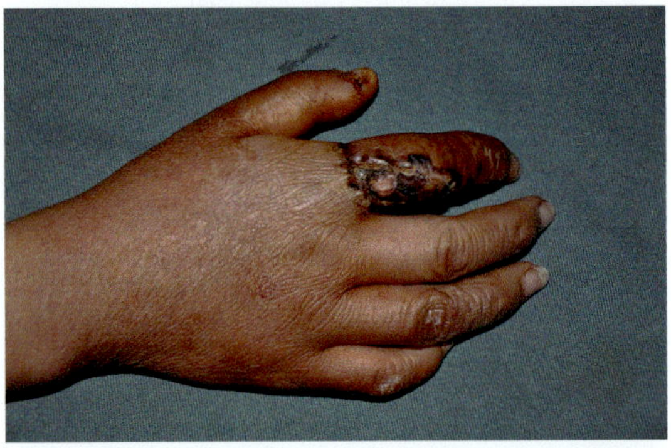

Fig. 22.16 The dorsal side 2 weeks later

uneven wounds, and bleeding. Successful debridement and replantation were performed under anesthesia under emergency conditions. The replanted fingers were red and had moderate tension after relaxing the tourniquet. They were packed with sterile gauze and padded with broken cotton yarn and the patient was brought back to the ward safely. He was given conventional treatments postoperatively, such as antibiotics, hormones, and antispasmodics. By 2 weeks later, the replanted fingers had successfully survived. The appearance and function were good after regular follow-up and functional exercise guidance, and the patient was satisfied (Figs. 22.17, 22.18, 22.19, 22.20, 22.21, 22.22, 22.23, 22.24, 22.25, 22.26, 22.27, 22.28, 22.29, 22.30, and 22.31).

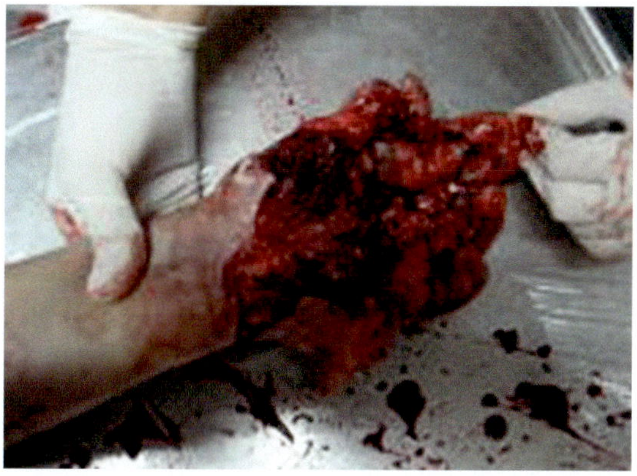

Fig. 22.17 The palm side of the left hand

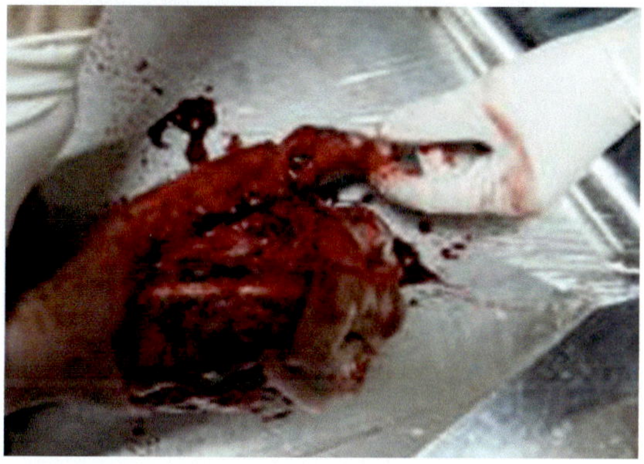

Fig. 22.18 The dorsal side of the left hand

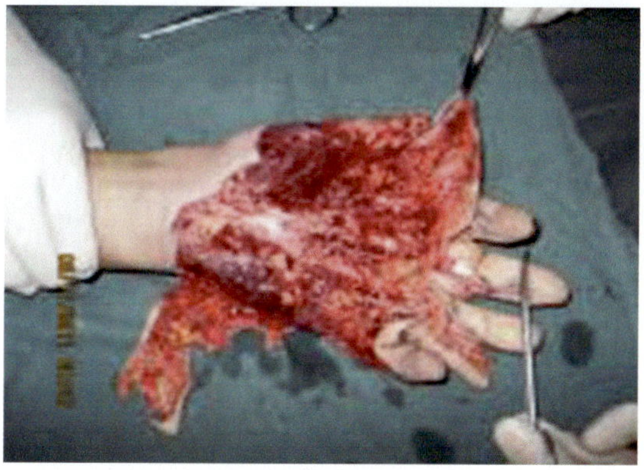

Fig. 22.19 The palm side during surgery

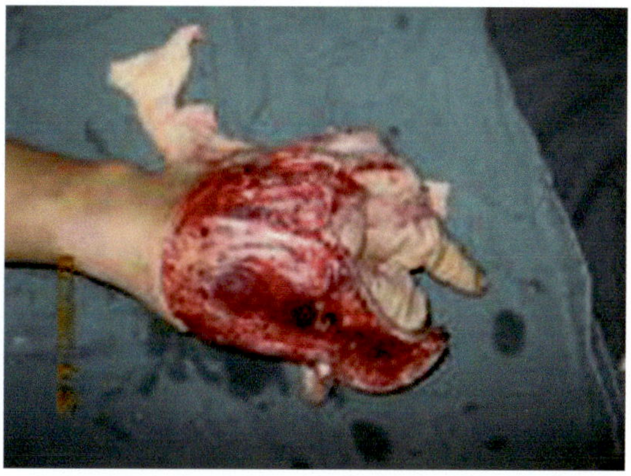

Fig. 22.20 The dorsal side during surgery

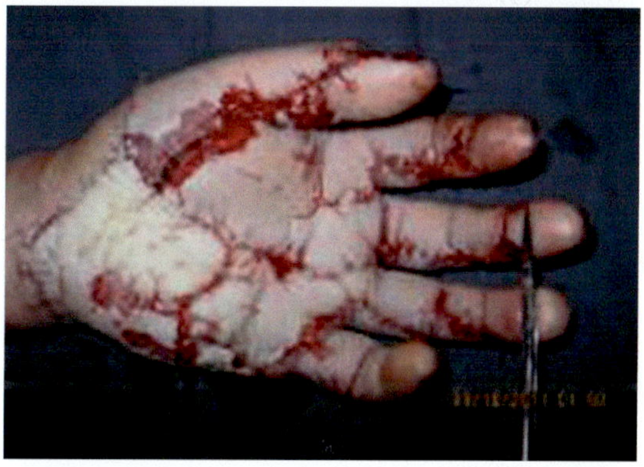

Fig. 22.21 The palm side after replantation

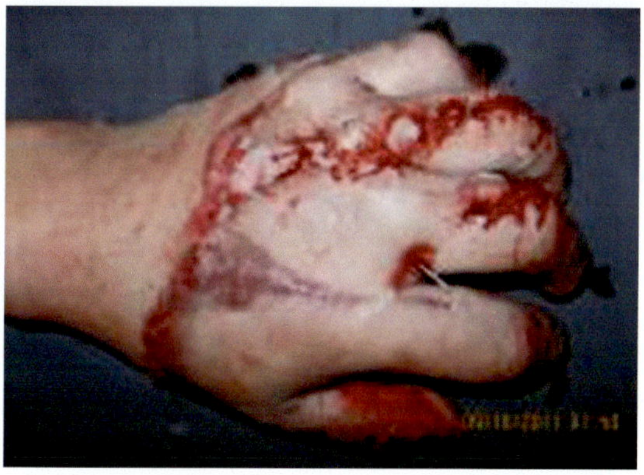

Fig. 22.22 The dorsal side after replantation

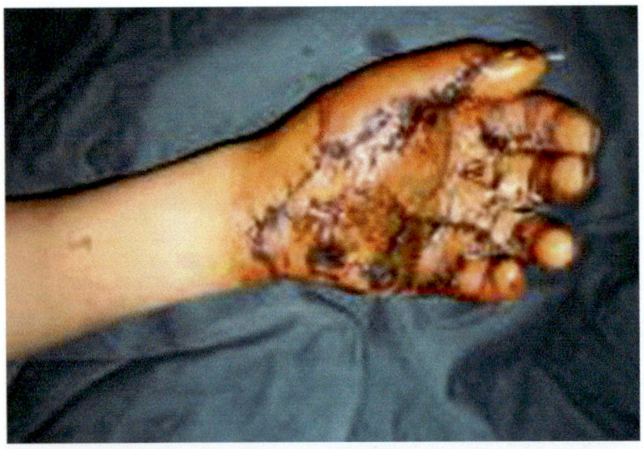

Fig. 22.23 The palm side 3 weeks later

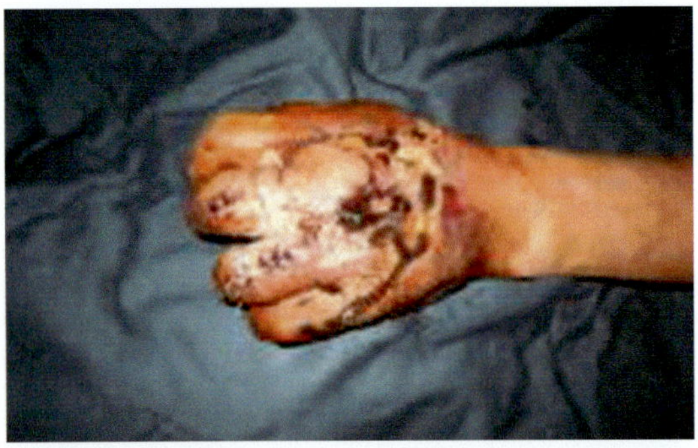

Fig. 22.24 The dorsal side 3 weeks later

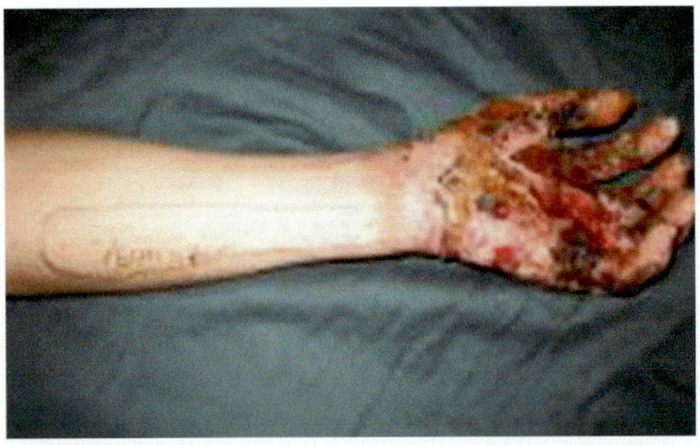

Fig. 22.25 The design of the flap

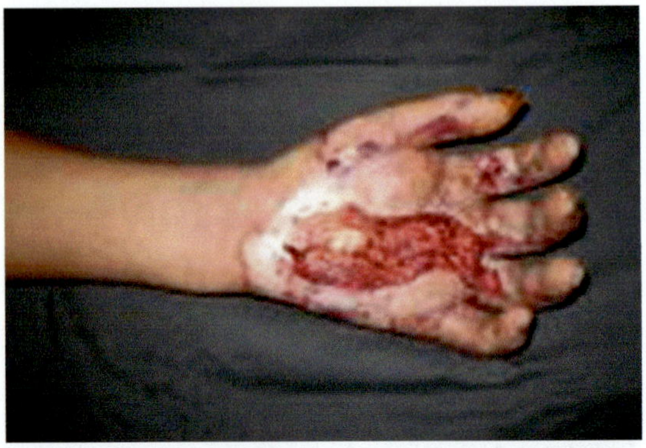

Fig. 22.26 The wound after debridement

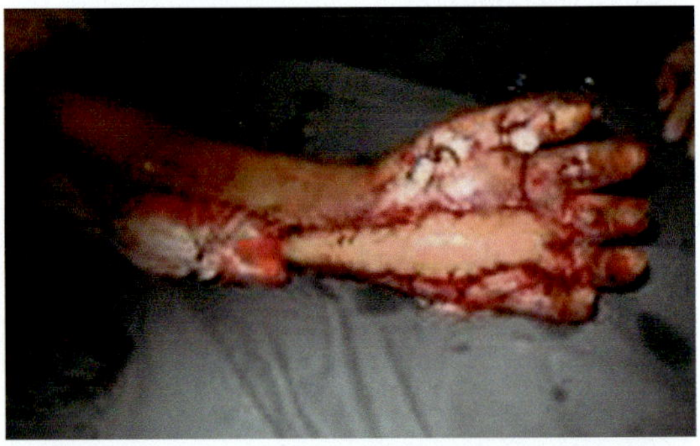

Fig. 22.27 The wound covered with the flap

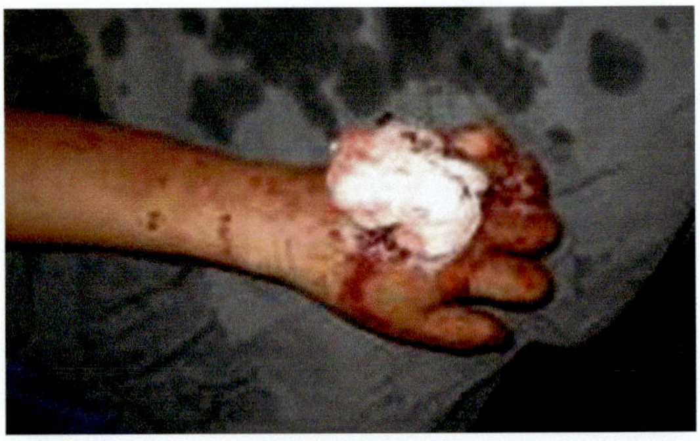

Fig. 22.28 The wound after a free skin graft

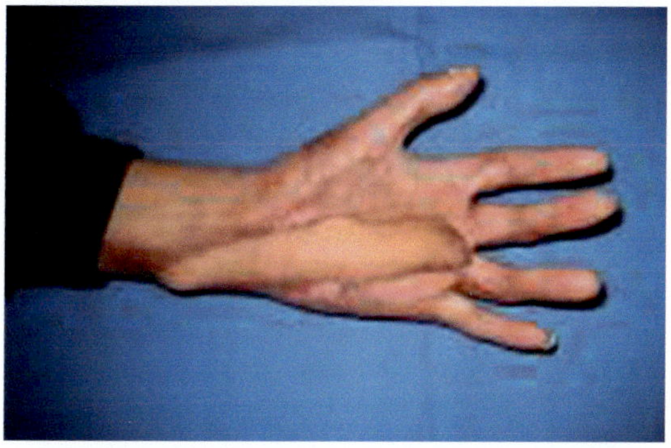

Fig. 22.29 The palm side 24 months later

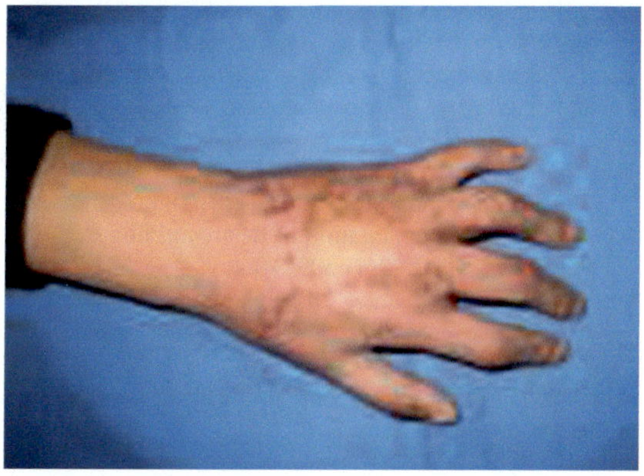

Fig. 22.30 The dorsal side 24 months later

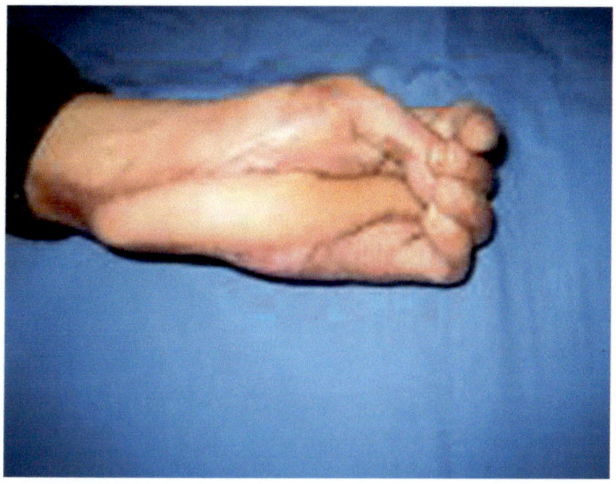

Fig. 22.31 Function 24 months later

22.3 Key Points in Surgery

(a) The key point for achieving success with this type of replantation is to reconstruct a good blood supply, based on the complete vascular bed, which can be tested by heparin–saline to assess whether it is worth replanting.

(b) Complete debridement is needed. The avulsed tissue could be opened longitudinally to find vessels that could be anastomosed under a microscope. Extend the incision at the proximal end; find and separate the vessels and nerves.

(c) Thorough debridement of the injured vessels and nerves under the microscope. It is better to repair them by means of transplantation, but do not leave the ones in which it is doubtful that they are injured.

(d) There are three methods for repairing vessel defects:

- If the defect of the vessels is short, the finger can be shortened and the vessels anastomosed directly.
- If the defect is mainly in the arteries, it could be repaired by transposition of the vascular nerve bundle of the nearby finger.
- Transplantation of vessels is suitable for defects of both the arteries and the veins.

(e) Multiple destroyed fingers are not suitable for transposition of nearby digital arteries, and could be spanned by transplanted veins.

(f) Arteries could be reconstructed by crossing, transposition, and transplantation. The dorsal digital vein could be repaired by transposition and transplantation.

(g) Tendon avulsed from the muscle belly could not be repaired directly and should be repaired by tendon transposition.

22.4 Announcements

(a) If it is not sure that the replanted finger will survive, the tendon defect could be left and handled in the second phase.
(b) Microincisions and drainage flap may be useful to improve venous return.
(c) To patients who are at a risk of hypercoagulability, postoperative anticoagulants are necessary and the blood coagulation system should be closely observed.
(d) The rate of vascular crisis is much higher in multiple destroyed fingers than in a single finger, and should be closely observed and handled.
(e) Defects of digital arteries could be repaired by transposition of the wrist vein or nearby digital vessels; it should be ensured that the veins are reversed during anastomosis. Defects of the dorsal digital veins could be repaired using the wrist vein directly.
(f) Postoperative rehydration of normal saline (500 mL) and heparin (100 mg) maintained for 24 h is useful for increasing the survival rate.
(g) It is necessary to take early, reasonable, and long-term functional exercise.

Suggested Reading

Chongshan J, Wang R, Qiang L. Clinical characteristics and replantation of avulsion severed finger. J Clin Orthopaed. 1999;01:17–9.

Gang Q, Wang W, Donghai L, et al. Replantation of whole avulsion severed thumb. Chin J Microsurg. 2007;30(6):475–6.

Guohu L. Clinical analysis of replantation of destroyed finger. J Bethune Mil Med Coll. 2014;5:470–1.

He R, Linge L, Peng C, et al. The experience of multiple avulsion severed fingers. Chin J Pract Hand Surg. 2014;3:338–9.

Hu H, Wang X, Hong C. Clinical analysis of 58 cases with degloved and avulsion severed thumb replantation. Chin J Pract Hand Surg. 2008;22(2):69–71.

Jie L. Nursing of replantation of complete avulsion severed thumb. Chin J Pract Hand Surg. 2006;3:159–65.

Liang Q, Xianzhong Z, Lu R, et al. The experience of replantation of destroyed thumb. Chin J Microsurg. 2011;34(5):417–8.

Mingcan Z. Situ replantation of skin avulsion of hand. Chin J Pract Hand Surg. 2001;17(3):183.

Pan X, Wang C. Replantation of destroyed finger. Chin J Microsurg. 1997;20(4):309–10.

Qulun Y, He S. 1 case of replantation of complete avulsion severed thumb. Chin J Pract Hand Surg. 2000;14(3):190.

Wang X, Ping Z, Zhu C, et al. Replantation of complete avulsion severed finger. J Pract Med. 2012;28(24):4200.